T0172908

METHODS & NEW FRONTIERS IN NEUROSCIENCE

Series Editors
Sidney A. Simon, Ph.D.
Miguel A.L. Nicolelis, M.D., Ph.D.

Published Titles

Apoptosis in Neurobiology
Yusuf A. Hannun, M.D., Professor of Biomedical Research and Chairman/Department
of Biochemistry and Molecular Biology, Medical University of South Carolina
Rose-Mary Boustany, M.D., tenured Associate Professor of Pediatrics and Neurobiology,
Duke University Medical Center

Methods for Neural Ensemble Recordings
Miguel A.L. Nicolelis, M.D., Ph.D., Professor of Neurobiology and Biomedical Engineering,
Duke University Medical Center

Methods of Behavioral Analysis in Neuroscience
Jerry J. Buccafusco, Ph.D., Alzheimer's Research Center, Professor of Pharmacology and
Toxicology, Professor of Psychiatry and Health Behavior, Medical College of Georgia

Neural Prostheses for Restoration of Sensory and Motor Function
John K. Chapin, Ph.D., Professor of Physiology and Pharmacology, State University of
New York Health Science Center
Karen A. Moxon, Ph.D., Assistant Professor/School of Biomedical Engineering, Science,
and Health Systems, Drexel University

Computational Neuroscience: Realistic Modeling for Experimentalists
Eric DeSchutter, M.D., Ph.D., Professor/Department of Medicine, University of Antwerp

Methods in Pain Research
Lawrence Kruger, Ph.D., Professor or Neurobiology (Emeritus), UCLA School of Medicine
and Brain Research Institute

Motor Neurobiology of the Spinal Cord
Timothy C. Cope, Ph.D., Professor of Physiology, Emory University School of Medicine

Nicotinic Receptors in the Nervous System
Edward D. Levin, Ph.D., Associate Professor/Department of Psychiatry and Pharmacology
and Molecular Cancer Biology and Department of Psychiatry and Behavioral
Sciences, Duke University School of Medicine

Methods in Genomic Neuroscience
Helmin R. Chin, Ph.D., Genetics Research Branch, NIMH, NIH
Steven O. Moldin, Ph.D, Genetics Research Branch, NIMH, NIH

Methods in Chemosensory Research
Sidney A. Simon, Ph.D., Professor of Neurobiology, Biomedical Engineering, and
Anesthesiology, Duke University
Miguel A.L. Nicolelis, M.D., Ph.D., Professor of Neurobiology and Biomedical Engineering,
Duke University

The Somatosensory System: Deciphering the Brain's Own Body Image
Randall J. Nelson, Ph.D., Professor of Anatomy and Neurobiology,
    University of Tennessee Health Sciences Center

New Concepts in Cerebral Ischemia
Rick C. S. Lin, Ph.D., Professor of Anatomy, University of Mississippi Medical Center

DNA Arrays: Technologies and Experimental Strategies
Elena Grigorenko, Ph.D., Technology Development Group, Millennium Pharmaceuticals

Methods for Alcohol-Related Neuroscience Research
Yuan Liu, Ph.D., National Institute of Neurological Disorders and Stroke, National Institutes
    of Health
David M. Lovinger, Ph.D., Laboratory of Integrative Neuroscience, NIAAA

In Vivo Optical Imaging of Brain Function
Ron Frostig, Ph.D., Associate Professor/Department of Psychobiology,
    University of California, Irvine

Primate Audition: Behavior and Neurobiology
    Asif A. Ghazanfar, Ph.D., Primate Cognitive Neuroscience Lab, Harvard University

Methods in Drug Abuse Research: Cellular and Circuit Level Analyses
    Dr. Barry D. Waterhouse, Ph.D., MCP-Hahnemann University

BIOMEDICAL IMAGING IN EXPERIMENTAL NEUROSCIENCE

Edited by Nick van Bruggen
Timothy Roberts

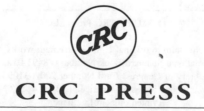

CRC PRESS

Boca Raton   London   New York   Washington, D.C.

Library of Congress Cataloging-in-Publication Data

Biomedical imaging in experimenal neuoscience / edited by Nick van Bruggen and
Timothy Roberts.
    p. cm. — (Methods & new frontiers in neuroscience)
    Includes bibliographical references and index.
    ISBN 0-8493-0122-X (alk. paper)
    1. Brain—Imaging. 2. Brain—Magnetic resonance imaging. I. van Bruggen, Nick. II.
Roberts, Timothy (Timothy P. L.) III. Methods & new frontiers in neuroscience series

QP376.6 .B55 2002
612.8′2—dc21   2002031093

Visit the CRC Press Web site at www.crcpress.com

© 2003 by CRC Press LLC

No claim to original U.S. Government works
International Standard Book Number 0-8493-0122-X
Library of Congress Card Number 2002031093
Printed in the United States of America 1 2 3 4 5 6 7 8 9 0
Printed on acid-free paper

Series Preface

Our goal in creating the Methods & New Frontiers in Neuroscience series is to present the insights of experts on emerging experimental techniques and theoretical concepts that are, or will be, at the vanguard of neuroscience. Books in the series cover topics ranging from methods to investigate apoptosis to modern techniques for neural ensemble recordings in behaving animals. The series also covers new and exciting multidisciplinary areas of brain research, such as computational neuroscience and neuroengineering, and describes breakthroughs in classical fields like behavioral neuroscience. We want these books to be the books every neuroscientist will use in order to get acquainted with new methodologies in brain research. These books can be given to graduate students and postdoctoral fellows when they are looking for guidance to start a new line of research.

Each book is edited by an expert and consists of chapters written by the leaders in a particular field. Books are richly illustrated and contain comprehensive bibliographies. Chapters provide substantial background material relevant to the particular subject. Hence, they are not only " methods books," but they also contain detailed "tricks of the trade" and information as to where these methods can be safely applied. In addition, they include information about where to buy equipment and about web sites helpful in solving both practical and theoretical problems.

We hope that as the volumes become available, the effort put in by us, by the publisher, by the book editors, and by individual authors will contribute to the further development of brain research. The extent that we achieve this goal will be determined by the utility of these books.

Sidney A. Simon, Ph.D.
Miguel A.L. Nicolelis, M.D., Ph.D.
Series Editors

Preface

The goals of experimental neuroscience research are fundamentally to gain mechanistic understanding of the pathology of disease in order to identify appropriate targets for potential pharmacological intervention and evaluation of putative therapies. With the advances in gene manipulation and transgene technologies, we have unprecedented ability to generate animal models of disease that more closely mimic the clinical conditions.

Noninvasive techniques capable of investigating altered pathophysiologies are now of paramount importance. Conventional methods that rely on histological and/or immunohistochemical staining demand the selective sacrifices of large cohorts of animals and include inherent assumptions of population homogeneity. Noninvasive imaging offers the obvious attractions of reducing sample sizes, use of individual data for internal baseline and control purposes, and consequent advantages in statistical power. It also offers opportunities to investigate behavior in individual animals that perhaps deviates from population norm expectations, i.e., to identify new and unanticipated behaviors.

Noninvasive imaging also offers accessibility to specific and dynamic physiological interactions that are amenable only at whole organism or system level, and cannot be addressed via single-time point, single-mechanism, *ex vivo* analysis. Advances in imaging methodologies provide increased physiological specificity at tissue, vascular, cellular, metabolic, and electrophysiological levels. Experimental neuroscience seeks to validate these specificities for their ultimate clinical value. On the other hand, once validated, these specificities can be expanded to characterize tissue, identify target pharmaceutical approaches, and evaluate novel mode-of-action-specific therapeutics.

This book is motivated by the rapidly advancing technologies of noninvasive imaging, the parallel rapid progress in developing genomic and other targeted pharmaceuticals, and the ongoing demand for greater understanding of diseases and therapies. Our target audience includes the biologists with interests in how advances in biomedical imaging may augment their *in vivo* research endeavors and clinical practitioners who seek deeper insights into the association between imaging results and disease pathophysiology.

We would like to thank the following for their assistance in preparing material for this book and their patience throughout this project: Evelyn Berry and Alison Bruce for help with manuscript preparation; and Simon Williams, Annie Ogasawara, Jed Ross, Joan Greve, Hope Steinmetz, Adrienne Ross, Kai Barck, and Lisa Bernstein for their support and patience. We are grateful for all our collaborators that provided data and illustrations — often at short notice! Finally, we thank our wives and children for their encouragement and tolerance.

Nick van Bruggen
Tim Roberts

Editors

Nick van Bruggen is a senior scientist at Genentech Inc. and head of the biomedical imaging group in the department of physiology. He earned a B.Sc in medicinal chemistry from University College London and a Ph.D in chemistry from Nottingham University, U.K. In 1987, while working in the laboratory of Professor David Gadian at The Royal College of Surgeons of England in London, he helped establish one of the earliest magnetic resonance imaging (MRI) systems dedicated to experimental biological research. In 1991, he was appointed to a lectureship position at Hunterian Institute and focused his research on developing novel MRI techniques for the investigation and understanding of pathophysiology, including the use of diffusion MR imaging and functional MRI for stroke research. In 1994, he moved to California to establish a biomedical imaging facility dedicated to *in vivo* experimental research for Genentech Inc., one of the original U.S. biotechnology companies.

Timothy P.L. Roberts is an associate professor in the department of medical imaging at the University of Toronto. He earned a B.A. and an M.A. in natural sciences from Cambridge University in England in 1988, and was granted a Ph.D. in MRI techniques at the Herchel Smith Laboratory for Medicinal Chemistry of Cambridge University in 1991. His postdoctoral research in the neuroradiology section of the laboratory of John Kucharczyk and Mike Moseley at the University of California at San Francisco (UCSF) focused on the quantitative use of high speed perfusion- and diffusion-sensitive MRI in animal models of cerebral ischemia, metabolic encephalopathies, and neonatal development. Dr. Roberts was appointed assistant professor of radiology at UCSF in 1994 as director of the biomagnetic imaging laboratory. He investigated electrophysiologic aspects of brain function using magnetoencephalography (MEG) and cellular and vascular responses using diffusion-weighted, perfusion-sensitive, and BOLD MRI. In 2002 Dr. Roberts moved to Canada where he holds the Canada Research Chair in Imaging Research.

He is a member of the International Society for Magnetic Resonance in Medicine, the American Society of Neuroradiology, the Cognitive Neuroscience Society, the Organization for Human Brain Mapping, the International Society of Cerebral Blood Flow and Metabolism, and the Institute of Physics. He has authored or co-authored over 150 journal articles and book chapters in the fields of physiological and functional MRI, magnetoencephalography, and magnetic source imaging.

Contributors

Helene Benveniste
Department of Anesthesiology
SUNY at Stony Brook
Stony Brook, NY

Stephen J. Blackband
University of Florida
Department of Biochemistry
Gainesville, FL

Fernando Calamante
Institute of Child Health
Unit of Biophysics
London, England

Richard Carano
Genentech Inc.
Department of Physiology
South San Francisco, CA

Yin-Ching I. Chen
Massachusetts General Hospital
MGH-NMR Center
Charlestown, MA

Simon Cherry
University of California
Department of Biomedical Engineering
Davis, CA

Alexander J. de Crespigny
Massachusetts General Hospital
MGH-NMR Center
Charlestown, MA

Elizabeth Disbrow
University of California at Davis
Center for Neuroscience
Davis, CA

Mathias Hoehn
Max Planck Institut
Neurologische Forschung
Köln, Germany

Bruce G. Jenkins
Massachusetts General Hospital
MGH-NMR Center
Charlestown, MA

Harley Kornblum
University of California
School of Medicine
Los Angeles, CA

Mark Francis Lythgoe
Institute of Child Health
Unit of Biophysics
London, England

Thomas M. Mareci
University of Florida
Department of Biochemistry
Gainesville, FL

Joseph B. Mendeville
Massachusetts General Hosp.
MGH-NMR Center
Charlestown, MA

Michel Modo
University of London
Institute of Psychiatry
Department of Psychology
London, England

Timothy P.L. Roberts
University of Toronto
Department of Medical Imaging
Toronto, Ontario

Nicola R. Sibson
University of Oxford
Department of Biochemistry
Oxford, England

David L. Thomas
University College London
Wellcome Trust High Field Laboratory
London, England

Nick van Bruggen
Genentech Inc.
Department of Physiology
South San Francisco, CA

Steven C.R. Williams
University of London
Institute of Psychiatry
Department of Clinical Neuroscience
London, England

Stephen R. Williams
University of Manchester
Imaging Science and Biomedical
  Engineering
Manchester, England

Table of Contents

1 Principles of MRI Contrast

Timothy P.L. Roberts and Nick van Bruggen

CONTENTS

1.1   INTRODUCTION

Magnetic resonance imaging (MRI) has become the mainstay of radiological techniques in diagnostic imaging and the technique of choice for assessing diseases of
the central nervous system. Its utility in experimental research using laboratory
animals has inevitably lagged behind its clinical counterpart due, in part, to equipment costs and requirements for qualified operators. However with technological
advances, increased availability, and deeper understanding of its physiological specificity and capabilities, the utility of MRI in experimental research is assured. Its
success in clinical practice and now in experimental research — an impressive
achievement considering MRI was introduced into clinical medicine a little over two

decades ago — is due to its flexibility and specificity to the altered pathophysiology of disease.

MRI affords a noninvasive imaging technique with high physicochemical (and ultimately, by inference, physiological) specificity, offering high anatomic resolution and a variety of controls over image appearance or contrast. While the development of imaging techniques in experimental models was a necessary precursor to its clinical implementation, the ongoing clinical application can be seen to motivate more rigorous and controlled experimental studies. Such feedback mechanisms promote advances in imaging methodology, clinical interpretation, and fundamental understanding of neuroscience.

The purpose of this chapter is to provide an overview of MRI, introduce the image contrasts attainable with the technology, and thus provide a backdrop to more detailed chapters that will expand on specific contrast mechanisms and their interpretation. A detailed description of the physics of MRI is beyond the scope of this chapter and can be found in numerous textbooks.

1.2 ORIGINS OF SIGNALS AND SENSITIVITY TO PHYSICAL FACTORS: MAKING A PHYSIOLOGICAL INFERENCE FROM A PHYSICAL TRUTH

In general, MRI investigations derive signals from the hydrogen nuclei (protons) of water molecules. Image intensity is modulated by the regional abundance (or local density) of water. The initial signal distribution is further altered by a variety of factors that reflect the local physicochemical microenvironment of the water molecules, such as their mobility or the presence of microstructural entities, macromolecules, and membranes. The utility and scope of MRI are related to the control over sensitivity to such modulatory influences; by observing the physical consequences of such factors on regional MRI signal intensity, we are led to *physiological* inferences that might account for *physical* changes.

1.2.1 Sources of Intrinsic Contrast: T_1, T_2, and T_2^* Relaxation Times

The physiological or physicochemical environment may influence signal intensity via a number of parameters, offering the opportunity of tailoring physiologically specific imaging approaches (or pulse sequences) by manipulating the image sensitivity to the individual parameters. The primary class of signal-influencing factors is composed of the relaxation time constants: T_1, T_2 and T_2^*. These characteristic times reflect aspects of the tissue environment and can allow physiologic interpretation of tissue features on a spatial scale orders of magnitude smaller than nominal digital imaging resolution.[†] While MRI pulse sequences may contain combined influences of T_1, T_2, and T_2^*, it is possible to focus an imaging strategy on one or

---

† Image resolution is typically defined by matrix size or number of square picture elements (pixels) spanning the field of view. For example, a 3-cm field of view divided into a 128×128 pixel matrix has an in-plane spatial resolution of 234 μm.

other of these relaxation time constants to generate, for example, a T_2-weighted image, with contrast or appearance dependent on regional (or pixel) T_2-values and relatively independent of the influences of T_1 and other differences from one image pixel to the next.

While the origin of tissue differences in relaxation time constants is the subject of many textbooks, it is worth a brief introduction as the basis of the "exquisite soft tissue contrast" so often associated with the MRI technique and to distinguish it from mere density-based noninvasive imaging approaches, such as x-ray computed tomography (CT).

1.2.1.1 Generation of Contrast Exploiting T_2*

In the generation of an MR image, the protons of water molecules are excited by a radiofrequency (RF) wave transmitted (via an RF transmitter coil) into the animal under investigation, positioned within a static, uniform, and strong magnetic field (typically several tesla, T, in magnitude — the *MR scanner*). There is no direct contact between the transmission coil and the animal, and radiofrequency waves constitute a nonionizing (low energy) form of radiation; thus the MR technology is regarded as noninvasive. The excited protons (often termed "nuclear *spins*," to reflect the underlying quantum mechanical origin of the nuclear magnetic resonance, NMR, effect) are subsequently detected as their magnetic orientation rotates about the axis of the strong, uniform external magnetic field of the MR scanner. Such magnetic rotation (or "precession") arises from the interaction of the external magnetic field with the proton's intrinsic magnetic moment, and occurs at a specific rate or frequency, *linearly dependent on the local external magnetic field*. This point (specifically that the local magnetic field determines precession rate) is critical to the understanding of a range of MR phenomena — from image formation through positional encoding (labeling or tagging) to signal loss associated with intrinsic or induced inhomogeneities (nonuniformities) of the static external magnetic field, as schematically illustrated in Figure 1.1. The latter, commonly termed "magnetic susceptibility related signal loss" (or "susceptibility artefact"), can be described in terms of a time constant, T_2*.

If differences in tissue magnetization or magnetic susceptibility lead to a spatially varying local magnetic field over a region, typically at the interface of entities of differing magnetic susceptibility, e.g., between tissue and bone (see Figure 1.1(a)), protons at different spatial locations in the region will precess at different rates, and over time will separate or diverge in terms of their magnetic orientations. A vector summation of individual proton magnetic orientations (reflected in the MRI intensity) will then decrease with increasing precession time, yielding signal attenuation and ultimately voiding. T_2* is a measure of the time taken for signal to be lost in such a manner and consequently can be considered as a measure of local magnetic field homogeneity. A short T_2* implies rapid signal loss, consequent to a widely varying or spatially heterogeneous magnetic field. Long T_2* values imply maintenance of signal intensity over long precession times, reflecting field uniformity. However, short T_2* values must not always be viewed as image artefacts arising from different intrinsic magnetic susceptibilities of neighboring tissues and leading

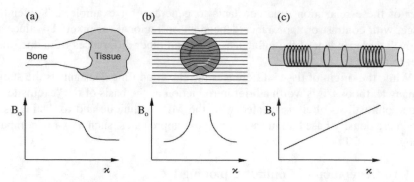

FIGURE 1.1 Field inhomogeneities (spatial variations) may be introduced by (a) intrinsic magnetic susceptibility differences between tissues (especially at interfaces between tissue and air or tissue and bone); (b) focal accumulation of a paramagnetic moiety (e.g., exogenous contrast containing Gd or Fe or endogenously present deoxyhemoglobin); or (c) application of a magnetic field gradient required for imaging, which causes a spatially varying magnetic field. A consequence of any of these mechanisms is that protons in differing positions will precess at different frequencies, and if their signals are summed, will rapidly lose signal coherence. Spectral lines will broaden and lose amplitude and image intensity will be attenuated.

to undesirable loss of signal at the tissue interface. Indeed, magnetic susceptibility *sensitivity* can also be exploited as a powerful form of MRI contrast (Figure 1.1(b)).

One of the primary applications exploiting T_2*-sensitivity is dynamic imaging (or tracking) of an intravenously administered bolus of exogenous contrast medium, typically containing a magnetic field-disturbing (T_2*-shortening) metal moiety (gadolinium, dysprosium, or iron). Confined to the vascular space, the agent leads to T_2* shortening and signal loss wherever it travels. By observing the kinetics of the transport of such a contrast agent bolus via highly temporal resolution, T_2*-weighted dynamic imaging, models of cerebral perfusion can be used to extract various timing and volume parameters of particular relevance in describing vascular physiology (see Chapter 2). This approach is used, for example, for stroke research in which ischemic territories are readily identified as regions immune from signal loss. While the fractional volume of the cerebral vasculature is small, it is worth considering the T_2*-shortening, field-disturbing effect of the contrast agent as a form of *sensitivity amplification*, since signal is lost from the intravascular compartment (containing the agent) and from the surrounding parenchyma (which experiences the contrast agent-mediated magnetic field disruption, despite its lack of contrast agent).

A further exploitation of magnetic susceptibility (or T_2* shortening) as source of contrast is the blood oxygenation level dependent (BOLD) mechanism, widely used in fMRI brain mapping investigations (see Chapters 4 and 5). Similar to the cerebral perfusion approach, dynamic T_2*-weighted imaging is performed to track transient changes in the magnetic field disturbances associated with the balance between oxyhemoglobin and deoxyhemoglobin in the blood. Deoxyhemoglobin, like the exogenous contrast agents used for bolus tracking perfusion studies, is paramagnetic. The presence of field gradients in and around the vessel (Figure 1.2)

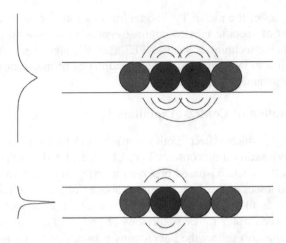

FIGURE 1.2 Susceptibility caused by blood. The paramagnetic nature of deoxygenated blood (dark spheres) generates magnetic field gradients in the blood vessels and in the surrounding tissues. These spatially varying local magnetic fields cause a loss of signal on the T_2^*-sensitive image.

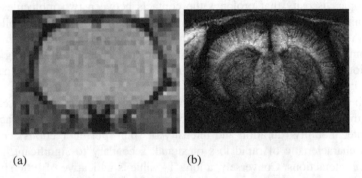

(a)   (b)

FIGURE 1.3 The increase in the relative amount of deoxyhemoglobin in the cerebral vessels can be visualized using a T_2^*-weighted imaging protocol. (a) A proton density coronal image acquired through the mouse brain. (b) After death induced by anoxia, the presence of deoxy-hemoglobin in the major vessels produces dramatic contrast using a T_2^*-weighted imaging protocol.

leads to local T_2^* shortening and signal loss. Thus changes in the relative amount of deoxyhemoglobin within the cerebral vasculature can be seen in a T_2^*-weighted MRI. Figure 1.3 shows a dramatic increase in the appearance of a T_2^*-weighted scan of the cerebral vasculature of the rodent brain following anoxia-induced death. Changes in the local concentration of deoxy-hemoglobin in the capillary bed also occur with neuronal activity elicited by peripheral stimulation or task performance. These phenomena can be observed, and their tissue substrates inferred, by tracking regional signal changes (see Chapter 4).

Final examples of the use of T_2* shortening as a form of beneficial contrast are the development of specific labeled contrast agents, analogous to the tracers used in nuclear medicine techniques such as PET (see Chapter 10), and exploiting the sensitivity amplification arising from the spatial extent of magnetic field disruption associated with paramagnetic moiety.

1.2.1.2 Generation of Contrast Exploiting T_2

In contrast to T_2*, which reflects both environmental features and intrinsic tissue properties, the relaxation time constant T_2 can be considered as relating specifically to the tissue itself. In fact T_2-based observation explicitly seeks to avoid spatially-dependent signal losses of the types discussed above (magnetic field inhomogeneity-related). This leads to a purer sensitivity of relaxation associated with magnetic interactions between water molecule protons (T_2 relaxation is often referred to as spin–spin relaxation, to reflect the interactions between water molecule protons or spins). Simply put, the tiny magnetic field associated with a given water molecule proton will influence the local magnetic field experienced by a neighboring (inter-acting) molecule.

The random Brownian motion (diffusion) of liquid state water molecules (as present in tissue) renders these interactions unpredictable and consequently irrecoverable. To the extent that such interactions are strong and/or sustained (e.g., due to microscopic viscosity that prolongs the contacts between two molecules) greater opportunity for net signal loss ensues. On the other hand, in a highly mobile milieu, spin–spin interactions may be fleeting and there may not be sufficient duration of field homogeneity disruption to lead to substantial signal loss. During such an interaction, the extra contribution to local magnetic field can be viewed as a transient form of inhomogeneity leading to signal loss.

Such random interaction or spin–spin relaxation-based signal loss is characterized by the time constant, T_2, which can be seen to reflect (among other factors) the local water mobility (duration and intensity of spin–spin interactions): a short T_2 value is characteristic of rapid loss of signal, secondary to significant, sustained spin–spin interactions. Conversely, a long T_2 value is indicative of little spin relaxation, probably secondary to a highly mobile water molecule environment such as cerebrospinal fluid (CSF) with only transient spin–spin interactions.

Image sensitivity to T_2 (as opposed to T_2*) is achieved by application of a class of MRI pulse sequences, based upon a concept known as *spin echo* (SE). The basic principles are illustrated in Figure 1.4. In spin echo formation, spatially dependent spin dephasing, as described above and characterized by the time constant T_2*, can be reversed by application of a second, 180° RF excitation pulse. This has the net effect of "flipping" the dephased spin magnetic orientation distribution in the transverse plane — an action analogous to tossing a pancake. The continued spatially-dependent precession rates lead to a *rephasing* of the distributed magnetic orientations, followed by an apparent recovery of signal intensity — the SE). In fact the reversal of T_2*-described signal loss in the formation of the SE is only partially successful.

The effects of random spin-spin interactions are, of course, irreversible by application of the 180° RF pulse (since identical interactions before and after the

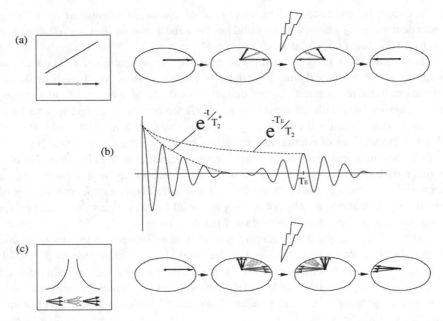

FIGURE 1.4 (a) In the presence of magnetic field heterogeneity (endogenous or via an applied external magnetic field gradient), excited nuclear spins acquire a resonant or precession frequency that depends on the external static magnetic field and on spatial position. Spatial coordinates with lower local magnetic fields will have lower frequencies (red arrows) and coordinates with higher local magnetic fields will have higher frequencies (blue arrows). An ensemble of such spins initially in phase (black arrow, far left cartoon) will subsequently dephase as individual spin vectors precess at these different frequencies (or rates). After application of a 180° RF pulse (jagged arrow), this dephased spin distribution has its magnetic orientation reversed in the transverse plane. Spins remain distributed in phase. However, spins continue to precess at a rate determined by their spatial coordinates. Since these remain unchanged, the divergent spin distribution will ultimately rephase, momentarily forming an echo of the initial in-phase distribution (black arrow, far right cartoon). (b) In terms of NMR signal intensity, the initial dephasing of spins leads to a damped oscillation, with signal intensity (vector sum of spin vector distribution) diminishing rapidly. If the source of dephasing is endogenous magnetic field variation only, this decaying signal is called the FID (free induction decay) and its envelope can be described by an exponential decay time constant, T_2^*. A long T_2^* value implies low field heterogeneity and persistent signal. A short T_2^* implies rapid signal loss associated with greater field heterogeneity. Application of the 180° pulse leads to a rephasing of this decaying signal, then to the formation of an echo (at the echo time, TE, a time after the 180° pulse equal to the time between initial excitation and application of the 180° pulse. The amplitude of this spin echo is considerably restored (compared to the decaying FID), but is nonetheless smaller than that of the initial FID because of the incomplete rephasing of the spin distribution. This is because the rephasing relies on the precession of each spin at exactly the same rate after the 180° pulse as it did in the interval between initial excitation and the 180° application. To the extent that random spin-spin interactions lead to additional dephasing during either period, the echo is imperfectly refocused. Thus, the echo amplitude is dependent on the echo time and the time constant T_2, describing random spin-spin interactions. This description is rendered even more complex by the process of Brownian motion or random water diffusion. Although spins have resonant frequencies related to their local magnetic fields as shown in (c), as they diffuse through magnetic field heterogeneity, they also become distributed in phase (e.g., diverging red arrows, at nominal low frequency locations). Since such diffusion is random, its effects also are imperfectly refocused (distributed black arrows, far right cartoon) by the mere 180° RF pulse and thus the spin echo amplitude is reduced further to an extent dependent on the rate of diffusion, the magnitude of field heterogeneities, and the echo time or TE. See Color Figure 1.4 following page 210.

pulse cannot be guaranteed). The amplitude of the SE is attenuated by a factor dependent on the T_2 time constant and on the time between initial excitation and SE formation (also known as echo time or TE).

Spin echo (SE) imaging, with T2-sensitivity or weighting, has become the mainstay of both clinical and investigational MRI studies. With high anatomic resolution (relative immunity to the deleterious effects of magnetic field inhomogeneities associated with the magnet or magnetic susceptibility differences between tissue structures) and with sensitivity to water mobility that commonly appears elevated in situations of edema, inflammation, etc.), the imaging approach provides reliable, sensitive and morphometrically precise identification and delineation of a number of pathophysiologies. The downside of such utility and sensitivity to a commonly indicated physical change, e.g., water mobility, is a concomitant lack of specificity. A number of physiologically plausible explanations can account for hyperintensity observed on T_2-weighted MRIs.

Although T_2-weighted SE imaging is described as insensitive to bulk magnetic susceptibility-related effects that lead to the signal loss characterized by $T_2{}^*$, such SE sequences retain a certain sensitivity to a type of magnetic susceptibility-related signal loss arising from the random diffusion of water molecules through magnetic field inhomogeneities (or local gradients) associated with magnetic susceptibility variations within tissue.

While this effect is generally negligible, it becomes of significance in two related settings of compartmentalized magnetic susceptibility difference. If the content of the intravascular space has a substantially different magnetic susceptibility to surrounding parenchyma, magnetic field gradients will extend beyond the capillaries into the surrounding tissues. Water molecules diffusing in this extravascular space will experience varying local magnetic fields and thus will have varying precession rates, ultimately leading to signal loss on ensemble averaging. The amount of signal loss will depend, in a somewhat complex fashion, on the freedom of water molecule diffusion, the microgeometric organization of vascular structures (capillaries and venules) and, of course, on the degree of magnetic susceptibility difference between intravascular and extravascular compartments.

T_2-weighted SE imaging is sensitive to this microscopic diffusion-related signal loss. On the other hand, $T_2{}^*$-weighted imaging is dominated by bulk magnetic susceptibility difference-related dephasing and is relatively insensitive to the additional diffusion-related contribution. This methodological difference becomes of interest when the intravascular space contains an exogenous magnetic susceptibility contrast agent or when the focus is on the $T_2{}^*$-shortening deoxyhemoglobin content of blood (as in fMRI; see Chapter 4).

Theoretical and experimental observations indicate that susceptibility-induced signal loss arising in the presence of a paramagnetic agent (an exogenous contrast agent or endogenous deoxyhemoglobin) within the vasculature depends on the microstructural environment of the vessels in the tissue of interest. Through a combination of pulse sequences with differing sensitivities to diffusion-mediated signal losses that are more pronounced at the capillary bed level, compared to a bulk susceptibility effect dominated by larger vessels, especially veins, it is possible to estimate the average vessel size with the voxel. By simultaneously or sequentially using both T_2- and T_2*-weighted imaging and observing the contrast agent-mediated and deoxyhemoglobin-mediated changes in relaxation rates (R_2 and R_2*), it becomes possible to infer information about vascular morphology and vessel size.

As vessel size increases so will the ratio of ΔR_2* to ΔR_2. This rationale has been used to estimate average vessel size within the voxel. Such approaches to vessel radius imaging show significant promise in the delineation and quantification of physiological processes such as neovascularization and angiogenesis associated with tumors, ischemia, inflammation, and wound healing.

In a similar vein, it has been proposed to use a spin-echo approach to the observation of deoxyhemoglobin concentration changes that underlie the BOLD contrast and fMRI method for functional brain mapping. As discussed above, while T_2*-weighted (gradient-recalled echo) sequences are indeed more sensitive to small fluctuations in field homogeneity, that sensitivity comes at a price: many gradient-recalled echo attempts to perform fMRI studies become dominated by larger vascular structures, particularly draining veins.

The fMRI method has been used in an attempt to map the distribution of neurons in tissues (not the vessels associated with them) — often called the "brain–vein debate." The SE approach with increased sensitivity to magnetic susceptibility changes in smaller (~10 μm) vascular structures (i.e., capillaries) is considered to yield a more spatially specific representation of active neuronal tissue. The balance between such specificity and adequate detection sensitivity to the BOLD contrast mechanism has largely resulted in the adoption of SE methods at higher magnetic field strengths (4 T and above). Interestingly, T_2 values for blood rapidly become shorter than those of surrounding tissue as external field strength increases (further diminishing confounding sensitivity to signal changes or apparent responses within the intravascular space).

1.2.1.3 Generation of Contrast Exploiting T_1

The other commonly encountered relaxation time constant in MRI is T_1. Since MRI acquisition depends on the successive excitation of water molecule protons within a slice or volume and the ultimate (digital) resolution is improved by increasing the number of such successive excitations (or phase encoding steps), it is clear that the interexcitation time interval (sequence repeat time or TR) is a key determinant of overall image acquisition time. For example, if an image matrix of 256 is called for, a TR of 1 sec would lead to a total acquisition time of over 4 min. If TR is reduced to 10 ms, image acquisition is reduced to 2.56 sec. What, however, is going on during the TR interval?

The answer is best illustrated by considering the RF energy imparted to the water molecules during RF excitation. They become excited and are no longer in their equilibrium, resting condition. In a vector description, they are often thought of as rotated from a magnetic orientation parallel to the external magnetic field to an orientation perpendicular to it (the transverse plane). Such excited transverse magnetic orientations then precess at a rate determined by the local magnetic field of their environment. At the same time, however, the excited spins no longer forced by RF excitation must relax or return to their equilibrium state. In a sense, they can be considered to pay back the energy imparted during excitation.

Another shared feature of both T_1-weighted and T_2-weighted images, compared with proton density-weighted images, and a general principle of physiologically specific MRI, is that this sensitivity to aspects of the physical microenvironment (soft tissue contrast) is gained at the expense of overall signal-to-noise-ratio. In performing T_1 or T_2 weighting, one selectively discards signals from long T_1 or short T_2 species, respectively, to gain contrast.The mechanisms behind such longitudinal (or spin-lattice) relaxation are complex, but in general it is reasonable to think that the relaxation is facilitated by the presence of microstructural elements, such as macromolecules, membranes, etc. (the lattice) that can can absorb via interactions the unwanted energy of the water molecule protons (spins). Consequently, tissue microenvironments that contain abundant microstructural entities to facilitate spin-lattice relaxation are associated with more rapid longitudinal recovery and thus more complete restoration of equilibrium during the sequence repeat (or interpulse) TR interval. They thus contribute more fully during subsequent RF excitation to signal collection. Their image intensity on a short-TR (T_1-weighted) image is thus hyper-intense compared to tissues that provide little opportunity for spin-lattice relaxation (and are characterized by longer T1 values). Thus both T_1-weighted and T_2-weighted images can be viewed as reflecting related (but not completely dependent) features of the physical microenvironment of the water molecules in tissue.

Manipulation of the imaging parameters to generate contrast and the effect of signal-to-noise ratio are shown in Figure 1.5. Sagittal images through the head of a mouse show the flat contrast in the proton density image (Figures 1.5A(a) and 1.5B(a)) can be enhanced by introducing T_2 (Figures 1.5A(b) and 1.5B(b)) or T_1 weighting (Figures 1.5A(c) and 1.5B(c)). Combining T_1 and T_2 weightings in the same protocol may produce high contrast, often with a loss of signal (Figure 1.5B(d)). This can be overcome with signal averaging to gain signal-to-noise improvement but at the expense of total imaging time (Figure 1.5A(d)).

A primary use of the T_1-weighted imaging sequence is in conjunction with a tissue-compartment specific exogenous contrast agent that locally shortens T_1. Typically based around the Gd^{3+} ion chelated into a water-soluble form, e.g., Gd-DTPA, such agents exert very spatially specific (short-range) T_1-shortening influences on local water molecules. On a T_1-weighted image, this leads to elevated signal (or signal enhancement) in the local environment of the contrast agent, due to the shortening of the longitudinal relaxation time constant, T_1.

Since the agent is generally administered intravenously and is retained in the intravascular space of the healthy brain by the tight junctions of the blood–brain barrier (BBB), such enhancement is limited to the small vascular space of the healthy brain. However, in pathologic situations such as malignant glioma and chronic stroke, in which the integrity of the BBB is compromised, the contrast agent will leave the intravascular space and accumulate in the extravascular milieu, leading to increased exposure to tissue water, and consequently more widespread T_1 shortening and pronounced signal enhancement. This is the basis of the commonly used clinical imaging approach of *T_1 post gad* for the sensitive detection of BBB disruption. In fact, gradations of BBB disruption can be assessed by rapid dynamic imaging of

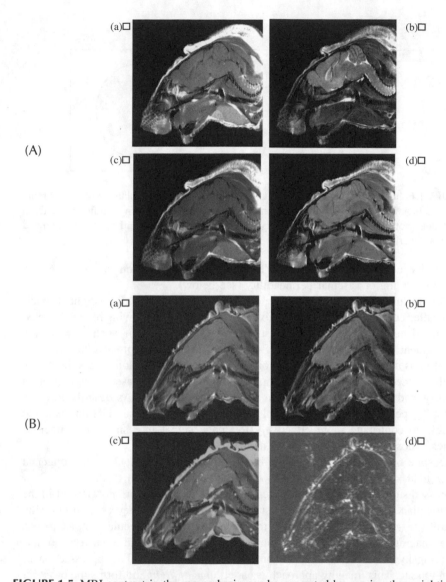

FIGURE 1.5 MRI contrast in the mouse brain can be generated by varying the weightings of the MRI protocol (T_1 and T_2). To illustrate this, sagittal sections through the mouse brain were recorded with different parameters. Image (a) was acquired with long repetition time (TR) and short echo time (TE) to minimize both T_1 and T_2 weighting and can be considered a proton density image. Image (b) is T_2-weighted since it was acquired with long TR and long TE. Note the improved CNS contrast and hyperintensity from the ventricles. Image (c) is T_1 weighted (short TR and TE) and (d) has degrees of both T_2 and T_1 weighting (short TR and long TE). Total image acquisition time was kept constant by increasing signal averaging. The same series of weightings was repeated for (a) through (d) of Figure 1.5B, but no compensation for the differences in imaging time as a result of altered TR was made. Note the signal washout in (d) in which the high contrast is negated by the loss of signal. (Image courtesy of Annie Ogasawara.)

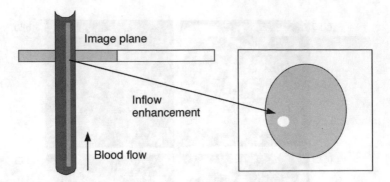

FIGURE 1.6 In-flow magnetic resonance angiography. The imaging plane experiences rapid RF excitation, leading to partial saturation (hypointensity/T_1 weighting). Inflowing arterial blood does not experience the slice-selective RF excitation train, and so is not saturated (appears hyperintense).

progressive enhancement post Gd-DTPA administration, often accompanied by kinetic modeling of vascular permeability (see below).

One feature of certain T_1-weighted images (particularly, the T_1-weighted gradient-recalled echo sequence) is the relative hyperintensity of inflowing blood, depicted as marked conspicuity of vascular structures. The origins of such flow-related enhancement lie in the mechanics of the image acquisition process in which T_1 weighting is achieved by the application of multiple RF excitation pulses, relatively closely spaced to only allow incomplete longitudinal (T_1-based) magnetization recovery, and thus yield T_1-dependent image signal intensity. As described above, shorter T_1 species recover more completely in a short interpulse (TR) interval, and are able to contribute more effectively to image signal intensity than longer T_1 species, whose image intensity is substantially suppressed.

Despite the relatively long T_1 of blood (approx 1.3 sec at 2 T and longer at higher field strengths), inflowing blood provides an exception to the "long T1 = suppressed signal" rule, since the water molecules of blood were not present in the imaging plane during the previous T_1-suppressing RF pulses. They were still flowing toward it (Figure 1.6). Consequently, the inflowing water molecule protons arrived at the imaging plane fully able to contribute to the image signal intensity, and thus appearing hyperintense relative to the stationary, somewhat T_1-suppressed background tissue. This imaging approach is called *time of flight* and forms the basis for magnetic resonance angiography. It is used routinely in clinical medicine to visualize blood vessels and has been used to good effect to image major vessels of the head in rats and mice (see Figures 1.7(a) and (b)).

1.2.2 SPIN GYMNASTICS: TAGGING, LABELING, AND SATURATION

1.2.2.1 Generation of Contrast Exploiting Diffusion

When excited (or transverse) spins lie in different magnetic fields, their magnetic orientations precess at different rates predicted by the local external magnetic field.

(a)   (b)

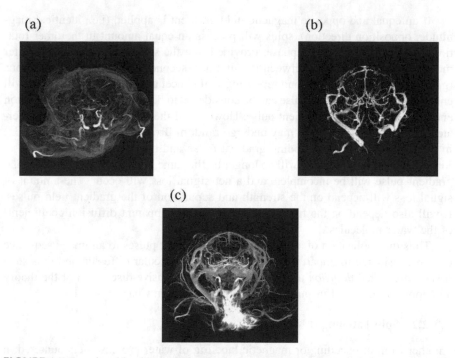

(c)

FIGURE 1.7 Imaging blood vessels in the mouse brain: several techniques can generate angiographic images of the cerebral vasculature. Three are shown here (all images are axial views of maximum intensity projections). The high signals seen in (a) and (b) are due to flow-related enhancement, the principle of which is illustrated in Figure 1.6. T_1 weighting is achieved by the application of multiple RF excitation pulses for a three-dimensional volume (slab-selective excitation) (a) or a slice-selection manner (b). Partial saturation of the signal occurs throughout the sample except in regions in which water molecules of flowing blood provide fresh unsaturated spins and therefore high signals. In (a), signal enhancement depends on the blood flow into the selected three-dimensional volume and therefore demonstrates a high degree of blood velocity dependence. The slice-selective version (b) reduces this sensitivity since the flowing blood must travel only a short distance. Greater definition of the vasculature anatomy is seen but an imaging time penalty is incurred. An alterative approach to generating angiographic information is through the use of a blood pool contrast agent (c). T_1 enhancement is achieved by use of contrast agents, in this case, Gd-DTPA conjugated to albumin, instead of the inflow effect. The conjugated contrast agent remains intravascular and its slow clearance allows high resolution imaging. In this case distinguishing between venous and arterial supply is not possible. (Image courtesy of Simon Williams.)

Over time, such precession at different rates leads to a loss of signal, as the magnetic orientation vectors progressively move out of sync or dephase. If a magnetic field gradient is imposed on the spin population so that the local magnetic field varies linearly with increasing spatial coordinate (in x, y, or z directions), the amount of precession or precession angle will depend on the spin position in the gradient field (i.e., its spatial coordinate). In a sense, the position of water molecules is thus *encoded* by the amount of precession and dephasing.

If an equal and opposite magnetic field gradient is applied (i.e., identical magnitude, opposition direction), spins will precess an equal amount in the other rotational sense, and will thus rephase. Provided that the spatial coordinate of a water molecule does not change between the first and second gradient field applications (gradient pulses), dephasing and rephasing will cancel and no net loss of signal will ensue. The second gradient pulse can be considered to decode the spatial information encoded during the first gradient pulse. However, if the gradient pulses are deliberately separated in time, spins may undergo random Brownian motion (or diffusion) in the time between the encoding gradient pulse and the decoding gradient pulse. Since their spatial coordinate will no longer be the same, rephasing during the second gradient pulse will be incomplete and a net signal loss will occur. The amount of signal loss will depend on the strength and separation of the gradient field pulses. It will also depend on the freedom of diffusion (or apparent diffusion coefficient) of the water molecules.

Thus the application of a matched pair of gradient pulses to an image sequence can be considered to impart image sensitivity to molecular diffusion and thus such images are called *diffusion weighted images*. An extensive discussion of the theory and applications of diffusion weighted MRI appears in Chapter 3.

1.2.2.2 Spin Labeling

Another form of encoding or magnetic labeling of water protons is encountered in the application of arterial spin labeling. Before application of an RF pulse for imaging, magnetic spins are considered in equilibrium (aligned with the external magnetic field). After excitation in the imaging process, they relax and return to equilibrium via T_1 mechanisms. However, prior to image acquisition, an additional form of magnetization preparation or manipulation can be performed: application of a certain type of RF pulse can cause the equilibrium spins to be inverted or adopt an anti-aligned magnetic orientation. Such an RF pulse is designated an inversion pulse. After the inversion pulse, the inverted spins must relax (via T_1 mechanisms) back to their equilibrium state.

If imaging is commenced during this relaxation process, its resultant intensity will be scaled by the degree of completion of such relaxation. This type of magnetization preparation can also be applied selectively, typically to a slice or slab of tissue. The inverted slice or slab may in fact not be identical to or even overlap the ultimately imaged region. This assumes relevance in the field of arterial spin labeling (ASL), in which a slab of tissue (tagged slab) distinct from the image target (imaged slice) and containing arterial vessels that feed the image slice is magnetically inverted before the imaged slice is imaged.

To the extent that intravascular arterial water spins become magnetically inverted and subsequently flow (or perfuse) into the imaged slice, the signal intensity arising from the imaged slice will differ compared to an otherwise similar image acquired without upstream arterial inversion (Figure 1.8). The subtraction of two such images reflects the degree of arterial blood supply to the imaged slice and can be used to estimate cerebral blood flow in quantitative units (see Chapter 2). In the absence of flow of inverted spins into the imaged slice, such spatially distinct spin inversion would essentially be irrelevant to intensity of the imaged slice (Figure 1.8).

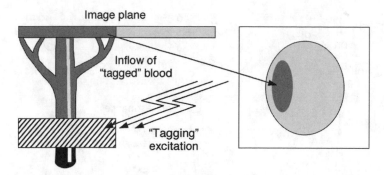

FIGURE 1.8 Principle of arterial spin labeling. Upstream blood experiences RF excitation, causing the magnetization to be tagged (typically, its magnetic orientation is inverted). Tagged blood then flows/perfuses into the imaging plane. Two experiments (with and without tagging) are subtracted to reveal perfused territory.

1.2.2.3 Magnetization Transfer

Another form of tagging or labeling of a spin population that might initially (and erroneously) be considered irrelevant to the imaged slice is exploited in the technique of magnetization transfer imaging (MTI). In this case, the irrelevant spin population is not upstream as in ASL; in fact, it lies within the image plane. The reason these spins might be ignored is that they are invisible under normal imaging conditions. This invisibility arises from the local physicochemical environment in which the protons are considered bound to large structural entities such as macromolecules or membrane elements. By virtue of their bound state, such protons are characterized by extremely short T_2 values (very restricted water mobility).

This principle is illustrated in Figure 1.9. On SE imaging, the protons suffer severe signal attenuation and effectively do not contribute to signal intensity. Associated with short T_2 values is a broad appearance (or resonance) in the spectral domain. The spectrum of a spin population reflects the effective resonant frequency distribution and uncertainty thereof, and is attained by Fourier transformation of the NMR signal response or free induction decay (FID) over time. While liquid state water protons in tissue may have spectra characterized by sharp peaks (with widths of tens of Hz), the corresponding spectral responses from the bound protons would be broader, lower in amplitude, and characterized by widths of many kHz.

Applying an RF pulse at a transmitted frequency somewhat distinct (e.g., 1 to 2 kHz) from the nominal liquid state water resonance peak would be expected to be irrelevant to the liquid state water protons with a narrow resonance extending over only tens of Hz. Indeed applying large amplitude of such off-resonance excitation to cause magnetic saturation or neutralization of protons whose resonant frequencies fell within such a range might initially be expected to be irrelevant since no liquid state water protons would be expected to be characterized by such resonant frequencies. However, the broad resonance response of the bound proton pool might well be expected to be affected by such an off-resonance pulse and thus might undergo magnetization saturation. This might still be regarded as irrelevant as these spins were not expected to contribute to image intensity by virtue of their short T_2 values.

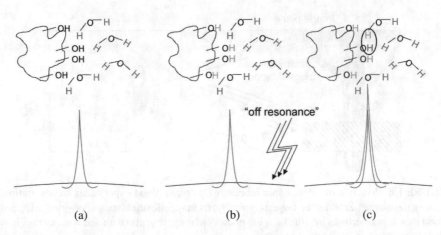

FIGURE 1.9 Principle of magnetization transfer: (a) Protons in tissue are modeled as existing in two pools (free water and macromolecular). Magnetic resonance signal is derived almost entirely from the free water pool that has sharp resonance, compared to the broad resonance (short T_2) of the bound protons. (b) Off-resonance RF irradiation does not directly affect the narrow free water resonance peak (*off resonance* is sufficiently shifted in frequency to minimally impact nominal water resonance); in practice this radiation is typically applied at a frequency 1 to 2 kHz offset. This radiation impacts the broad resonance of the bound pool, leading to magnetic saturation of the protons. (c) Under appropriate chemical conditions (e.g., in myelin), protons from the bound pool and free water exchange carry saturated, noncontributory magnetization into the free pool and decrement the free water proton count available to generate the signal, leading to signal loss and diminished spectral peak. The process is called magnetization transfer and exists only when both (1) a macromolecular bound pool exists and (2) conditions are appropriate for proton exchange. The degree of magnetization transfer related signal loss can be quantified, e.g., as an index of myelin content. See Color Figure 1.9 following page 210.

In one situation, such off-resonance saturation is not irrelevant to image intensity: if the physicochemical environment is appropriate, protons from the bound pool may undergo chemical exchange with protons from interacting free water molecules. This can be considered "swapping" of protons from the large molecule to the small one. This is facilitated in a number of settings, but exposed protons on hydroxyl (OH) groups of macromolecules may be favored candidates for such exchanges. If such off-resonance saturation pulses are applied to the broad resonance-bound pool, the exchange removes a potential signal-generating proton from the free water, liquid state pool, and binds it in a magnetically invisible fashion on the macromolecule. At the same time, the proton is replaced in the free water pool by a proton that has undergone magnetic saturation or neutralization during its tenure on the macromolecule (and during off-resonance RF irradiation) and is unable to contribute to image intensity in the way other free water protons do.

The combined effect of off-resonance irradiation and chemical exchange of protons leads to signal loss on subsequent imaging. This phenomenon is termed *magnetization transfer*. The extent of signal loss depends on the density of the macromolecularly bound protons and the rate or freedom of proton exchange. Quantitation of the difference between images acquired with and without such off-resonance irradiation (MT pulses) leads to the construction of the magnetization transfer ratio (MTR) — a parameter reflecting density and exchange features. MTR is mathematically equal to the normalized signal loss accompanying application of off-resonance irradiation pulses.

While a number of biological settings (e.g., collagen in cartilage) offer MT effects as a characterizing principle, the most widespread application in neuroscience lies in the MT effects of myelin in white matter. MT effects (quantified by MTR) may be used to study myelin formation and white matter maturation during development, as well as demyelinating diseases such as multiple sclerosis, in which progressive disease is seen as progressive reduction in MTR from values of ~0.5 to 0.6 in normal white matter to ~0.3 in severe demyelinating diseases.

1.2.3 WHEN INTRINSIC CONTRAST IS INSUFFICIENT: CONTRAST MEDIA

Despite the abundance of physiological sensitivities available with native MRI methodology, additional physiologic specificity analogous to that obtained with nuclear medicine techniques can be achieved with the application of exogenous tracers or contrast media.

1.2.3.1 Low Molecular Weight Gadolinium-Based Contrast Agents

In a clinical MRI setting, choice of contrast media is limited by regulatory approval to the class of nonspecific, low molecular weight extracellular fluid (ECF) agents, typically organic cage-like structures of ~500 Da size chelated to the Gd^{3+} ion. Water accesses the Gd^{3+} ion, which enhances longitudinal or spin-lattice relaxation; T_1 is locally shortened. Thus such agents are commonly associated with increased signal intensity (enhancement) on T_1-weighted images. Since even a 500-Da molecule is retained intravascularly by an intact blood brain barrier (BBB), these agents have been adopted as markers of BBB disruption revealed as tissue enhancement after intravenous Gd administration.

For example, regional disruption of the BBB associated with CNS neoplasia is frequently used as a marker of disease burden in clinical and preclinical efficacy studies (Figure 1.10). The use of these agents is not limited to positive enhancement. In addition to shortening T_1 (providing positive enhancement on T_1-weighted images), the magnetic properties of the Gd^{3+} ion disturb local magnetic field homogeneity and thus can be considered as shortening T_2^*. The added sensitivity offered by exploiting T_2^* shortening (which extends over a wider spatial scale than T_1 shortening) was used in the dynamic tracking of bolus injection of Gd-based contrast media for the assessment of cerebral perfusion (see Chapter 2).

1.2.3.2 Other Elements: Dysprosium and Iron

Indeed, without the requirements for regulatory approval, alternative moieties are considered in experimental imaging of neuroscience models. For example, replacing

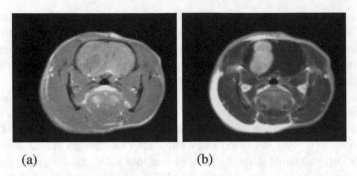

(a)   (b)

FIGURE 1.10 Contrast-enhanced MRI using low molecular weight contrast agents (e.g., Gd-DPTA) can be used to demonstrate regional disruption of the blood–brain-barrier. In this example, U87 cells were inoculated into the striatum of a CD1 nude mouse, resulting in a tumor that is only just evident from the conventional MRI scan (a). Following intravenous injection of Gd-DTPA, the T_1-weighted image clearly delineates the tumor burden as evident from the regional barrier disruption and accumulations of contrast agent. (Image courtesy of Annie Ogasawara and Simon Williams.)

Gd with Dy (dysprosium) offers near two-fold increased sensitivity (the magnetic moment of Dy is considerably greater than that of Gd; its field disturbance is more pronounced), while the potentially contaminating coincident effect of T_1 shortening is considerably less pronounced.

Similarly iron (Fe)-based agents can be tracked dynamically. Where signal loss is delayed or absent, one can infer abnormal or diminished cerebral perfusion. Indeed, using dynamic imaging, it is possible to probe the progressive nature of enhancement associated with BBB disruption conventionally examined only as one time point, "T_1 post Gad." By observing signal changes on dynamically acquired images and applying appropriate tracer kinetic models, it is possible to model the microvascular hyperpermeability associated with BBB breakdown or neo-angiogenesis. By observing progressive enhancement over time in brain tissue despite clearance from plasma, one can infer transport rates from the intravascular to the extravascular space.

The quantification of microvascular permeability has proven efficacious in models of cerebral neoplasm, inflammation, and ischemia. However, perhaps its most exciting utility is rapid assessment of novel pharmaceuticals, whose modes of action in combating angiogenesis, for example, might reduce vascular permeability by blocking the effects of vascular endothelial growth factor (VEGF), also known as vascular permeability factor (VPF). This leads to consideration of imaging-based, physiologically specific indicators of pharmaceutical action and efficacy and ultimately to the suggestion of physiologically specific, imaging-derived surrogate outcome markers.

1.2.3.3 Macromolecular Contrast Agents

Freed from the regulatory restriction requiring low molecular weight agents (preferred mainly because of their clinically acceptable elimination profiles), macromolecular and particulate agents can be contemplated. Such agents can be synthesized (e.g., by conjugating to albumin) such that the enhancing moiety (Gd, Dy, or Fe) is retained intravascularly and at near-constant concentrations over extended periods.[†] The degree of signal enhancement can be related quantitatively to the fractional tissue blood volume. Variations in CBV can thus be tracked dynamically, e.g., during experimental manipulation of pO_2 and pCO_2.

Cerebral blood volume (CBV) changes accompanying neural activity (fMRI; see Chapters 4 and 5) can be tracked quantitatively and *with specificity* (eliminating confounding consideration of CBF (cerebral blood flow) changes and changes in the balance of oxyhemoglobin and deoxyhemoglobin exploited in BOLD imaging). Intravascular agents can be used also for high resolution (T_1-weighted) MRIs of cerebral vessels without requiring sensitivity to vascular flow that may be compromised in stenotic vessels. Due to the success of noncontrast or timed GdDTPA-enhanced magnetic resonance angiography (MRA) methodologies and difficulties distinguishing arterial and venous enhancement with intravascular contrast media methods, this potential application is less widespread. Nevertheless, in small animal studies in which high resolution is essential, blood pool contrast agents allow for long imaging times necessary to achieve sufficient signal-to-noise ratio for the resolution required. Using this technique, MRAs from the mouse brain can be obtained as illustrated in Figure 1.7(c).

1.2.3.4 Targeted Contrast Agents

Highly specific magnetic resonance-visible molecular probes provide an additional opportunity for neuroscientific imaging in animal models. Overcoming inherent sensitivity limitations, seeking methods of molecular amplification, and exploiting the advantages of high magnetic field images led to significant developments in the molecular MRI field (see Chapter 10).

1.3 CONCLUSION

In summary, MRI provides a powerful array of physiologic sensitivities. The combined interpretations of MRIs with different sensitivities can allow considerable inference into the workings of the physicochemical, and hence physiological microenvironment. By exploiting the intrinsic sensitivities of the NMR signal or in conjunction with exogenous contrast media, the reader is invited in subsequent chapters to explore in more detail the opportunities offered by MRI and identify its place in small animal settings in conjunction with alternative imaging modalities, such as positron emission tomography (PET). Especially in the context of preclinical evaluation of novel therapies the roles of imaging in the processes involved in drug development are vital. Beyond the identification of candidate pathways for pharmaceutical investigation, the use of imaging is critical for characterizing tissue with physiologic specificity and also for monitoring the modes of action and efficacies of treatments with both volumetric (morphometric) and physiological parametric analysis.

---

† Rodent plasma disappearance half-lives for covalently bound albumin-GdDTPA are typically quoted on the order of 3 hours. Thus, effectively near-constant plasma concentration of Gd can be maintained over 30- to 60-minute periods (1/6 to 1/3 half-life).

ACKNOWLEDGMENT

Tim Roberts gratefully acknowledges the Canada Research Chair program/Canadian Institute for Health Research for the Canada Research Chair in Imaging Research.

2 MRI Measurement of Cerebral Perfusion and Application to Experimental Neuroscience

Mark F. Lythgoe, David L. Thomas, and Fernando Calamante

CONTENTS

0-8493-0122-X/03/$0.00+$1.50

2.1 MEASURING CEREBRAL BLOOD FLOW: BRIEF HISTORY

The importance of blood flow to the brain has been recognized since antiquity. Even though its true function remained elusive, it was acknowledged that cerebral blood flow (CBF) deserved close investigation. Around 450 B.C., Pythagoras distinguished two types of vessels. He recognized the ebb and flow of blood in the veins and stressed the importance of circulation for mental function (Bell, 1987).

Diogenes of Apollonia (460 B.C.) professed that pleasure and pain resulted from blood aeration, and emphasized the intellectual value of the spirit of life or *pneuma*, the shimmering steam that rose from the shed blood of a sacrificed victim. Through-out the fourth century B.C., Aristotle and others thought that the brain was a secondary organ that served as a cooling agent for the heart. Hippocrates, a Greek physician born in 460 B.C., suggested that thoughts, ideas, and feelings came from the brain and not from the heart as others believed. He attempted to document the condition known as apoplexy or stroke of God's hand (an early term for stroke) and noted, "During spasm, the loss of speech for a long time is unfortunate; if present for a short time, it proclaims a paralysis of the tongue, of the arm, or parts situated on the right side." He attributed the underlying causes to the flow of "black bile" into the head caused by heating of the blood vessels.

Galen of Pergamus (131–201 A.D.), a renowned anatomist and physiologist, was first to describe the *rete mirabile* (marvelous net) as a place where the "vital spirit" ascended from the heart to the brain. He also divided apoplexy into four varieties, the worst of which included stertor and foaming at the mouth. He rightly attributed death in such cases to failure of respiration.

During the Renaissance and the era of the great anatomists, Leonardo da Vinci and Andreas Vesalius described in detail the architecture of the cerebral vessels. In 1664, Thomas Willis demonstrated the existence of blood vessels in the brain by injecting a dark-colored dye. He noted an arterial circle at the base of the brain, now referred to as the Circle of Willis. In the 17th century, Wepfer applied William Harvey's concept of the circulation of blood through the body to Willis's finding and established that a stroke could be caused by a blood clot in the arteries that stopped the flow of vital spirits into the brain.

One of the first reports of direct CBF investigation was by Frans Donders in 1850. He observed pial vessels through a glass window sealed in the calvarium and saw variations in calibers of vessels in different states, especially during asphyxia when they were dilated. In 1890, Roy and Sherringham, while using measurements of the vertical diameter of the brain in the open cranium, were the first to suggest intrinsic local control of CBF that corresponded to functional activity: "…the chemical products of cerebral metabolism contained in the lymph which bathes the walls of the arterioles of the brain can cause variations of the calibre of the cerebral vessels; that in this reaction the brain possesses an intrinsic mechanism by which its vascular supply can be varied locally in correspondence with local variations of functional activity" (Bell, 1987). This work paved the way for modern functional imaging and the need to monitor blood flow to the brain

Over the past 100 years, a number of techniques have been devised to measure CBF. From the early invasive measurements of pressure and thermoelectric effects to the development of indicator fractionation and clearance methods such as autoradiography, hydrogen clearance, and positron emission tomography (PET), clinical and experimental needs for effective CBF assessment have been met by some efforts to develop such quantification techniques (Bell, 1984). Nevertheless, the goal of developing a noninvasive method that facilitates the mapping of CBF with high temporal and spatial resolution over a wide range of relevant blood flows has not yet been attained.

2.2 MAGNETIC RESONANCE IMAGING TECHNIQUES

The advantage of using magnetic resonance imaging (MRI) to assess perfusion is that, in addition to being noninvasive, it may be used in combination with other nuclear magnetic resonance (NMR) techniques (e.g. diffusion-weighted imaging, metabolite spectroscopy, tissue relaxometry). This allows concurrent longitudinal assessment of tissue perfusion, morphology, metabolism and function, thus providing a more complete understanding of developing pathophysiology. The sensitivity of NMR to the movement of spins in flowing liquids was noted at a very early stage (Singer, 1959) and led to the important radiological technique of magnetic resonance angiography (MRA) (Potchen et al., 1993).

Efforts to image perfusion have been dogged by the relatively low volume and velocity of moving spins in capillary beds. The initial work of Le Bihan et al. (1986) and Turner (1988) used the dephasing of randomly perfusing water protons (intravoxel incoherent motion or IVIM) in magnetic field gradients as an index of tissue perfusion. In the succeeding years, two distinct MRI techniques have appeared, both with well supported claims to provide quantitative assessments of CBF. These methods differ with regard to use of exogenous and endogenous MRI-visible tracers. The first technique, dynamic susceptibility contrast (DSC) MRI, is not entirely noninvasive, in that it requires injection of a contrast agent. The second method, arterial spin labeling (ASL), uses radio frequency (RF) pulses to label moving spins in flowing blood.

In recent years, methods for measuring perfusion using MRI have been used in an increasing number of applications (Calamante et al., 1999b; Thomas et al., 2000). This chapter outlines the techniques and applications of magnetic resonance perfusion imaging in the research environment for the detection of blood flow changes during neuroimaging studies.

2.3 MEASURING PERFUSION USING DYNAMIC SUSCEPTIBILITY CONTRAST MRI

Dynamic susceptibility contrast (DSC) MRI, also known as bolus tracking MRI, is a powerful technique for measuring physiological parameters related to cerebral blood flow. The technique involves injection of a bolus of a paramagnetic contrast agent (e.g., gadolinium DTPA) and the rapid measurement of the MRI signal loss due to spin dephasing (i.e., decrease in T_2 and T_2^*) during its passage through the tissue (Villringer et al., 1988).

Since the transit time of the bolus through the tissue is only a few seconds, a fast imaging technique (typically echo planar imaging [EPI] or fast low angle shot [FLASH] is required to obtain sequential images during the wash-in and wash-out of the contrast material (Figure 2.1). In a brain region with an intact blood–brain barrier (BBB), the compartmentalization of the contrast agent leads to a significant drop in signal that dominates the more local T_1 relaxation enhancement (Gillis and Koenig, 1987; Villringer et al., 1988).

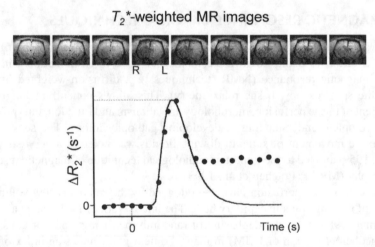

FIGURE 2.1 Sequential T_2^*-weighted MR images obtained with high temporal resolution during the first passage of a bolus of paramagnetic contrast agent, together with the time course of the R_2^* change (proportional to the concentration of the contrast agent). The images show the signal intensity decrease associated with the passage of a bolus. Time course data are fitted to a γ-variate function to remove the contrast agent recirculation. DSC-MRI (FLASH sequence, flip angle 15°, repetition time = 11 ms, echo time = 7 ms) was performed on a coronal rat brain slice 1 hour after occlusion of the left middle cerebral artery. Images were acquired with a time resolution of 0.7 seconds. (Modified from Dijkhuizen, R.M., Magnetic Resonance Imaging and Spectroscopy in Experimental Cerebral Ischaemia, Thesis, University of Utrecht, Netherlands, 1998b.)

2.3.1 QUANTIFICATION: KINETIC MODEL

Assuming a linear relationship between the change in relaxation rate $R_2 = 1/T_2$ (or R_2*) and the concentration of contrast agent ($C(t)$), and assuming changes in signal intensity are caused solely by contrast agent-dependent changes in R_2/R_2*, $C(t)$ can be calculated on a pixel-by-pixel basis (Villringer et al., 1988; Rosen et al., 1990; Boxerman et al., 1995):

$$C(t) = \kappa_{tissue} \cdot \Delta R_2 = -\frac{\kappa_{tissue}}{TE} \cdot \ln\left(\frac{S(t)}{S_0}\right) \qquad (2.1)$$

where $S(t)$ is the signal intensity at time t, S_0 is the baseline, i.e., the signal intensity before contrast administration, and TE is the echo time of the pulse sequence. The proportionality constant κ_{tissue} depends on the tissue, the contrast agent, the field strength, and the pulse sequence parameters.

The model used to quantify perfusion is based on the principles of tracer kinetics for nondiffusible tracers (Zierler, 1965; Axel, 1980), and relies on the assumption that the contrast material remains intravascular. The concentration of tracer in the tissue can be expressed (Østergaard et al., 1996; Calamante et al., 1999b) as:

$$C(t) = \left(\frac{\rho}{k_H}\right) \cdot CBF \cdot \left(C_a(t) \otimes R(t)\right) = \left(\frac{\rho}{k_H}\right) \cdot CBF \int_0^t C_a(\tau) R(t - \tau) d\tau \qquad (2.2)$$

where $C_a(\tau)$ is the arterial input function (AIF), i.e., the concentration of tracer entering the tissue at time τ, $R(t - \tau)$ is the residue function describing the fraction of contrast agent remaining in the tissue at time t after injection of an ideal instantaneous bolus (i.e., a δ function) at time t, and $\otimes$ indicates the mathematical convolution operation. The constant ρ is the density of brain tissue, and $k_H = (1 - H_{art})/(1 - H_{cap})$ accounts for the difference in hematocrit (H) between large vessels (*art*) and capillaries (*cap*), since only plasma volume is accessible to the tracer.

The convolution operation in Equation 2.2 accounts for the fact that part of the spread in the concentration time curve for a nonideal bolus is due to the finite length of the actual bolus (Perthen et al., 2002). Equation 2.2 can be interpreted by considering the AIF as a superposition of consecutive ideal boluses $C_a(\tau)d\tau$ injected at time τ. For each ideal bolus, the concentration still present in the tissue at time t will be proportional to $C_a(\tau)R(t-\tau)d\tau$, and the total concentration $C(t)$ will be given by the sum (or integral) of all these contributions. In order to calculate CBF, Equation 2.2 must be deconvolved (see Østergaard et al., 1996) to isolate $CBF \cdot R(t)$, and the flow obtained from its value at time $t = 0$ (since $R(t = 0) = 1$, i.e., by definition, no tracer has left the tissue at $t = 0$).

2.3.2 QUANTIFICATION OF CEREBRAL BLOOD VOLUME AND MEAN TRANSIT TIME

The compartmentalization of the contrast agent within the intravascular space can also be used to obtain information about cerebral blood volume (CBV). For an intact BBB, CBV is proportional to the normalized total amount of tracer:

$$\text{CBV} = \left(\frac{k_H}{\rho}\right) \cdot \frac{\int C(t)dt}{\int C_a(t)dt} \qquad (2.3)$$

The normalization to the AIF accounts for the fact that, independent of the CBV, a greater concentration will reach the tissue if more tracer is injected.

The CBF and CBV are related through the central volume theorem (Stewart, 1894; Meier and Zierler, 1954): MTT = CBV/CBF, where MTT is the mean transit time. MTT can be calculated if CBF and CBV are known. MTT represents the average time required for a given particle of tracer to pass through the vascular bed defined by CBV after an ideal instantaneous bolus injection. Based on the classical outflow experiment (concentration in the venous output, $C_{OUT}(t)$, is measured and the MTT is calculated directly from the first moment of tracer concentration; Axel, 1995), many studies have calculated MTT from the first moment of $C(t)$ measured in tissue. However, as noted by Weisskoff et al. (1993), the first moment of $C_{OUT}(t)$ is different from the first moment of $C(t)$:

$$\text{MTT} \neq \frac{\int tC(t)dt}{\int C(t)dt} \qquad (2.4)$$

It is important to note that MTT cannot be calculated without first solving Equation 2.2. The first moment of $C(t)$ is only an approximation and depends on the topology of the vasculature (Weisskoff et al., 1993). Some studies used the central volume theorem to estimate a perfusion index (CBF$_i$) from the ratio of the CBV to the first moment of concentration time curve (used as an approximation to MTT). However, apart from the dependency on the underlying vascular structure, the perfusion index is influenced by the shape of the bolus (Perthen et al., 2002).

This technique can provide, in principle, CBF in absolute units (ml/100 g/min). The values of the constants in the above equations (ρ, k_H, κ_{tissue} and κ_{aif}) must be estimated (Rempp et al., 1994; Gückel et al., 1996; Schreiber et al., 1998; Vonken et al., 1999; Smith et al., 2000). Alternatively, a cross-calibration to a gold standard technique can be used to calibrate the DSC-MRI measurement (Østergaard et al., 1998; Wittlich et al., 1995). Although the values obtained in normal subjects are consistent with expected CBF values, some concerns still exist regarding accuracy under various physiological conditions (Calamante et al., 2002; Sorensen, 2001).

2.3.3 DECONVOLUTION VS. SUMMARY PARAMETERS

Analysis of DSC data using deconvolution is time consuming and computationally intensive, but can produce *direct* information about CBF, CBV, and MTT. The main drawback is that it requires measurement of the AIF in order to solve Equation 2.2 (Østergaard et al., 1996). The AIF is generally estimated from the signal time curve from pixels within a major artery (e.g., the middle cerebral artery or internal carotid artery), assuming an equivalent relationship to Equation 2.1 with a proportionality constant κ_{aif}.

Although this is possible in small animals (Perman et al., 1992; Porkka et al., 1991), proper characterization is not straightforward. Furthermore, the measured bolus can be further delayed and dispersed on its transit from artery to tissue (Østergaard et al., 1996; Calamante et al., 2000). This is sometimes observed in cases of abnormal vascular distribution, such as occlusion, stenosis, or collateral flow. The additional delay and dispersion are interpreted by the model as occurring *within* tissue. This leads to underestimation of CBF, overestimation of MTT, and potential underestimation of CBV (Calamante et al., 2000).

An alternative approach to analyzing and quantifying DSC-MRI data involves measurement of summary parameters calculated directly from the profile of the $C(t)$ curve as *indirect* perfusion measures. The more common parameters used are bolus arrival time (BAT), time to peak (TTP), i.e., time until the maximum of $C(t)$, maximum peak concentration (MPC), i.e., maximum value of $C(t)$, first moment of $C(t)$, and area under the peak (see Figure 2.2 and Equation 2.4).

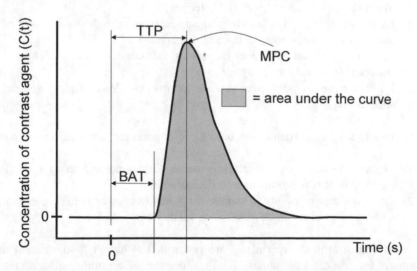

FIGURE 2.2 Representation of the concentration curve following injection of a paramagnetic contrast agent. Several summary parameters may be calculated from the profile of the curve as indirect perfusion measures. Bolus arrival time (BAT); time to peak (TTP), i.e., time until the maximum of $C(t)$; maximum peak concentration (MPC), i.e., maximum value of $C(t)$; and area under the peak are shown.

This type of indirect analysis is widely used because it involves minimal post-processing and does not require AIF measurement. However, apart from the area under the peak (which is proportional to CBV; see Equation 2.3), all other summary parameters provide only indirect measures of perfusion since they can be affected also by CBV and MTT (Weisskoff et al., 1993). Furthermore, they can be influenced by injection conditions (volume injected, injection rate, cannula size, etc.), vascular geometry, and cardiac output. While they may be effective in the identification of abnormal regions (see Section 2.6.1), the interpretation of such abnormality in terms of perfusion is not straightforward (Weisskoff et al., 1993, Perthen et al., 2002). In particular, AIF differences between individuals can produce variability in the summary parameters larger than that due to the abnormality under investigation (Perthen et al., 2002). Therefore, their use for setting up thresholds, for comparisons of individuals, and in follow-up studies can produce misleading results that should be interpreted with caution.

2.3.4 LIMITATIONS OF HUMAN VS. ANIMAL STUDIES

Many assumptions, limitations, and problems in quantifying DSC-MRI data in human studies are less important in animal experiments because of differences in size, cardiac output, blood flow, and bolus volume. The main advantages of DSC-MRI quantification in animal experiments are:

1. Smaller effect due to bolus delay and dispersion
2. Much sharper injected bolus (i.e., sharper AIF)
3. Easier access to bolus injection in an artery proximal to the tissue of interest (minimizes bolus delay and dispersion)
4. Fewer dose-related limitations (at present, maximum dose in adult human studies is 0.3 mmol/kg body weight)
5. Minimum movement artefacts (experiments done under general anaesthesia)

On the other hand, certain issues have more importance in animal experiments:

1. Increased difficulty in identifying voxels within major arteries for AIF measurement (distortions and partial volume)
2. Small number of points to sample the bolus (narrower bolus): potential sources of errors with deconvolution methods

Finally, most animal experiments are performed at higher field strength than commonly used in clinical studies (1.5 T). Since the susceptibility effects created by the bolus of contrast agent are approximately linear with magnetic field strength, higher magnetic field allows for smaller doses. Alternatively, for the same dose, thinner slices or smaller voxels can be used, but one effect that should be considered is associated T_1 prolongation at higher field. Although this is advantageous for ASL (see next section), it decreases the signal-to-noise ratio (SNR) of the DSC-MRI (less relaxation recovery for a fixed repetition time).

2.4 MEASURING PERFUSION USING ARTERIAL SPIN LABELING

Arterial spin labeling (ASL) is a tissue perfusion measurement method that uses magnetically labeled blood water as an endogenous tracer. It is appealing because it does not require injection of exogenous tracers and places no limitation on the number of repeat measurements that can be made in a single study. This makes ASL well suited for the continuous monitoring of CBF over experimental courses of minutes or hours, e.g., to monitor the heterogeneous evolution of tissue perfusion after experimental ischemia and reperfusion in animal models. The images generated with ASL can be converted into CBF maps (ml/100 g/min) as long as certain other MR parameters are also measured.

2.4.1 GENERATING PERFUSION-WEIGHTED IMAGES USING ASL

Inflowing blood water is labeled by inversion of its spin magnetization. Two images must be acquired: the labeled image obtained by spin labeling and the control image for which no labeling is performed. The difference between the two images is proportional to the amount of labeled blood that enters the imaging slice during the time between labeling and image acquisition, and therefore is proportional to CBF. Spin labeling can be achieved via several approaches, which has given rise to a number of ASL techniques.

2.4.1.1 Continuous ASL

Continuous ASL (CASL) is so named because the magnetization of inflowing arterial blood water is continuously inverted as it passes through a plane in the neck over a period of several seconds, allowing a build-up of labeled water in the perfused cerebral tissue. This approach is illustrated in Figure 2.3. The most important features of continuous ASL are:

1. The application of a magnetic field gradient along the slice-select direction, causing ^1H water spins to resonate at a frequency dependent on their position in this direction. See Figure 2.3(b).
2. Concurrently, a radio frequency pulse with a frequency corresponding to ^1H water spins in the neck (typically 5 to 10 kHz offset from the main field frequency) is applied. This causes the inversion of flowing spins as they pass through this frequency range. See Figure 2.3(c). The process responsible for spin inversion is known as flow-induced adiabatic inversion (Dixon et al., 1986). For the control image, the frequency offset of the pulse is reversed so that the location of the affected plane does not coincide with arteries supplying blood to the brain. See Figure 2.3(a). The pulse duration is typically 1 to 3 seconds.
3. Following the labeling or control RF pulse, an image is acquired using a fast imaging technique (such as EPI or FLASH) with minimal T_2 or T_2^* weighting, to avoid confounding BOLD effects.

The result is a pair of images that can be used to calculate a map of CBF.

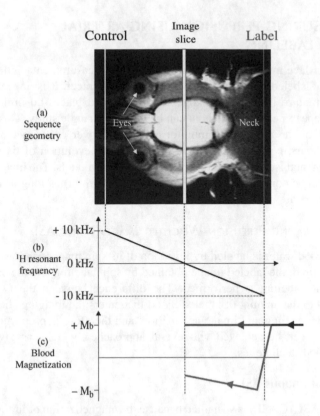

FIGURE 2.3 Continuous arterial spin labeling using flow-induced adiabatic fast passage. (a) Axial MR image through the rat brain shows the relative positions of the imaging (coronal) slice and the inversion (red) and control (green) planes. (b) The application of a magnetic field gradient causes the resonant frequency of water protons to constitute a linear function of position (over the range ~ −10 kHz to +10 kHz). (c) By simultaneously applying a −10-kHz off-resonance RF pulse, blood water spins are inverted as they flow through the inversion plane (spin labeling). The control plane does not intersect any major arteries and does not cause blood spin labeling. See Color Figure 2.3 following page 210.

2.4.1.2 Pulsed ASL

In pulsed ASL (PASL), the label also takes the form of spin inversion. Blood magnetization is labeled by a short (~10 ms) frequency-modulated RF pulse that inverts all spins in a selected region simultaneously. By selecting different regions of inversion and allowing inflow time before image acquisition, flow-sensitive images can be generated. For example, a pair of inversion recovery images can be acquired in which one image follows a slice-selective inversion pulse and the other image follows a global (nonselective) inversion pulse. See Figure 2.4a.

In both cases the inversion time *TI* is the same, and so signal from static tissue in the imaging slice is the same. The difference between the images comes from the difference in magnetization of inflowing blood in the two acquisitions: in the slice-selective inversion recovery (ssIR) image, inflowing blood is fully relaxed and so

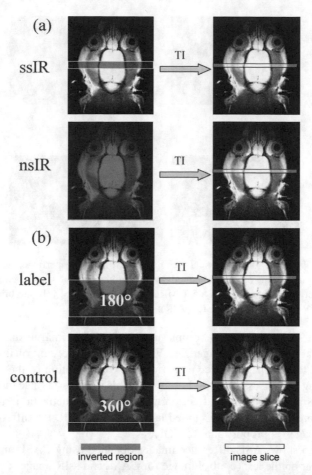

FIGURE 2.4 Pulsed arterial spin labeling using spatially restricted inversion pulses. (a) The flow-sensitive alternating inversion recovery [FAIR] approach acquires a pair of images, one following a slice-selective inversion pulse (upper) and the other following a global (nonselective) inversion pulse (lower). A difference between the images is caused by the difference in magnetization state of the inflowing blood water. (b) EPISTAR also acquires a pair of images, although the difference in inflowing magnetization state is generated by inverting a volume of blood immediately proximal to the imaging slice (upper) or by applying a 360° pulse to this volume (leaving it effectively unaltered; lower). Images were acquired at a time *TI* after application of the inversion pulse. See Color Figure 2.4 following page 210.

increases the apparent relaxation rate of the tissue water; in the global (nonselective) inversion recovery (nsIR) image, inflowing blood is initially inverted and subsequently relaxing during *TI* and so its effect on the relaxation rate of the tissue water is small. The difference in signal intensity between the two images is proportional to CBF. This technique is known as flow-sensitive alternating inversion recovery or FAIR (Kwong et al., 1992; Kim, 1995).

An alternative PASL approach, known as echo planar imaging and signal targeting with alternating radio frequency or EPISTAR (Edelman et al., 1994; Edelman

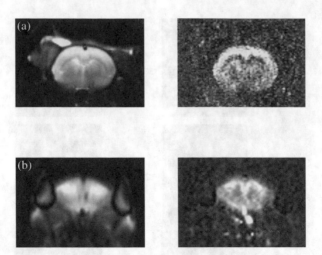

FIGURE 2.5 Examples of anatomical (left) and corresponding perfusion-weighted images (right) of normal rodent brains generated by the subtraction of spin-labeled from control images. (a) Rat brain obtained in a 8.5 T MR scanner using CASL. (b) Gerbil brain obtained in a 2.35 T MR scanner using PASL (FAIR).

and Chen, 1998), is to invert a volume immediately proximal to the imaging slice to generate a spin labeled image. See Figure 2.4(b). The control image inverts a region distal to the imaging slice or performs a 360° rotation of the magnetization in the labeling region, as shown in Figure 2.4. This is necessary because the labeling RF pulse has another indirect effect on tissue water magnetization known as magnetization transfer. It will be discussed later. As with FAIR, the difference between these two images is proportional to CBF.

Figure 2.5 shows ASL difference images obtained using CASL and FAIR. Base images appear on the left (control image for CASL and ssIR image for FAIR); those on the right are the CBF-weighted subtraction images.

2.4.1.3 Generating CBF Maps from ASL Images

Quantification of CBF using ASL images is based on modelling each voxel as a single well mixed compartment. The rate of change of the longitudinal relaxation of brain tissue water magnetization is classically described by the Bloch equation:

$$\frac{dM_b(t)}{dt} = \frac{M_b^0 - M_b(t)}{T_1} \tag{2.5}$$

where $M_b(t)$ is the longitudinal magnetization per gram of tissue at time t, M_b^0 is the fully relaxed value of $M_b(t)$, and T_1 is the longitudinal relaxation time. In the presence of flow, this equation can be modified by the addition of two extra terms:

$$\frac{dM_b(t)}{dt} = \frac{M_b^0 - M_b(t)}{T_1} + f \cdot M_a(t) - f \cdot M_v(t) \tag{2.6}$$

The first added term ($f \cdot M_a(t)$) represents the gain of magnetization by the tissue caused by inflow. The second added term ($f \cdot M_v(t)$) accounts for the loss of magnetization due to outflow. $M_a(t)$ is the magnetization of the inflowing (arterial) blood per ml. $M_v(t)$ is the magnetization of the outflowing (venous) blood per ml, and f is blood flow (ml/g/second). If we consider brain tissue and microvasculature to constitute a well mixed compartment, the magnetization of the venous blood is related to that of the brain tissue via the blood–brain partition coefficient of water or λ (Herscovitch and Raichle, 1985) by:

$$M_v(t) = \frac{M_b(t)}{\lambda} \tag{2.7}$$

and so Equation 2.2 can be written as:

$$\frac{dM_b(t)}{dt} = \frac{M_b^0 - M_b(t)}{T_1} + f \cdot M_a(t) - \frac{f}{\lambda} \cdot M_b(t) \tag{2.8}$$

By manipulating the state of arterial magnetization or M_a, one can modify the apparent relaxation and magnetization of the brain tissue water. If the state of the inflowing blood water is known and the change of magnetization of the tissue water is measured, solving Equation 2.8 for f will allow the calculation of blood flow. As described, arterial magnetization is labeled in ASL by spin inversion.

For CASL, the inflowing magnetization is continuously inverted for several seconds prior to image acquisition ($M_a(t) = -1$), allowing the build-up of a steady state so that Equation 2.8 can be solved (Williams et al., 1992) to yield:

$$f = \frac{\lambda}{T_{1app}} \frac{\left(M_b^{cont} - M_b^{label}\right)}{2M_b^{cont}} \tag{2.9}$$

where M_b^{cont} and M_b^{label} are the control and spin labeled tissue magnetizations, respectively, and T_{1app} is the longitudinal relaxation time of brain tissue including the effect of flow:

$$\frac{1}{T_{1app}} = \frac{1}{T_1} + \frac{f}{\lambda} \tag{2.10}$$

Equation 2.10 is a fundamental equation of ASL, showing how the apparent longitudinal relaxation time is directly related to perfusion. Inspection of Equation 2.9 shows that CBF is directly proportional to the ASL difference signal (control minus label), and can be directly calculated if T_{1app} and λ are known or measured. Figure 2.6 shows images used to create a perfusion map with CASL.

For PASL, where all inflowing magnetization is inverted at a single point in time ($TI = 0$ seconds), the tissue magnetization difference signal at later TI is:

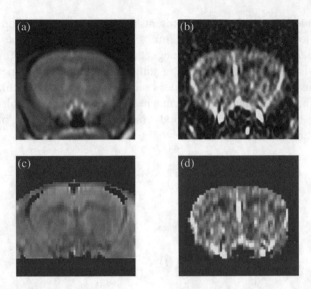

FIGURE 2.6 Examples of images used to create a CASL perfusion map. (a) Control image of the CASL perfusion image pair. (b) The result of subtracting the spin-labeled image from the control image. A T_1 map (c) is then combined with these images according to Equation 2.9 to produce a quantitative perfusion map (d).

$$\Delta M = 2M_b^0 \cdot TI \cdot \frac{f}{\lambda} \cdot \exp\left(-\frac{TI}{T_1}\right) \tag{2.11}$$

if we assume blood and tissue have the same longitudinal relaxation times (see next section). This difference signal maximizes at $TI \sim T_1$, at which point the PASL signal is a factor of e^{-1} less than the CASL signal, showing the greater theoretical sensitivity of CASL. However, a number of practical issues make the comparison of CASL and PASL less straightforward; they are discussed in the next section.

2.4.1.4 Factors Affecting Quantification of CBF with ASL

Several factors affect the accuracy of the quantification of CBF using ASL with the tissue model described above.

Inversion efficiency — Ideally, all spin labeled water will have its magnetization fully inverted, i.e., $M_a = -M_a^0$ where M_a^0 is the equilibrium arterial water magnetization. In practice, however, this will not be the case. In CASL, spin inversion is achieved by flow-induced adiabatic inversion that relies on blood flowing at a certain rate or greater, as defined by the adiabatic condition: $1/T_{1a}, 1/T_{2a} << (1/B_1) \cdot G \cdot v << \gamma B_1$ where T_{1a} and T_{2a} are the longitudinal and transverse relaxation times of arterial blood water, respectively, B_1 is the amplitude of the applied RF field, G is the amplitude of the magnetic field gradient, v is the velocity of flow, and γ is the magnetogyric ratio.

For the typical values of parameters used in animal studies, this condition is generally satisfied in the major arteries. However, flow through the arteries is laminar; a certain proportion of the blood water will flow at subthreshold velocities. Not all the arterial water magnetization will be inverted. This will produce a lower perfusion signal difference between the labeled and control images.

In order to account for this effect, a parameter known as inversion efficiency (α) is introduced. The α value ranges from 0 (no inversion) to 1 (full inversion) and enters the CBF quantification by appearing in the denominator of the right hand side of Equation 2.9, i.e., $2M_b^{cont}$ becomes $2\alpha\, M_b^{cont}$. The value of α can be measured by observing the effect of the spin labeling RF pulse on the intravascular signal just downstream from the labeling plane (Zhang et al., 1993). For flow-induced adiabatic inversion, the value is usually 0.7 to 0.8. Similarly, the inversion pulses used in PASL do not produce 100% inversion. It is appropriate to introduce the inversion efficiency as a multiplying factor on the right side of Equation 2.11. However, the efficiency of short, frequency modulated inversion pulses is generally quite high ($\alpha \sim 0.95$).

Transit time — Following spin inversion, blood water travels through the vascular tree until it reaches the capillary bed and exchanges into the cerebral tissue. In theory, the time taken for the transit of blood from the point where it is labeled to the point where it exchanges into the brain is short relative to the longitudinal relaxation time of the blood water (T_{1a}). In other words, the labeled blood enters the tissue in a state defined by its initial degree of inversion (α). In practice, T_{1a} is 1 – 2 seconds and the transit time can be of the same order, especially in larger animals or humans. This has a direct effect on the accuracy of quantification, since the calculated value of CBF is directly proportional to α (see previous paragraph).

Transit time effects are particularly problematic in CASL, where the labeling plane is necessarily a certain distance from the imaging slice so that it coincides with a major artery. With PASL, transit times tend to be smaller because the labeled region can be placed immediately adjacent to the imaging slice. In order to deal with transit time effects, one of two approaches can be adopted. The transit time can be measured (Ye et al., 1997) or the pulse sequence can be modified so as to minimize the effects of transit time on CBF quantification (Alsop and Detre, 1996; Wong et al., 1998). Using the former approach, an effective inversion efficiency (α') that incorporates transit time (Δ) can be defined:

$$\alpha' = \alpha \exp\left(\Delta/T_{1a}\right) \tag{2.12}$$

The α' is the degree of inversion of spin labeled water when it exchanges from blood into tissue. Acquiring maps of transit times is a time-consuming and noise-prone process. For this reason, the second approach described above is more common, and the method for reducing the sensitivity of ASL to transit times is to insert a delay between the end of the spin labeling period and image acquisition. The theoretical justification for this approach is beyond the scope of this book (interested readers should consult the relevant references), but it can be shown that inclusion of a sufficiently long postlabeling delay changes the equation for CBF quantification to:

$$f = \frac{\lambda \left(M_b^{cont} - M_b^{label} \right)}{2\alpha M_b^0} C \left(T_{1ns}, T_{1s}, T_{1a}, T_{ex}, \Delta \right)$$ (2.13)

for CASL (where T_{1ns} and T_{1s} are tissue T_1 values in the absence and presence of off-resonance radiation, respectively (see the magnetization transfer section below), T_{ex} is the time between when a spin is labeled and when it crosses the BBB, and C is a scaling factor to account for relaxation effects). Similarly,

$$f = \frac{\left(M^{cont} - M^{label} \right)}{2\alpha M_0 TI_1 \exp \left[-TI_2 / T_{1a} \right]} \cdot Q \left(T_{1a}, T_1, T_{ex}, f, \lambda, TI_2 \right)$$ (2.14)

for the QUIPSS (quantitative imaging of perfusion using a single subtraction) II (Wong, Buxton, and Frank, 1998) version of PASL where TI_1 is the inversion time during which spin labeled blood enters the imaging slice, TI_2 is the inversion time plus the delay before image acquisition, and Q is a scaling factor accounting for relaxation. In both cases (Equations 2.13 and 2.14), the scaling factors C and Q are approximately constant for a given set of relaxation times and sequence parameters (which are measured and user-defined, respectively), making the CBF calculation dependent only on the measured ASL signals. The major drawback of transit time-insensitive ASL methods involving postlabeling delays is that the measurement sensitivity is reduced due to decay of the label during the delay.

Intravascular signal — In the original model for CBF quantification using ASL, it was assumed that all signal emanates from the brain tissue, and thus all the signal in the ASL difference image comes from water exchanged from the vasculature into the brain. This assumption may be incorrect for two reasons. First, a certain amount of spin labeled blood may have entered the imaging slice toward the end of the labeling period (for CASL) or inversion time (for PASL) and may not have had sufficient time to exchange out of the capillary bed. Second, spin labeled blood may be passing through the imaging slice en route to perfusing a different region of the brain.

The effect of preexchange intracapillary blood on the ASL signal can be incorporated into the theoretical model. However, if the labeled blood does not perfuse tissue in the same voxel, its contribution to the ASL difference signal is not desired. In order to eliminate the signal from these larger vessels, flow-sensitive crusher gradients can be used (Detre et al., 1992; Ye et al., 1997). Alternatively, the transit time-insensitive techniques in which a delay is inserted between the end of the labeling period and the image acquisition allow most of the faster moving blood to wash out of the imaging slice before image acquisition. In this way, vascular artefacts are eliminated, except in regions where very long transit times cause spin labeled blood to remain in the vasculature (e.g., regions with collateral flow) at the time of image acquisition.

Magnetization transfer — The 5- to 10-kHz off-resonance RF pulse used to achieve spin inversion exerts a secondary effect on brain tissue magnetization. This is because the hydrogen nuclei of larger molecules or water molecules resonate with a range of frequencies, including the 5- to 10-kHz off-resonance. The magnetization of these nuclei is directly saturated by the spin labeling pulse. Magnetization transfer between the saturated nuclei and the MR-visible free water causes the MR signal to decrease. Consequently, the signal in the ASL images decreases for reasons not related to CBF.

Proper quantification of perfusion requires MT effects to be accounted for (Zhang et al., 1992; Mclaughlin et al., 1997). The most important consequence relates to acquiring the control ASL image. For the control image to experience exactly the same MT effects as the spin labeled image, an off-resonance RF pulse must be applied prior to its acquisition. This is usually done with the magnetic field gradient reversed in polarity, so that the plane of inversion for the control image is positioned above the head of the subject, and no blood water inversion results. See Figure 2.3.

Although smaller for PASL, the same effects also occur with EPISTAR, necessitating a 360° RF pulse designed to have the same MT characteristics as the inversion pulse without net effect on magnetization of the inflowing blood. See Figure 2.4(b). Since the RF pulses used in FAIR (Figure 2.4a) have the same bandwidth (the only difference being whether the slice-select gradient is on or off during the play-out of the pulse), MT effects automatically cancel out.

Signal-to-noise issues — For typical normal values of CBF (and because the half life of the spin label is limited by T_1 relaxation to 1 to 2 seconds), the total signal difference in an ASL image is expected to be 1 to 5% of the base image signal intensity. Therefore, the SNRs of the base images must be high (>100) for the quality of the difference images to be acceptable. The precision of calculated CBF values is directly related to the SNR of the ASL difference image, and often a compromise must be made between temporal resolution of CBF measurement and signal averaging to ensure adequate SNR for precise quantification.

Multislice ASL — Due to the need for equivalent MT effects in both the spin labeled and control CASL images, multislice acquisition using this technique is complicated. Two methods have been proposed. In the first method (Silva et al., 1995), an RF surface coil with a small spatial range is placed on the neck and used to perform spin labeling. The B_1 field generated by the coil does not reach the imaging slices and thus causes no MT effect. This method is effective but needs specific hardware. In the second approach (Alsop and Detre, 1998), the control RF pulse is modified so that it acts as a 360° double inverter, producing identical MT effects to the inversion pulse throughout the whole brain but without causing spin inversion (*cf.* EPISTAR control image acquisition).

The efficacy of a flow-induced adiabatic double inversion pulse has yet to be definitively assessed; however, the methods hold future promise if CASL is to become a practical research tool. The implementation of multislice PASL is more straightforward. FAIR requires a widening of the slice-selective inversion to encompass all the imaging slices, and EPISTAR requires that the inversion slab is placed proximally to all imaging slices. The most important implications of multislice PASL are the inevitably long transit times for slices furthest from the spin labeled regions that can compromise accuracy and sensitivity.

Accuracy of theoretical model — The single-compartment, freely diffusible tracer model for water in the brain clearly represents a simplification. More complex

models that treat the intravascular and extravascular spaces separately and allow for
the limited diffusivity of water have been suggested (St. Lawrence et al., 2000; Zhou
et al., 2001; Parkes and Tofts, 2001). The technique involves adding more variables
such as CBV and the extraction fraction of water from the capillary bed into the
brain tissue into the models.

While these models describe the physical system more accurately than the single-
compartment model, their practical application to interpretation and quantification
of ASL data, which is inherently limited in quantity and by relatively low SNR, may
be difficult due to their complexity. Some errors of the single-compartment model
tend to cancel each other out, particularly in gray matter, for example, an extraction
fraction of less than unity is at least partially compensated for by the presence of
intravascular signal, so the value obtained using the simple model is reasonably
accurate (St. Lawrence, Frank, and Mclaughlin, 2000). This concurs with the experimental validations comparing the results of ASL measurements to those obtained
using other CBF methods and generally showing good correlation among different
techniques (Walsh et al., 1994; Hoehn et al., 1999; Ye et al., 2000; Pell et al., 1999c).

2.5 COMPARISON OF DSC AND ASL FOR USE IN
SMALL ANIMAL CEREBRAL PERFUSION STUDIES

For the neuroscientist wanting to include perfusion measurements within a battery
of MR data scans, the decision whether to use DSC or ASL will depend on the
requirements of the experiment. We now examine the ways each technique offers
benefits over the others in certain situations.

The main advantages of DSC are the speed of measurement, the large signal
change induced by the passage of the bolus (high contrast-to-noise), and the potential
to measure CBV and MTT in addition to CBF. For this reason, if a single, rapid
perfusion-weighted image is required, DSC is likely to be the preferred approach.
Also, as discussed earlier, bolus delay and dispersion effects are minimal in small
animals, making perfusion quantification reliable (with the caveat that the arterial
input function is difficult to measure accurately and the bolus passage occurs more
quickly and may not be very well sampled). Multiple measurements at different time
points can be made, although the number and frequency are limited by the clearance
time of the contrast agent from the blood. In addition, DSC should be performed
after other imaging sequences because the paramagnetic contrast agent can affect
T_2, T_1, and apparent diffusion coefficient (ADC) values.

ASL offers the advantage of noninvasiveness. ASL minimizes animal preparation
time and surgery, improves postprocedure recovery, and allows a series of CBF
measurements to be made with relatively high temporal resolution. It is therefore
useful for monitoring hemodynamic time courses. The main limitation on temporal
resolution is determined by the amount of data averaging necessary to achieve
acceptable signal-to-noise level. For typical small animal experiments, the averaging
timescale and temporal resolution are on the order of a minute. As with DSC, the
deleterious effects of transit time delays are small in comparison with the human
brain, making CBF quantification reliable in the normal brain.

Unfortunately, the reliability of cerebral perfusion measurements made using both DSC and ASL is reduced in situations of compromised flow, e.g., during ischemia. Since bolus delay and transit times are increased, the assumptions made for flow quantification may be violated. It is important to be aware of this when interpreting the CBF data. For example, the perfusion-based signal changes in both DSC and ASL are reduced by genuine reduction in CBF and also by an increase in delay and transit time. The CBF reduction may be overestimated if delay effects are not accounted for. Similarly, flow increases may be overestimated if accompanied by simultaneous and significant decreases in delay and transit times.

In DSC, a changing delay time can be measured by allowing it to be a variable in the time course fit, although this decreases the accuracy of the other fitted parameters. Accounting for changes in bolus dispersion is not straightforward. In ASL, a changing transit time can be measured at the cost of reduced time resolution (≥ 5 minutes). In summary, while perfusion MRI can be used in the study of cerebral hemodynamics, it is currently necessary to exercise caution when interpreting quantitative CBF values in the severely abnormal brain.

2.6 APPLICATION OF MR PERFUSION IMAGING

2.6.1 DSC APPLICATIONS

2.6.1.1 Cerebral Ischemia

One of the first applications of the DSC technique was the study of cerebral ischemia in experimental animal models. Unlike conventional MRI (T_1, T_2, and proton density) that is insensitive to acute ischemia, diffusion-weighted imaging (DWI) and DSC-MRI were shown to detect a stroke within minutes of the event. While DWI may provide unique information about the effect of an ischemic insult as early as a few minutes postictus, it is clearly desirable to obtain information about the integrity of the vascular bed.

Pioneering studies in the late 1970s using a hydrogen clearance technique to measure CBF in a primate model showed that a reduction of CBF below 12 ml/100 g/min for >2 hours produces focal infarction or nonrecoverable tissue, demonstrating a link between degree and duration of ischemia and eventual tissue injury (Morawetz et al., 1979). Prompted by this work, much of the interest in the earlier MRI studies related to acute identification of ischemic regions (Moseley et al., 1990; Wendland et al., 1991; Kucharczyk et al., 1991; Finelli et al., 1992; Maeda et al., 1993). However, since the area with a perfusion deficit was found to be larger than the area depicted by DWI (Roberts et al., 1993), the emphasis moved toward the use of DSC-MRI to complement and help interpret changes observed using conventional MRI and DWI, with the ultimate aim of identifying and characterizing ischemic penumbra (Astrup et al., 1981).

Combined diffusion and DSC-MRI summary parameters were used to identify a severe ischemic central area surrounded by a more moderately affected peripheral area in transient middle cerebral artery occlusion (MCAO) studies in rats (Muller et al., 1995a) and in permanent MCAO studies in cats (Moseley et al., 1990, 1993) and rats (Quast et al., 1993; Pierce et al., 1997; Dijkhuizen et al., 1997). Pierce et al.

(1997) showed that the ADC was linearly correlated with maximum peak (MP) signal in the periphery, and suggested that their combined study could be useful for quantitative assessment of the variable flow gradients in focal ischemia, including areas at risk in the ischemic periphery.

A similar approach was used to identify different levels of ischemia in a cat model of partial MCAO. The combination of high speed ADC measurements and MP signal allowed the differentiation of mild (no change in ADC and slight reduction in the MP), moderate (slight reduction in ADC and reduced MP), and severe cerebral hypoperfusion (marked drop in ADC and almost complete absence of contrast agent passage) (Roberts et al., 1993, 1996). DSC summary parameters were also used to study the reperfusion state in transient MCAO in the cat (Kucharczyk et al., 1993), distinguishing between successful and failed reperfusion and identifying delayed reperfusion injury.

In a study of transient focal ischemia in cats (Caramia et al., 1998), DSC summary parameters were used to identify the hemodynamic spatial heterogeneity in response to ischemia and reperfusion. In particular, a peripheral area of increased vascular transit time (VTT = TTP minus BAT) was observed and interpreted as a mismatch between CBF and CBV. The area had a different response to reperfusion compared to the core region. Comparison of CBF, CBV, and MTT maps in a permanent MCAO piglet model also demonstrated regions of tissue heterogeneity (Figure 2.7). In areas of mild ischemia (CBF > 30 ml/100 g/minute) that had potential to proceed onto infarction, MTT maps indicated a flow-volume mismatch due to vasodilation from the reduced perfusion pressure.

In regions of more severe ischemia (<30 ml/100 g/minute), CBV declined with CBF and the MTT maps indicated the area destined for infarction (Sakoh et al., 2000). Using gradient and spin echo steady state contrast imaging to estimate total and microvascular CBV, together with ASL to measure CBF, Zaharchuk et al. (2000) demonstrated that microvascular CBV progressively decreased with duration of the insult as the tissue became irreversibly damaged. Differing levels of CBF and total CBV reduction were observed in infarcted and spared tissue. To gain further insight into identification of the ischemic penumbra, Carano et al. (2000) used a multispectral analysis of MRI data during cerebral ischemia in the rat. It indicated that combining both diffusion and perfusion parameters may provide a better estimate of nonrecoverable tissue than ADC alone.

Another application where DSC summary parameters were used is the determination of the relationship between apoptosis and perfusion deficits during transient cerebral ischemia in cats. Vexler et al. (1997) showed that a significantly higher number of apoptotic cells were observed in areas that experienced 2.5 hours of severe perfusion deficit (regardless of the state after reperfusion), as compared with the number in areas with moderate hypoperfusion during occlusion, and maintained perfusion on reperfusion. These results suggest that the apoptotic process is induced in the ischemic core and contributes to degeneration of neurons associated with transient ischemia.

In a study of delayed tissue damage in a model of temporary hypoxia–ischemia in the rat, ADC alone was a bad predictor of long term outcome (Dijkhuizen et al., 1998a). Measurements of ADC, T_2-weighted imaging, DSC summary parameters

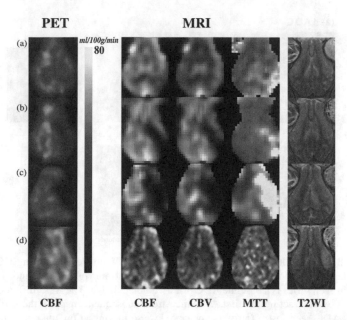

FIGURE 2.7 Comparison of CBF, CBV, and MTT maps produced from DSC-MRI and CBF images obtained by PET 6 hours after permanent MCAO or reperfusion. (a) Mild ischemia (CBF >30 ml/100 g/minute in the ischemic cortex). (b) Moderate ischemia (CBF 12 to 30 ml/100 g/minute in the ischemic cortex). (c) Severe ischemia (CBF <12 ml/100 g/minute in the ischemic cortex). (d) Postischemic hypoperfusion. Note the reliable correlation of DSC-MRI and PET. MTT clearly shows hemodynamic compromise. (Sakoh, M. et al., 2000, *Stroke*, 31, 1958. With permission.) See Color Figure 2.7 following page 210.

(MP, TTP, and PA), laser–Doppler flowmetry, and histology were used to demonstrate regional responses to reperfusion and associated tissue-specific sensitivities to delayed damage. Other studies also demonstrated delayed decreases in ADC. After ischemia and reperfusion in a rat model, estimates of CBF index were similar in both normal and tissue with delayed damage (Li et al., 2000), although another study suggested that the progress of delayed cell death was accompanied by an increase in CBV (van Lookeren-Campagne et al., 1999).

2.6.1.2 Cortical Spreading Depression

DSC summary parameters (rCBV and TTP) have also been used to study cortical spreading depression. By following ADC changes in ischemia-induced spreading depression, Röther et al. (1996a, 1996b) showed that the transient ADC changes originated in the border of the core region that had a moderate perfusion deficit (increased bolus transit time). The variation in ADC recovery time in the ischemic periphery reflected the severity of the tissue perfusion deficit.

De Crespigny et al. (1998) studied the changes in rCBV and ADC during spreading depression in rats but did not use DSC techniques (Figure 2.8). Steady state CBV measurements using a blood pool contrast agent were performed simultaneously with high speed ADC mapping. They found a transient increase in regional CBV (with subsequent rCBV decrease in 50% of animals) that followed the ADC

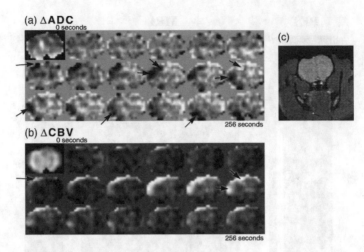

FIGURE 2.8 Serial ADC difference images (a) and rCBV images (b) during KCl-induced spreading depression in rat brain. Time runs top left to bottom right, 16 seconds/image. The first image in each series is a baseline ADC or T_2-weighted image. The ADC difference images were formed by subtracting the first ADC map from subsequent maps in the series. A dark area of low ADC seen in (a) (arrows) appears close to the initiation site and spreads along the cortex up toward midline and down to the base of the brain. Bright cortical areas in the rCBV images (b) indicating increased blood volume show a similar propagation pattern. A higher resolution gradient echo image of the same coronal slice is shown for anatomical reference (c). The dark indentation at the top left side of the brain is a magnetic susceptibility artefact caused by the silver recording electrode. (de-Crespigny, A. et al., *J. Cereb. Blood Flow Metab.*, 18, 1008, 1998. With permission.)

changes with a variable delay (average value of ~16 seconds), thought to be a consequence of the elevated energy requirements during the repolarization after spreading depression.

2.6.1.3 Therapeutic Evaluation

The combined use of DSC-MRI and DWI provides an excellent tool to investigate effects of new therapeutic interventions in models of embolic stroke in animals. Reith et al. (1996) assessed the effects of thrombolytic therapy using rt-PA in a rat model. Yenari et al. (1997) examined the combined effects of rt-PA and direct antithrombin therapy using hirulog in rabbits. Röther et al. (1996c) studied the effects of rt-PA in a model of cerebral venous thrombosis.

Bolus tracking techniques have also been used to evaluate the cerebroprotective effects of noncompetitive NMDA antagonists (Minematsu et al., 1993; Pan et al., 1995) and treatment with the free radical scavenger U74389G (Muller et al., 1995b) in temporary focal ischemia in rats. Other applications include the evaluation of the neuroprotection using NBQX in permanent focal cerebral ischemia in the rat (Lo et al., 1997) and the assessment of the efficacy of intravenous (as compared to intraarterial) therapy with prourokinase in a model of embolic stroke in rats (Takano et al., 1998). In all these studies, serial measurements of diffusion and perfusion were performed in treated and control animals. Based on these studies and others, it is clear that the measurement of perfusion can be used to assess several aspects of a therapeutic study. Reproducibility of the insult and quality of reperfusion may be judged by the initial degree of ischemia and subsequent level of recirculation. Assessment of the effects of therapy on the improvement of blood flow and relationship between blood flow and final outcome or other measured parameters is possible using longitudinal measurements (Beaulieu et al., 1998).

2.6.2 ASL APPLICATIONS

Since the establishment of the ability of techniques to reflect tissue perfusion status, ASL has been used increasingly as an experimental tool in several areas of investigation. The quantitative accuracy of the flow measurements of pulsed and continuous techniques has been investigated using animal and human studies. While pulsed ASL has almost exclusively been used in the field of functional MRI (see Section 2.6.1.6), continuous ASL has also been successfully applied in experimental neuropathology studies.

2.6.2.1 Cerebrovascular Disease

Soon after CASL was proposed, Detre et al. (1993) used it to demonstrate the redistribution of blood flow through anastomoses after unilateral occlusion of the common carotid artery in the rat. They labeled blood flowing through the unoccluded artery only and showed the effective territory of the artery and how the territory changed after occlusion of the other artery. Jiang et al. (1994) monitored the effect of whole body hypothermia on the recovery of perfusion after transient MCAO. CBF was measured quantitatively by CASL with a time resolution of 8.5 minutes using a standard spin echo imaging approach. The degree of postischemic hypoperfusion was reduced if hypothermic conditioning was applied.

More recently, Jiang et al. (1998b) used CASL to study reperfusion levels after antiintercellular adhesion molecule 1 antibody treatment of MCAO in the rat and investigate the thrombolysis of embolic stroke after administration of rt-PA (Figure 2.9) in the rat brain (Jiang et al., 1998a). Busch et al. (1998) also studied the effect of rt-PA on an embolic stroke insult and compared the results from ASL perfusion with ADC measurements. Their results showed that an improvement in blood flow as shown by the ASL perfusion maps led to a slowly progressing reversal of ADC changes in the periphery of the ischemic territory, indicative of tissue recovery.

In an experiment examining acute changes of tissue relaxation parameters following MCAO, Calamante et al. (1999a) used ASL perfusion mapping to identify the extent and the severity of ischemia in the affected middle cerebral artery (MCA) territory. Lythgoe et al. (2000) used CASL to characterize changes observed in a rat model of oligemic perfusion using partial occlusion of the MCA (Figure 2.10). FAIR has also been used during cerebral ischemia to detect regional changes in CBF following permanent proximal and distal occlusion of MCA in a rat model (Tsekos et al., 1998). As expected, proximal occlusion of the MCA reduced CBF in both cortex and striatum, whereas distal occlusion only decreased CBF in the cortex.

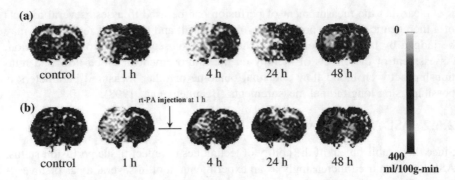

FIGURE 2.9 Cerebral blood flow (CBF) maps of coronal sections of an untreated (a) and a recombinant tissue activator (rt-PA)-treated (b) animal showing the evolution of changes in CBF, obtained before and during ischemia at 1, 4, 24, and 48 hours after embolization. After onset of embolization, a rapid decline in CBF was observed in the occluded MCA territory in both animals. CBF remained lower during the acute phase of ischemia (a). A return of CBF was observed in the cortex 48 hours after embolization (a). A rapid return of CBF was demonstrated (Jiang, Q. et al., *J. Cereb. Blood Flow Metab.*, 18, 758, 1998a) after treatment with rt-PA 1 hour after injection of clot (b); rt-PA was administered 1 hour after embolization. See Color Figure 2.9 following page 210.

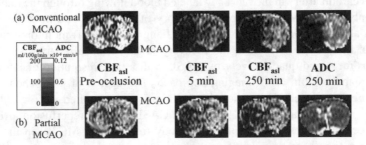

FIGURE 2.10 (a) Conventional MCAO in the rat; concomitant CBF measured using ASL (CBF_{asl}) and ADC decline. (b) Partial occlusion of the MCA; moderate CBF_{asl} decrease without energy failure; no ADC decrease. (Lythgoe, M.F., et al., *Mag. Res. Med.*, 44, 706, 2000. With permission.)

Instead of using a permanent model, Olah et al. (2001) investigated perfusion, ADC, and ATP changes following 1 hour of ischemia and used the perfusion image as an indicator of successful recirculation on deocclusion. Pell at el. also used FAIR perfusion imaging in the study of global ischemia and reperfusion time courses (Pell et al., 1999a, 1999b). Perfusion was measured with a time resolution of 4 minutes, allowing definition of a period of acute postischemic recovery of flow followed by a prolonged period of hypoperfusion (Figure 2.11). The combination of CBV and CBF measurements with contrast agent MRI and CASL, respectively, was made possible by the development of a novel, long half-life magnetopharmaceutical contrast agent with modified susceptibility characteristics (Zaharchuk et al., 1998). The technique allows the estimation of total and microvascular CBV, CBF, and water

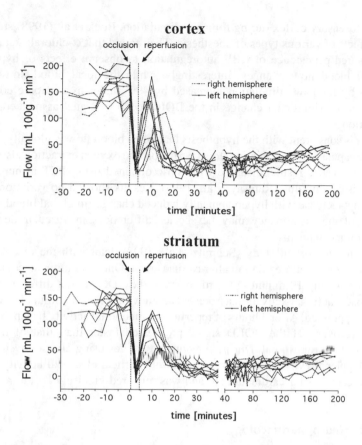

FIGURE 2.11 CBF time courses measured using ASL from cortex and striatum before, during, and after 4 minutes of bilateral common carotid artery occlusion in a gerbil forebrain ischemia model. Time = 0 minutes is set at the moment of occlusion. Recirculation was initiated at time = 4 minutes. (Pell, G.S. et al., *Stroke*, 30, 1999a. With permission.)

extraction, and has been applied to the measurement of CO_2 reactivity and cerebral ischemia (Zaharchuk et al., 1998, 1999, 2000).

Although most studies were performed on rats, it is also feasible to investigate perfusion changes in mice (Hesselbarth et al., 1998). Recirculation following 1 hour of ischemia in mice can result in slow recovery of perfusion, which is heterogeneous, incomplete, and may account for damage in selective regions (van Dorsten et al., 1999). All the studies cited demonstrate the ability of ASL to provide time courses of perfusion measurements with good temporal resolution in a series of individual subjects.

2.6.2.2 Functional ASL Studies in Animals

A number of scientists now use ASL to investigate functional neuronal activation and the neurophysiological basis of BOLD contrast which remains unclear. Kerskens et al. (1996) adapted a rat model and showed increases in blood flow using CASL in somatosensory cortex during forepaw stimulation. Bock et al. (1998) studied the CBF effects of various types of anesthesia. They found that α-chloralose anesthesia best ensured persistence of CBF autoregulation to observe effects of hypercapnia on local blood flow changes. Interestingly, while the local blood flow increase induced by forepaw stimulation increased by 40% under hypercapnic conditions, they noted no significant change in the BOLD contrast signal associated with the stimulation.

This is consistent with the hypothesis that when blood flow is globally increased by hypercapnia during activation, local perfusion and oxygen extraction also increase in parallel. These results disagree with those obtained using PET in human brain with a visual stimulus (Ramsay et al., 1993). Results showed no variation of local blood flow increase with hypercapnically induced changes in global blood flow. The sources of the discrepancy may be species differences in vascular density and regulation mechanisms.

Another important study (Schmitz et al., 1998) dealt with the recovery of rat cerebral vascular autoregulation after cardiac arrest. One hour after successful resuscitation following 10 minutes of cardiac arrest, the ADC did not differ from control levels, but functional activation associated again with forepaw stimulation was completely suppressed. After 3 hours of reperfusion, functional activity began to reappear but the recovery of the BOLD signal progressed faster than that of the CASL perfusion-weighted signal. During previous rat studies using electrophysiology and laser–Doppler flowmetry, this group found that cortical electrical activity was also slow to recover after cardiac arrest, and was mirrored precisely by the recovery in rCBF.

2.6.2.3 Neuropharmacology

Silva et al. (1995) were the first to perform pharmacological fMRI using perfusion techniques, in a rat model. They examined the CBF response to amphetamine, using the two-coil CASL method, and found that amphetamine causes significant and spatially specific increases in perfusion in many areas of the brain including the cortex, cingulate, and caudate putamen, in agreement with previous results using deoxyglucose uptake to monitor brain activation.

This pioneering study indicates the power of perfusion methods to indicate the localization of the effects of psychopharmaceuticals in the brain. Care must always be taken to control for any global effects on blood flow due to the crude vasoactive properties of such drugs. Later work from the same laboratory (Forman et al., 1998) used picrotoxinin (a GABA antagonist) to stimulate rat brain. Perfusion was measured by CASL and brain glutamate was independently assayed using microdialysis. After 30 minutes of picrotoxinin-induced stimulation, glutamate levels decreased. CBF was found to remain elevated, suggesting that additional factors modulate the relationship of neuronal neurotransmitters and hemodynamics at these later stages. More recently arterial spin labeling was used to assess the effects of locally injected agents on CBF. Parenchymal infusion of 2-chloroadenosine, a strong vasodilator, demonstrated a potent, dose-dependent, and sustained vasodilatation over large areas of the brain (Kochanek et al., 2001). See Figure 2.12.

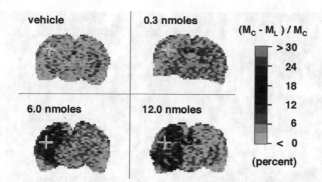

FIGURE 2.12 Pseudocolor images reflecting $100 \cdot (M_C - M_L) \cdot M_C - 1$ (where M_C is the magnetization intensity from the control image and M_L is the magnetization from the labeled image) of a coronal slice at ~90 minutes after injection of saline vehicle or 2-chloroadenosine at 0.3, 6.0, or 12 nmoles. Injection of saline and 0.3 nmoles of 2-chloroadenosine produced no apparent effect on local perfusion. In contrast, injection of 6 nmoles of 2-chloroadenosine produced an obvious local increase in perfusion. Injection of 12 nmoles produced a marked increase in perfusion encompassing almost the entire hemisphere ipsilateral to injection. Plus signs indicate approximate locations of injection sites (Kochanek, P.M. et al., *Mag. Res. Med.*, 45, 924, 2001. With permission.). See Color Figure 2.12 following page 210.

2.6.3 OTHER APPLICATIONS USING MR CONTRAST AGENTS OR ASL

2.6.3.1 Head Injury and Cerebral Ischemia (CO₂ Reactivity and Hyperglycemia)

Both DSC-MRI and arterial spin labeling have been applied to investigate disturbances of cerebral blood flow that are common sequelae of traumatic brain injuries. MRI perfusion imaging was performed after closed head injury (Assaf et al., 1999) and controlled cortical impact (Hendrick et al., 1999) in rats. Early perfusion changes were observed in both models, indicating a reduction in CBF or rCBV (Assaf et al., 1999) in the region of brain injury 2 to 4 hours after the initial insult.

Assaf et al. (1999) followed the time course of the rCBV and demonstrated a heterogeneous pattern at 24 hours and normalization after 1 week, although they concluded that rCBV was less informative than T_1 and ADC in terms of final histological damage. Further assessment of CBF following head injury was made by Forbes et al. (1997), using hyperventilation to decrease $PaCO_2$ and assess vascular reactivity. Hypocarbia reduced CBF in normal tissue and large cortical regions, but not within the area of contusion-enriched tissue, indicating a loss of vascular reactivity in this region.

In addition to using CO_2 reactivity to investigate head injury, Olah et al. (2000) used ASL to measure CBF and CO_2 reactivity during transient cerebral ischemia (Figure 2.13). They suggest that severe ischemia is followed by a prolonged disturbance of CO_2 reactivity, despite already normalized energy metabolism. A study investigating the pathophysiology of cerebral ischemia using bolus tracking documented reduced CBF in hyperglycemic compared with normoglycemic

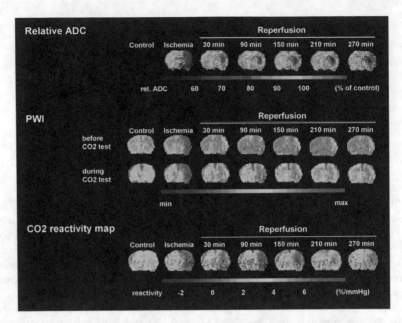

FIGURE 2.13 Time course of relative ADC (top row), PWI (middle row) before and during CO_2 reactivity, and quantitative CO_2 map (bottom row), during middle cerebral artery occlusion (ischemia), and at different time points of reperfusion. Note the inverse or low cerebrovascular reactivity during ischemia and the slow, incomplete improvement during reperfusion (Olah, L. et al., *Stroke*, 31, 2236, 2000. With permission.). See Color Figure 2.13 following page 210.

animals and suggested microvascular damage exacerbated by hyperglycemia as the primary culprit (Quast et al., 1997).

2.7   CONCLUSION

The challenge for perfusion imaging is the measurement of CBF in a noninvasive fashion with high temporal and spatial resolution. The chosen technique should be widely available, suited to both experimental and clinical conditions, and applicable to a variety of physiological states and flow values. MRI perfusion techniques have become important tools in the research environment and are used routinely by increasing numbers of research facilities every day.

It is clear that CBF imaging techniques provide measures of perfusion to tissue that are related to the function status of the tissue. Since MRI is noninvasive, the measurements may be repeated to follow tissue changes over time scales of seconds, minutes, days, or even years.

This unique information, when combined with high resolution structural images using standard MR methods, MR spectroscopy, or functional MRI, may lead to better understanding of the complex relationship of measurements of perfusion and the functional status of tissue, the accurate delineation of at-risk tissue, and improved prognostic measures in both experimental and clinical settings.

ACKNOWLEDGMENTS

The authors acknowledge the Wellcome Trust for its support of the work carried out at the Department of Radiology and Physics, Institute of Child Health and Great Ormond Street Hospital for Children NHS Trust, London. The authors also thank A. de Crespigny, M. Chopp, M. Sakoh, G.S. Pell, K.S. Hendrich, and M. Hoehn for contributing figures to this chapter.

REFERENCES

Alsop, D.C. and Detre, J.A. (1996). Reduced transit time sensitivity in noninvasive magnetic resonance imaging of human cerebral blood flow. *J. Cereb. Blood Flow Metabol.,* 16, 1236.

Alsop, D.C. and Detre, J.A. (1998). Multisection cerebral blood flow MR imaging with continuous arterial spin labeling. *Radiology,* 208, 410.

Assaf, Y. et al. (1999). Diffusion and perfusion magnetic resonance imaging following closed head injury in rats. *J.Neurotrauma,* 16, 1165.

Astrup, J., Siesjo, B.K. and Symon, L. (1981). Thresholds in cerebral ischaemia: the ischaemic penumbra. *Stroke,* 12, 723.

Axel, L. (1980). Cerebral blood flow determination by rapid-sequence computed tomography. *Radiology,* 137, 676.

Axel, L. (1995). Methods using blood pool tracers, in *Diffusion and Perfusion Magnetic Resonance Imaging,* Le Bihan, D., Ed., Raven Press, New York, 205.

Beaulieu, C. et al. (1998). Polynitroxyl albumin reduces infarct size in transient focal cerebral ischemia in the rat: potential mechanisms studied by magnetic resonance imaging. *J. Cereb. Blood Flow Metabol.,* 18, 1022.

Bell, A.B. (1987). Early study of cerebral circulation and measurement of cerebral blood flow, in *Cerebral Blood Flow,* Wood, J.H., Ed., McGraw-Hill, New York, 3.

Bell, B.A. (1984). A history of the study of the cerebral circulation and the measurement of cerebral blood flow. *Neurosurgery,* 14, 238.

Bock, C. et al. (1998). Functional MRI of somatosensory activation in rats: effect of hypercapnic up-regulation on perfusion and BOLD imaging. *Mag. Res. Med.,* 39, 457.

Boxerman, J.L. et al. (1995). MR contrast due to intravascular magnetic susceptibility perturbations. *Mag. Res. Med.,* 34, 555.

Busch, E. et al. (1998). Reperfusion after thrombolytic therapy of embolic stroke in the rat: magnetic resonance and biochemical imaging. *J. Cereb. Blood Flow Metabol.,* 18, 407.

Calamante, F., Gadian, D.G., and Connelly, A. (2002). Quantification of perfusion using bolus tracking MRI in stroke: assumptions, limitations, and potential implications for clinical use. *Stroke,* 33, 1146.

Calamante, F., Gadian, D.G., and Connelly, A. (2000). Delay and dispersion effects in dynamic susceptibility contrast MRI: simulations using singular value decomposition. *Mag. Res. Med.,* 44, 466.

Calamante, F. et al. (1999a). Early changes in water diffusion, perfusion, T_1 and T_2 during focal cerebral ischemia in the rat studied at 8.5 T. *Mag. Res. Med.,* 41, 479.

Calamante, F. et al. (1999b). Measuring cerebral blood flow using magnetic resonance techniques. *J. Cereb. Blood Flow Metabol.,*19. 701.

Caramia, F. et al. (1998). Mismatch between cerebral blood volume and flow index during transient focal ischemia studied with MRI and GD-BOPTA. *J. Mag. Res. Imaging,* 16, 97.

Carano, R.A. et al. (2000). Multispectral analysis of the temporal evolution of cerebral ischemia in the rat brain. *J. Mag. Res. Imaging,* 12, 842.

de Crespigny, A. et al. (1998). Magnetic resonance imaging assessment of cerebral hemodynamics during spreading depression in rats. *J. Cereb. Blood Flow Metabol.,* 18, 1008.

Detre, J.A. et al. (1992). Perfusion imaging. *Mag. Res. Med.,* 23, 37.

Detre, J.A. et al. (1993). Redistribution of cerebral blood flow following unilateral carotid occlusion: noninvasive determination by perfusion imaging with selective labeling of arterial water. *Proc. Soc. Mag Res. Med.,* 12th Annl. Mtg., New York, Abstract, 247.

Dijkhuizen, R.M. et al. (1997). Regional assessment of tissue oxygenation and the temporal evolution of hemodynamic parameters and water diffusion during acute focal ischemia in rat brain. *Brain Res.,* 750, 161.

Dijkhuizen, R.M. et al. (1998a). Dynamics of cerebral tissue injury and perfusion after temporary hypoxia–ischemia in the rat: evidence for region-specific sensitivity and delayed damage. *Stroke,* 29, 695.

Dijkhuizen, R.M. (1998b). Magnetic resonance imaging and spectroscopy in experimental cerebral ischaemia. Thesis, University of Utrecht, Netherlands.

Dixon, W.T. et al. (1986). Projection angiograms of blood labeled by adiabatic fast passage. *Mag. Res. Med.,* 3, 454.

Edelman, R.R. and Chen, Q. (1998). EPISTAR MRI: multislice mapping of cerebral blood flow. *Mag. Res. Med.,* 40, 800.

Edelman, R.R. et al. (1994). Qualitative mapping of cerebral blood flow and functional localization with echo-planar MR imaging.and signal targeting with alternating radio frequency. *Radiology,* 192, 513.

Finelli, D.A. et al. (1992). Evaluation of experimental early acute cerebral ischemia before the development of edema: use of dynamic, contrast-enhanced and diffusion-weighted MR scanning. *Mag. Res. Med.,* 27, 189.

Forbes, M.L. et al. (1997). Assessment of cerebral blood flow and CO_2 reactivity after controlled cortical impact by perfusion magnetic resonance imaging using arterial spin labeling in rats. *J. Cereb. Blood Flow Metabol.,* 17, 865.

Forman, S.D. et al. (1998). Simultaneous glutamate and perfusion fMRI responses to regional brain stimulation. *J. Cereb. Blood Flow Metabol.,* 18, 1064.

Gillis P. and Koenig, S.H. (1987). Transverse relaxation of solvent protons induced by magnetized spheres: application to ferritin, erythrocytes, and magnetite. *Mag. Res. Med.,* 5, 323.

Gückel F.J. et al. (1996). Cerebrovascular reserve capacity in patients with occlusive cerebrovascular disease: assessment with dynamic susceptibility contrast-enhanced MR imaging and the acetazolamide stimulation test. *Radiology,* 201, 405.

Hendrick, K.S. et al. (1999). Early perfusion after controlled cortical impact in rats: quantification by arterial spin-labelling MRI and the influence of spin lattice relaxation time heterogeneity. *Mag. Res. Med.,* 42, 673.

Herscovitch, P. and Raichle, M.E. (1985). What is the correct value for the blood–brain partition coefficient for water? *J. Cereb. Blood Flow Metabol.,* 5, 65.

Hesselbarth, D. et al. (1998). High resolution MRI and MRS: a feasibility study for the investigation of focal cerebral ischemia in mice. *NMR Biomed.,* 11, 423.

Hoehn, M. et al. (1999). Validation of arterial spin tagging perfusion MR imaging: correlation with autoradiographic CBF data. *Proc. ISMRM 7th Annl. Mtg.,* 1843.

Jiang, Q. et al. (1994). Effect of hypothermia on transient focal ischemia in rat brain evaluated by diffusion- and perfusion-weighted NMR imaging. *J. Cereb. Blood Flow Metabol.*, 14, 732.

Jiang, Q. et al. (1998a). Diffusion-,T_2-, and perfusion-weighted nuclear magnetic resonance imaging of middle cerebral artery embolic stroke and recombinant tissue plasminogen activator intervention in the rat. *J. Cereb. Blood Flow Metabol.*, 18, 758.

Jiang, Q. et al. (1998b). Diffusion, perfusion, and T_2 magnetic resonance imaging of anti-intercellular adhesion molecule 1 antibody treatment of transient middle cerebral artery occlusion in rat. *Brain Res.*, 788, 191.

Kerskens, C.M. et al. (1996). Ultrafast perfusion-weighted MRI of functional brain activation in rats during forepaw stimulation: comparison with T_2-weighted MRI. *NMR in Biomed.*, 9, 20.

Kim, S.G. (1995). Quantification of relative cerebral blood flow change by flow-sensitive alternating inversion recovery (FAIR) technique: application to functional mapping. *Mag. Res. Med.*, 34, 293.

Kochanek, P.M. et al. (2001). Assessment of the effect of 2-chloroadenosine in normal rat brain using spin-labeled MRI measurement of perfusion. *Mag. Res. Med.*, 45, 924.

Kucharczyk, J. et al. (1991). Diffusion/perfusion MR imaging of acute cerebral ischemia. *Mag. Res. Med.*, 19, 311.

Kucharczyk, J. et al. (1993). Echo-planar perfusion-sensitive MR imaging of acute cerebral ischaemia. *Radiology*, 188, 711.

Kwong, K.K. et al. (1992). Dynamic magnetic resonance imaging of human brain activity during primary sensory stimulation. *Proc. Natl. Acad. Sci. U.S.A.*, 89, 5675.

Le Bihan, D. et al. (1986). MR imaging of intravoxel incoherent motions: application to diffusion and perfusion in neurologic disorders. *Radiology*, 161, 401.

Li, F. et al. (2000). Transient and permanent resolution of ischemic lesions on diffusion-weighted imaging after brief periods of focal ischemia. *Stroke*, 31, 946.

Lo, E.H. et al. (1997). Neuroprotection with NBQX in rat focal cerebral ischemia: effects on ADC probability distribution functions and diffusion-perfusion relationships. *Stroke*, 28, 439.

Lythgoe, M.F. et al. (2000). Acute changes in MRI diffusion, perfusion, T_1 and T_2 in a rat model of oligemia produced by partial occlusion of the middle cerebral artery. *Mag. Res. Med.*, 44, 706.

Maeda, M. et al. (1993). Acute stroke in cats: comparison of dynamic susceptibility-contrast MR imaging with T_2- and diffusion-weighted MR imaging. *Radiology*, 189, 227.

McLaughlin, A.C. et al. (1997). Effect of magnetization transfer on the measurement of cerebral blood flow using steady-state arterial spin tagging: a theoretical investigation. *Mag. Res. Med.*, 37, 501.

Meier, P. and Zierler, K.L. (1954). On the theory of the indicator dilution method for measurement of blood flow and volume. *Appl. Physiol.*, 6, 731.

Minematsu, K. et al. (1993). Diffusion and perfusion magnetic resonance imaging studies to evaluate a noncompetitive N-methyl-D-aspartate antagonist and reperfusion in experimental stroke in rats. *Stroke*, 24, 2074.

Morawetz, R.B. et al. (1979). Regional cerebral blood flow thresholds during cerebral ischaemia. *Fed. Proc.*, 38, 2493.

Moseley, M.E. et al. (1993). Early detection of regional cerebral ischemia using high speed MRI. *Stroke*, 24, 160.

Moseley, M.E. et al. (1990). Diffusion-weighted MR imaging of acute stroke: correlation with T_2-weighted and magnetic susceptibility-enhanced MR imaging in cats. *Am. J. Neuroradiol.*, 11, 423.

Muller, T.B. et al. (1995a). Combined perfusion and diffusion-weighted magnetic resonance imaging in a rat model of reversible middle cerebral artery occlusion. *Stroke*, 26, 451.

Muller, T.B. et al. (1995b). Perfusion and diffusion-weighted MR imaging for *in vivo* evaluation of treatment with U74389G in a rat stroke model. *Stroke*, 26, 1453.

Olah, L. et al. (2000). CO_2 reactivity measured by perfusion MRI during transient focal cerebral ischemia in rats. *Stroke*, 31, 2236.

Olah, L., Wecker, S., and Hoehn, M. (2001). Relation of apparent diffusion coefficient changes and metabolic disturbances after 1 hour of focal cerebral ischemia and at different reperfusion phases in rats. *J. Cereb. Blood Flow Metabol.*, 21, 430.

Østergaard, L. et al. (1998). Absolute cerebral blood flow and blood volume measured by magnetic resonance imaging bolus tracking: comparison with positron emission tomography values. *J. Cereb. Blood Flow Metabol.*, 18, 425.

Østergaard, L. et al. (1996). High resolution measurement of cerebral blood flow using intravascular tracer bolus passages I. Mathematical approach and statistical analysis. *Mag. Res. Med.*, 36, 715.

Pan, Y. et al. (1995). Quantitative and dynamic MRI of neuroprotection in experimental stroke. *J. Neurol. Sci.*, 131, 128.

Parkes, L.M. and Tofts, P.S. (2001). Modelling of arterial spin labelled perfusion data with varying delay time, including permeability effects. *Proc. ISMRM 9th Annl. Mtg.*, 100.

Pell, G.S. et al. (1999a). Reperfusion in a gerbil model of forebrain ischemia using serial magnetic resonance FAIR perfusion imaging. *Stroke*, 30, 1263.

Pell, G.S. et al. (1999b). Implementation of quantitative FAIR perfusion imaging with a short repetition time in time course studies. *Mag. Res. Med.*, 41, 829.

Pell, G.S. et al. (1999c). Validation of the FAIR technique of perfusion quantification with hydrogen clearance. *Proc. ISMRM 7th Annl. Mtg.*, 599.

Perman, W.H. et al. (1992). Simultaneous MR acquisition of arterial and brain signal time curves. *Mag. Res. Med.*, 28, 74.

Perthen, J.E. et al. (2002). Is quantification of bolus tracking MRI reliable without deconvolution? *Mag. Res. Med.*, 47, 61.

Pierce, A.R. et al. (1997). MRI measurements of water diffusion and cerebral perfusion: their relationship in a rat model of focal cerebral ischemia. *J. Cereb. Blood Flow Metabol.*, 17, 183.

Porkka, L. et al. (1991). Arterial input function measurement with MRI. *Proc ISMRM 10th Annl. Mtg.*, 120.

Potchen, E.J. et al. (1993). *Magnetic Resonance Angiography*, Mosby, St, Louis.

Quast, M.J. et al. (1993). The evolution of acute stroke recording by multimodal magnetic resonance imaging. *Mag. Res. Imaging*, 11, 465.

Quast, M.J. et al. (1997). Perfusion deficit parallels exacerbation of cerebral ischemia/reperfusion injury in hyperglycemic rats. *J. Cereb. Blood Flow Metabol.*, 17, 553.

Ramsay, S.C. et al. (1993). Changes in global cerebral blood flow in humans: effect on regional cerebral blood flow during a neural activation task. *J. Physiol.*, 471, 521.

Reith, W. et al. (1996). Monitoring of tissue plasminogen activator treatment with multislice diffusion mapping and perfusion imaging in a thromboembolic stroke model. *Int. J. Neuroradiol.*, 2, 397.

Rempp, K.A. et al. (1994). Quantification of regional cerebral blood flow and volume with dynamic susceptibility contrast-enhanced MR imaging. *Radiology*, 193, 637.

Roberts, T.P. et al. (1996). Sensitivity of high-speed perfusion-sensitive magnetic resonance imaging to mild cerebral ischemia. *Eur. Radiol.*, 6, 645.

Roberts, T.P. et al. (1993). High speed MR imaging of ischemic brain injury following stenosis of the middle cerebral artery. *J. Cereb. Blood Flow Metabol.*, 13, 940.

Rosen, B.R. et al. (1990). Perfusion imaging with NMR contrast agents. *Mag. Res. Med.,* 14, 249.

Röther, J. et al. (1996a). MR detection of cortical spreading depression immediately after focal ischemia in the rat. *J. Cereb. Blood Flow Metabol.,* 16, 214.

Röther, J. et al. (1996b). Recovery of the apparent diffusion coefficient after ischemia-induced spreading depression relates to cerebral perfusion gradient. *Stroke,* 27, 980.

Röther, J. et al. (1996c). Experimental cerebral venous thrombosis: evaluation using magnetic resonance imaging. *J. Cereb. Blood Flow Metabol.,* 16, 1353.

Sakoh, M. et al. (2000). Cerebral blood flow and blood volume measured by magnetic resonance imaging bolus tracking after acute stroke in pigs. *Stroke,* 31, 1958.

Schmitz, B. et al. (1998). Recovery of the rodent brain after cardiac arrest: a functional MRI study. *Mag. Res. Med.,* 39, 783.

Schreiber, W.G. et al. (1998). Cerebral blood flow and cerebrovascular reserve capacity: estimation by dynamic magnetic resonance imaging. *J Cereb Blood Flow Metabol.,* 18, 1143.

Silva, A.C. et al. (1995). Multislice MRI of rat brain perfusion during amphetamine stimulation using arterial spin labeling. *Mag. Res. Med.,* 33, 209.

Singer, J.R. (1959). Blood flow rates by nuclear magnetic resonance measurements. *Science,* 130, 1652.

Smith, A.M. et al. (2000). Whole brain quantitative CBF and CBV measurements using MRI bolus tracking: comparison of methodologies. *Mag. Res. Med.,* 43, 559.

Sorensen, A.G. (2001). What is the meaning of *quantitative* CBF? *Am. J. Neuroradiol.,* 22, 2356.

Stewart, G.N. (1894). Researches on the circulation time in organs and on the influences which affect it. Parts I–III. *J. Physiol.* (London), 15, 1.

St. Lawrence, K.S., Frank, J.A., and McLaughlin, A.C. (2000). Effect of restricted water exchange on cerebral blood flow values calculated with arterial spin tagging: a theoretical investigation. *Mag. Res. Med.,* 44, 440.

Takano, K. et al. (1998). Efficacy of intra-arterial and intravenous prourokinase in an embolic stroke model evaluated by diffusion–perfusion magnetic resonance imaging. *Neurology,* 50, 870.

Thomas, D.L. et al. (2000). Measurement of diffusion and perfusion in biological systems using magnetic resonance imaging. *Phys. Med. Biol.,* 45, R97.

Tsekos, N.V. et al. (1998). Quantitative measurements of cerebral blood flow in rats using the FAIR technique: correlation with previous iodoantipyrine autoradiographic studies. *Mag. Res. Med.,* 39, 564.

Turner, R. (1988). Perfusion studies and fast imaging, in *Cerebral Blood Flow,* Rescigno, A. and Boicelli, A., Eds., Plenum Publishing, New York, 245.

van Lookeren-Campagne, M. et al. (1999). Secondary reduction in the apparent diffusion coefficient, increase in cerebral blood volume and delayed neuronal death following middle cerebral artery occlusion and early reperfusion in the rat. *J. Cereb. Blood Flow Metabol.,* 1999, 1354.

van Dorsten, F.A. et al. (1999). Diffusion- and perfusion-weighted MR imaging of transient focal cerebral ischaemia in mice. *NMR Biomed.,* 12, 525.

Vexler, Z.S. et al. (1997). Transient cerebral ischemia: association of apoptosis induction with hypoperfusion. *J. Clin. Invest.,* 99, 1453.

Villringer, A. et al. (1988). Dynamic imaging with lanthanide chelates in normal brain: contrast due to magnetic susceptibility effects. *Mag. Res. Med.,* 6, 164.

Vonken, E.P.A. et al. (1999). Measurement of cerebral perfusion with dual-echo multislice quantitative dynamic susceptibility contrast MRI. *J. Mag. Res. Imaging,* 10, 109.

Walsh, E.G. et al. (1994). Radioactive microsphere validation of a volume localised continuous saturation perfusion measurement. *Mag. Res. Med.,* 31, 147.

Weisskoff, R.M. et al. (1993). Pitfalls in MR measurement of tissue blood flow with intravascular tracers: which mean transit time? *Mag. Res. Med.,* 29, 553.

Wendland, M.F. et al. (1991). Detection with echo-planar MR imaging of transit of susceptibility contrast medium in a rat model of regional brain ischemia. *J. Mag. Res. Imaging,* 1, 285.

Williams, D.S. et al. (1992). Magnetic resonance imaging of perfusion using spin inversion of arterial water. *Proc. Natl. Acad. Sci. U.S.A.,* 89, 212.

Wittlich, F. et al. (1995). Quantitative measurement of regional blood flow with gadolinium diethylenetriaminepentaacetate bolus track NMR imaging in cerebral infarcts in rats: validation with the iodo[C-14]antipyrine technique. *Proc. Natl. Acad. Sci. U.S.A.,* 92, 1846.

Wong, E.C. et al. (1998). Quantitative imaging of perfusion using a single subtraction (QUIPSS and QUIPSS II). *Mag. Res. Med.,* 39, 702.

Ye, F.Q. et al. (2000). $H_2^{15}O$ PET validation of steady-state arterial spin tagging cerebral blood flow measurements in humans. *Mag. Res. Med.,* 44, 450.

Ye, F.Q. et al. (1997). Correction for vascular artifacts in cerebral blood flow values measured by using arterial spin tagging techniques. *Mag. Res. Med.,* 37, 226.

Yenari, M.A. et al. (1997). Improved perfusion with rt-PA and hirulog in a rabbit model of embolic stroke. *J. Cereb. Blood Flow Metabol.,* 17, 401.

Zaharchuk, G. et al. (1998). Continuous assessment of perfusion by tagging including volume and water extraction (CAPTIVE): a steady-state contrast agent technique for measuring blood flow, relative blood volume fraction, and the water extraction fraction. *Mag. Res. Med.,* 40, 666.

Zaharchuk, G. et al. (1999). Cerebrovascular dynamics of autoregulation and hypoperfusion: an MRI study of CBF and changes in total and microvascular cerebral blood volume during hemorrhagic hypotension. *Stroke,* 30, 2197.

Zaharchuk, G. et al. (2000). Is all perfusion-weighted magnetic resonance imaging for stroke equal? The temporal evolution of multiple hemodynamic parameters after focal ischemia in rats correlated with evidence of infarction. *J. Cereb. Blood Flow Metabol.,* 20, 1341.

Zhang, W., Williams, D.S., and Koretsky, A.P. (1993). Measurement of rat brain perfusion by NMR using spin labeling of arterial water: *in vivo* determination of the degree of spin labeling. *Mag. Res. Med.,* 29, 416.

Zhang, W. et al. (1992). Measurement of brain perfusion by volume-localized NMR spectroscopy using inversion of arterial water spins: accounting for transit time and cross-relaxation. *Mag. Res. Med.,* 25, 362.

Zhou, J.Y. et al. (2001). Two-compartment exchange model for perfusion quantification using arterial spin tagging. *J. Cereb. Blood Flow Metabol.,* 21, 440.

Zierler, K.L. (1965). Equations for measuring blood flow by external monitoring of radioisotopes. *Circ. Res.,* 16, 309.

3 MRI Measurement of Cerebral Water Diffusion and Its Application to Experimental Research

Richard A.D. Carano, Nick van Bruggen, and Alex J. de Crespigny

CONTENTS

0-8493-0122-X/03/$0.00+$1.50
© 2003 by CRC Press LLC

3.1 INTRODUCTION

Contrast in magnetic resonance imaging (MRI) can be generated by exploiting a variety of physiochemical processes including molecular diffusion. Diffusion-weighted MRI (DWI) provides a unique approach to generating contrast in MRI experiments. *Diffusion* is the random Brownian motion of water molecules. In the course of their random travel through cerebral tissues, water molecules encounter a number of structures in the intracellular, extracellular, and vascular compartments. As a result, the rate of water diffusion depends on the microscopic structural environment in the tissue. Measurement of this parameter can yield valuable insights into the regional metabolic and structural changes occurring in disease states.

MRI is uniquely capable of measuring this parameter noninvasively. Sensitizing the MRI protocol to the diffusion properties of water allows unique anatomical and functional information to be revealed — information that may not be revealed by conventional imaging techniques. DWI is sensitive to the acute events associated with tissue ischemia and alterations in axonal myelination. Its sensitivity and specificity to pathophysiology make it uniquely suited for neuroscience research and clinical diagnosis of conditions as diverse as stroke and schizophrenia.

Diffusion-weighted imaging provides information about the underlying natures of pathologies along with identification and localization of diseases. This chapter describes both the theory and methodology for MRI diffusion quantification in the brain and applications of this technology to experimental neuroscience research.

3.2 WATER DIFFUSION IN BIOLOGICAL TISSUES

The measurement of water diffusion using nuclear magnetic resonance (NMR) was established several decades ago. Classical approaches for the measurement of diffusion rely on measuring the displacement of a tagged molecule over time, for example, isotope deposition and wash-out techniques. The MRI approach follows a similar theory. The tag for an NMR experiment is provided by a magnetic field gradient or pulsed gradient that produces a phase shift of the transverse magnetization relative to the static field. This technique provides a particularly elegant method for labelling water and other molecules.

Although NMR techniques for measuring diffusion of molecules were first described in the 1960s,[1,2] it was not until the mid 1980's before diffusion-weighted MRI experiments were performed.[3] This resurgence of interest in diffusion was, to a large part, prompted by the proposal that, because the movement of blood through the randomly oriented capillary could be viewed as a pseudo-random process and as such resembles Brownian motion, that MRI could measure tissue perfusion.[3–5]

The ability to monitor tissue perfusion nondestructively represents a "Holy Grail" in physiology. The notion was that the tissue bed could be modeled as a two-compartment system, consisting of the extracellular and intracellular spaces constituting one compartment and the capillary bed the other. Theory predicted that the capillary compartment would have a diffusion coefficient that was much greater than that of the extravascular tissue. Accurate MRI measurements of the diffusion coefficient of water should yield values for the two compartments together with their volumes.[6] Further, it was shown that if a model for the geometry of the capillary network is known for the tissue in question, then it is possible to convert the measurement from the diffusion imaging into perfusion rate (having units of ml min^{-1} g^{-1}).[7]

A considerable effort was made to develop perfusion imaging and a number of variants of the initial method were tested. Despite the elegant theory, successful practical application of these imaging techniques to perfusion imaging remains to be realized and may not be feasible.[8,9] Nevertheless, because of the intense research activity in the arena of DWI, many important advances that exerted major impacts in the clinical diagnosis and experimental research area have been realized.

Diffusion weighted imaging is sensitive to the translation of water molecules undergoing random Brownian motion over short distances (i.e., diffusion). Although molecules move very rapidly at body temperature, they constantly collide with each other and with membranes and other tissue structures. This means their average net progress is quite slow. During typical observation times of the MRI technique (40 to 100 ms), these distances are on the order of 5 to 20 μm.[10] Figure 3.1(a) illustrates this situation for two-dimensional free diffusion. The average diffusion distance, L, is given by the Einstein relationship. If the water molecules encounter barriers (cell membranes, etc.; Figure 3.1(b)), the measured diffusion is greater parallel to the barriers than perpendicular to them. This is known as diffusion anisotropy, and will be discussed in a later section.

In general, most membranes encountered by the water molecules are semipermeable and have complex shapes, so that water motion is hindered rather than truly restricted by the barriers. Changes in the permeability, density, or geometry of the barriers can produce significant changes in the rate of water diffusion. Thus, tissue water diffusion is very sensitive to the tissue microstructure and this gives us a new source of MRI contrast in a range of disease conditions.

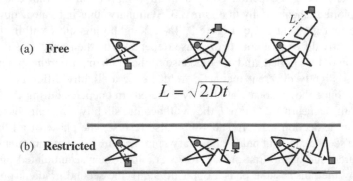

(a) **Free**

$$L = \sqrt{2Dt}$$

(b) **Restricted**

FIGURE 3.1 Water diffusion in free space (a) and with restrictive boundaries (b). The mean diffusion length L over time t is given by the Einstein relationship, where D is the diffusion coefficient. In (b), diffusion is anisotropic, i.e., faster parallel to the barriers than perpendicular to them.

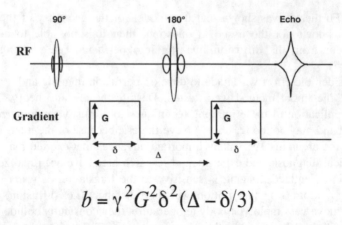

$$b = \gamma^2 G^2 \delta^2 (\Delta - \delta/3)$$

FIGURE 3.2 Stejskal-Tanner pulse sequence for NMR diffusion measurement. The degree of diffusion weighting is defined by the b value that depends on the gradient strengths and timings.

3.3 *IN VIVO* MEASUREMENT OF WATER DIFFUSION

In vivo measurement of water diffusion using NMR relies on the fact that water proton spins moving through a magnetic field gradient acquire phase at a rate depending on both the strength of the gradient and the velocity of the spins. Diffusion is typically measured using a spin echo pulse sequence similar to that shown in Figure 3.2. The method utilizes a pair of strong gradient pulses placed symmetrically around the 180° refocusing pulse in a spin-echo sequence[2] as outlined in Chapter 1. The b value[3] is a measure of the degree of diffusion weighting that depends on the strength and duration of the applied gradient pulses and their separation. The b value is typically expressed in units of seconds/mm².

The phase changes experienced by a small group of spins within one imaging voxel are plotted schematically in Figure 3.3. Stationary spins in tissue acquire phase during the first gradient pulse (Figure 3.3(a)). Neighboring spins within the voxel acquire slightly different amounts of phase depending on their exact position along the direction of the applied gradient. Because of the gradient, different spin positions results in a slightly different magnetic field, hence a slightly different resonance frequency. Since they resonate at slightly different frequencies during the gradient pulse over the same time duration t, they will acquire slightly different phase angles. See Chapter 1, Section 1.2.2.1. The 180° pulse reverses the phase of all the spins. During the second gradient pulse, stationary spins acquire the same amount of phase they acquired during the first pulse. However, since their accumulated phase was reversed by the pulse (same phase, opposite sign), the second gradient pulse only serves to unwind the phase accumulation from the first pulse. At the end of the sequence, all the spins are refocused to zero phase and add up to form an echo.

If the spins are moving, for example if the whole sample is undergoing uniform motion, or the spins are in blood flowing coherently in a vessel, then they acquire phase quadratically during the first gradient pulse, Figure 3.3(b). During the second

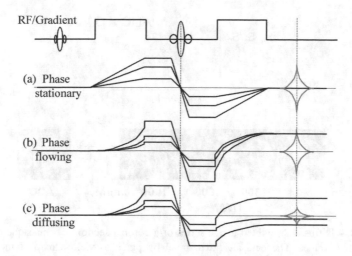

FIGURE 3.3 Evolution of spin phase for three neighboring spins within a voxel as a function of time during Stejskal-Tanner diffusion pulse sequence. (a) Stationary spins are refocused to form an echo. (b) Spins in bulk motion (e.g., flowing blood) are refocused with a net phase shift. (c) Diffusing spins experience differing phase shifts due to their different random walk paths and are incompletely refocused.

gradient pulse, their phase is 'unwound' at the same rate relative to each other (since they are all moving together) but there is a different overall phase change because the spins have moved and are now in a different magnetic field than during the first pulse (because of the applied gradient). Thus they still refocus to form an echo but with a net phase shift compared to stationary tissue. This is the basis of flow measurement by MRI (magnetic resonance angiography, MRA).

Spins undergoing microscopic random motion (i.e., diffusion; Figure 3.3(c)) also acquire phase quadratically in proportion to their rate of motion. The phases accrued during the first and second gradient pulses are different because the spins have moved the same way as flowing spins. In this case, each spin with a voxel takes a different random path through space and thus ends up with a different amount of phase at the end of a sequence. Since the magnetization vectors of all spins in the voxel are added vectorially to form the acquired echo detected by the scanner, the dispersion in spin phase due to random motion results in a reduction in the *magnitude* of the echo signal.

Signal intensity in a DWI is inversely related to the water diffusion coefficient D and the strength, duration, and separation of the applied magnetic field gradients described by the b factor. For a given diffusion coefficient, the signal decreases exponentially with increasing b value according to:

$$S_b = S_o \, e^{-bD}$$

where S_b is the DW signal intensity and S_o is the signal with no diffusion gradients applied. Acquiring multiple DWI scans with incremented b values permits the

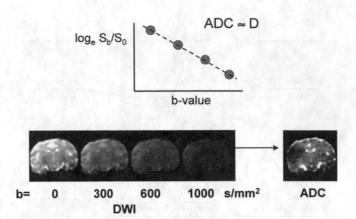

FIGURE 3.4 Diffusion-weighted image series of a coronal section in a macaque brain with incremental b values. The data are fitted, pixel by pixel, to yield a map of the apparent diffusion coefficient. Bright pixels indicate fast diffusion (e.g., CSF); dark pixels indicate slower diffusion (e.g., lesion).

calculation of the diffusion coefficient D by fitting the pixel data to this equation (Figure 3.4).

The apparent diffusion coefficient (ADC) measured in MRI experiments can be affected by other processes such as magnetic susceptibility and motion (CSF pulsations, respiration, head motion). In fact, for *in vivo* MRI of the central nervous system (CNS), the major confounding factor of DW imaging is motion. For humans, involuntary head motion and cardiac-induced cerebrospinal fluid (CSF) and brain pulsations result in phase changes due to bulk motion (Figure 3.3(b)) and signal changes due to diffusion. In anesthetized animals, respiratory-induced motion is often a problem unless a robust stereotactic frame (that may not be practical in all cases) is used. Because the motion is irregular, the motion-induced phase changes are different between each phase encoded step in a conventional spin echo (SE) sequence, and produces severe ghosting artefacts in the resulting image (Figure 3.5(a)). Although the motion can be corrected to a degree, for example, by using navigator echoes (Figure 3.5(b)),[11,12] a more reliable approach is using snapshot echo planar imaging (EPI; Figure 3.5(c)), a technique used widely for diffusion imaging.[13,14] With EPI, all phase-encoded steps are rapidly acquired in a single excitation. Motion-induced phase changes may still occur, but the phase information in the image is generally discarded after processing, and only the magnitude information displayed. Since EPI is so fast, many different diffusion b values and gradient directions may be acquired in a reasonable total acquisition time. However, an important limitation to EPI is its sensitivity to magnetic susceptibility variations. For example, the air–tissue interfaces around sinus cavities produce local magnetic field gradients due to the differences in magnetic susceptibility between air and tissue. These field gradients extend into the surrounding tissue and can cause significant geometric distortion and signal drop-outs in the images. At high magnetic fields (3 T and above) this effect can severely limit the use of EPI for certain parts

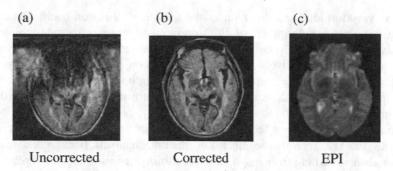

(a)	(b)	(c)
Uncorrected	Corrected	EPI

FIGURE 3.5 Motion-induced ghosting in diffusion weighted spin-echo images (a) can be corrected to a degree (b) using navigator echoes. A more robust approach is diffusion-weighted echo planar imaging (c).

of the brain and spine. This prompted the development of multishot diffusion-weighted EPI sequences,[15] but this step reintroduced motion sensitivity.

3.4 FACTORS INFLUENCING ADC IN TISSUE

The typical dimensions of a voxel in an MRI are ~0.25 × 0.25 × 1 mm. With voxel volumes in the 0.02 to 0.2 mL range, it is clear that each voxel will contain large populations of differing cell types, along with vascular structures, blood, CSF, fatty tissue, etc., depending on voxel location. Thus, in spite of the fact that water molecule diffusion samples dimensions are on the order of typical cell sizes during the echo time of the MRI image, the large ensemble of cells and structures sampled in each voxel means that the resulting diffusion weighted image signal, or ADC value, can depend upon a range of physiological processes operating on the microscopic and macroscopic level. This is both a strength and a weakness for DWI. It provides good sensitivity to functional changes in tissues, but specificity may be poor unless very careful experimental control is exerted.

The most important determinant of tissue water ADC is water mobility. While the T_2 and T_1 relaxation parameters depend on water mobility on the nanosecond to microsecond time scales (translational and rotational motions of the water molecule and their interaction with other water molecules and macromolecules), ADC depends on water mobility on a millisecond time scale. For example, in cerebral ventricles, water diffusion is relatively unimpeded and CSF has a high diffusion coefficient, about 2.1×10^{-3} mm^2/second (near that of pure water) and appears bright in ADC maps of the brain (Figure 3.4). Normal gray and white matter has lower ADC values (0.8 to 1.0×10^{-3} mm^2/second) than pure water because of its complex tissue structure.

Factors that impede water diffusion in tissue include increased viscosity (due to various dissolved compounds and macromolecular content), membrane permeability (during the typical MRI diffusion measurement time, typically less than 100 ms, water molecules must cross many intracellular membranes and cell walls) and tortuosity (although extracellular space is in communication with CSF space, it has a highly complex shape; water diffusion paths, even if they remain extracellular, become very tortuous and this reduces the measured diffusion coefficient). Temperature is a major determinant of diffusion in many systems, including biological organisms. However in living tissues, temperature variations are generally small since temperature is actively controlled to maintain biochemical stability. As a result, temperature changes are not generally thought to be major factors in ADC measurements in the CNS, except in specific circumstances (e.g., death or during cryosurgery).

In addition to factors affecting true diffusion of water, diffusion measured by MRI (i.e., the ADC) can also be affected by other mechanisms. Background magnetic field gradients resulting from magnetic susceptibility variations, metal implants, and deoxygenated blood from a hemorrhage will add to or subtract from the ADC weighting gradient pulses to reduce the measured ADC value. This effect can be mitigated by careful pulse sequence design.[16]

Perhaps more importantly, microscopic fluid flow can lead to an increase in ADC not related to true Brownian motion of the water molecules. In large vessels, flow results in a signal phase shift if the voxel is located within a vessel. If located away from major vessels, a tissue voxel may encompass many randomly oriented capillaries. While flow within each capillary may be uniform, their random orientation results in a signal drop resembling the one caused by true diffusion. This so-called intravoxel incoherent motion (IVIM) concept was initially proposed as a method to measure perfusion in tissue.[3] It has not been widely used because of the small dynamic range of the effect.

Probably the greatest impact of diffusion MRI has been in the area of stroke imaging. Brain water ADC is measurably slower in regions of acute ischemia compared to normal brain. The ischemic damage can be identified acutely, prior to any other detectable changes using conventional imaging approaches. The use of diffusion imaging in the study of pathology is summarized in the following section.

3.5 DIFFUSION WEIGHTED MRI AND CEREBRAL PATHOLOGY

In 1990, Moseley et al.[17] published a seminal paper demonstrating that DWI could be used for the early detection of cerebral ischemia. In a cat model of focal cerebral ischemia, MRI was performed 45 minutes following onset of ischemia. DWI showed a dramatic hyperintensity in the brain in a region consistent with the ischemic territory. Conventional MRI sequences, in which contrast is based upon changes in T_1 or T_2 relaxation times (see Chapter 1), failed to identify the acute pathology. Furthermore, the acute changes observed with DWI preceded histological evidence of infarction.

The ability to detect tissue responses before the appearance of pathology is an exciting observation. The same study indicated that white matter tracts exhibit an image intensity dependent on the relative orientation of the applied field gradient. This so-called anisotropic behavior is attributed to the presence of structural material that restricts the diffusion of water in a direction perpendicular to the white matter tracts, but allows water to diffuse relatively freely in the parallel direction. These observations opened the floodgates for intense activity exploiting these observations in the study of acute cerebral injury and fiber orientation. Moseley's paper introduced the concept of MRI as a functional imaging technique for investigating pathophysiology and led to a new era in the utility of MRI for the study of disease.

3.5.1 STUDIES IN CEREBRAL ISCHEMIA

Cerebral ischemia is the term for a state of reduced blood flow to the brain tissue. The most prevalent cause is cardiovascular disease related to hypertension and atherosclerosis. The ischemia may be global, as in the case of cardiac arrest, or focal, as occurs in stroke. CNS tissue has minimal energy reserves and is dependent on high rates of blood flow (typically 60 to 75 ml/100 g/minute). The degree of cell damage related to a stroke is dependent on the duration and amount of reduction in cerebral blood flow (CBF). As CBF falls, the brain will initially compensate by increasing oxygen extraction to maintain near-normal metabolism.

Upon further reduction of blood flow to rates approaching 18 to 25 ml/100 g/minute, the compensatory mechanism is no longer adequate to maintain neuronal function. If the stroke is focal, neurological impairment will result. Although neurons become quiescent, this level of blood flow is sufficient to prevent loss of ion homeostasis and preservation of the internal mileau. The brain has a critical blood flow below which ATP is depleted and Na^+/K^+ ATPase is impaired, leading to an increase in extracellular potassium. The first event is a gradual increase in K^+ conductance followed by a more dramatic and rapid efflux. The rise in extracellular K^+ depolarizes voltage-dependent Ca^{2+} channels and causes an increase in intracellular Ca^{2+}. This initiates a cascade of biochemical events, including activation of proteolytic enzymes and loss of mitochondrial membrane function, that ultimately culminates in loss of cellular function and death.

In a focal stroke arising from the occlusion of a large feeding vessel, collateral blood flow can respond to increase blood flow to the periphery of the ischemic region. Since tissue damage depends on both the duration and severity of the blood flow reduction, injury from a focal or multifocal stroke occurs in a graded fashion from the core of the infarct. This observation led Astrup et al. in 1981[18] to introduce the concept of the *ischemic penumbra* — an area of tissue that, although electrically silent, has sufficient CBF for the maintenance of cell membrane integrity. The term is currently used to imply zones of potentially viable and salvageable tissue (if treated with appropriate intervention). As a result, the concept of ischemic penumbra has influenced our thinking and directed our search for an imaging technique capable of defining this region.

3.5.1.1 Cell Swelling

There is now strong evidence to link the disruption of the ion homeostasis that occurs following stroke to the decrease in ADC. Ionic gradients across the cell membrane are maintained by active processes and are dependent upon membrane-bound ATPases. Disruptions of electrochemical gradient, and the high permeability of mammalian cells, result in dramatic cell swelling.[19] It has been estimated that during conditions of anoxic depolarization the interstitial space is decreased from 20 to less than 6%.

Once the blood flow falls below the critical threshold for maintaining Na^+/K^+ ATPase activity, large amounts of intracellular potassium are lost to the extracellular space, and sodium and osmotically obliged water move into the cell, resulting in cell swelling (a stage often called cellular or cytotoxic edema). In a model of global cerebral ischemia produced by occlusion of the common carotid artery (CCA) in the gerbil, Busza et al.[20] demonstrated that DWI signal enhancement only occurred when the cerebral blood flow fell below 15 to 20 ml/100 g/minute. This is similar to the critical flow threshold for maintenance of tissue high-energy metabolites[21] and ion homeostasis. Furthermore, a number of studies, using high speed imaging techniques in which ADC can be measured every few seconds, have revealed the immediate temporal changes in ADC that occur upon induction of ischemia. In models of cardiac arrest[22] as well as focal cerebral ischemia[23] it was found that the temporal profile for the changes in ADC were very similar to the known time course of K+ conductance,[24] namely, a slow gradual increase initially followed by a rapid phase lasting 2–3 minutes in total and presumably reflecting true pump failure. Conditions that preserve high levels of ATP, either by hypothermia or hyperglycaemia,[22] delay the onset of the rapid phase and the ADC decline alike.

The consensus that the ADC changes reflect cellular swelling is further supported by studies in which cell volume changes occur in the absence of severe ischemia. For example, ouabain, a specific inhibitor of membrane-bound Na^+/K^+ ATPase administered directly into the hippocampi of anesthetized rats produced a local reduction in ADC to about 33% of the control value — a reduction similar to that observed during cerebral ischemia.[25]

Dramatic cellular swelling, but with preservation of blood flow and without ischemia occurs during spreading depression. Leao first described spreading depression (SD) in 1944 when he observed, following the cortical stimulation of the brain of an anesthetized rabbit, a slow moving depression of cortical activity.[26] The changes in cortical interstitial space during SD are similar to those that occur in anoxia and are related to ion movement.[24] Spreading depression can be initiated readily in the cerebral cortex of a rat by topical administration of KCl. It is seen as a wave of cellular depolarization that spreads from the site of origin, propagating with velocity of about 3-6 mm/minute, and invades the entire cortex, affecting each area profoundly for only about 2 minutes. It is not known whether SD occurs in humans, but it has been purported to be involved in a number of neurological disorders, including migraine, stroke, and trauma. Since this phenomenon is associated with a transient but profound disruption of cell volume regulation, it represents an attractive alternative to tissue ischemia to elicit the DWI response.[27] DWI has been employed to demonstrate changes in the diffusivity of water due to an episode of SD. Diffusion maps show an area of reduced diffusivity approximately 2 mm in size, propagating away from the site of initiation at approximately 3 mm/minute, consistent with the known physiology of SD.[28,29] It has also been shown that that waves of cortical SD can be initiated by the core of the ischemic infarction in models of focal cerebral ischemia,[30] presumably due to the relative high levels of extracellular potassium. It has been suggested that the repetitive waves of depolarization that travel through the penumbral zone contribute to the gradual depletion of high-energy metabolism and contribute to the expansion of the ischemic lesion.[30] Takano et al. demonstrated that ischemia-related and induced SDs increase the size of the ischemic lesion, supporting the hypothesis for a causative role of SD in extending focal ischemic injury.[31] DWI has been used to study ischemia-induced SD in the brain of rodents.[31-35]

The link of high energy metabolism, blood flow, and DWI response has been a focus of much experimental attention. Autoradiographic techniques for measuring CBF combined with bioluminescence and fluoroscopic methods for quantifying ATP, glucose, lactate, and pH have been used to identify the spatial relationship of DWI changes, CBF, and metabolism after occlusion of the middle cerebral artery.[36,37] During the early phase of cerebral ischemia the area of hyperintensity seen on the DW images was significantly larger than the region of ATP depletion, although it matched the area exhibiting tissue acidosis. The difference became progressively smaller with the evolution of the lesion. After 7 hours, the area of tissue damage indicated by DW images was identical to the region of ATP depletion and infarction defined by subsequent histology. This is an important observation since it appears to contradict previous findings that linked ATP depletion and the consequential cellular swelling to a reduction in ADC. Other factors can lead to cellular swelling in the acute phase of cerebral ischemia, for example, anaerobic production of metabolites including lactate can contribute to the development of cytotoxic edema.[37,38] In support of this argument, good agreement is seen between lactate production and signal intensity changes revealed by DWI following cardiac arrest induced in experimental animals.

It is clear that DWI is sensitive to altered pathophysiology as diverse as SD, ischemia, and excitotoxicity. A reduction in interstitial space is common to all those conditions. It seems likely that this morphological event is central to the DWI response. The underlying mechanism, however, responsible for the decrease in ADC has been the subject of several investigations, as discussed below.

Attempts have been made to provide a more definitive description of the ADC response in terms of changes in extracellular volume fraction. Changes in the fraction can be estimated *in situ* by measuring the electrical impedance of the brain. Electrical conductance occurs mainly via the extracellular space and changes in the extracellular volume fraction are accompanied by conductance changes. Parallel experiments using DWI and measurements of conductance showed a remarkable correlation between the evolution of DW hyperintensity and changes in impedance following the intrastriatal injection of the NMDA neurotoxin and the subsequent recovery after MK-801 treatment.[39]

3.5.1.2 Diffusion Weighted MRI and Therapeutic Intervention

The ability to demonstrate ischemic damage acutely prior to infarction has important implications for the assessment of putative therapies aimed at reducing stroke damage. It is well established that prompt, adequate restoration of CBF to the ischemic territory will reduce the size of the ultimate infarction that would have resulted from permanent occlusion. In clinical practice, thrombolysis remains an effective therapy if administered within a few hours of stroke onset. This is consistent with the concept of ischemic penumbra — a region of ischemic but potentially viable tissue surrounding a core of infarction in which tissue viability is maintained by adequate perfusion from collateral circulation through the formation of anastomoses.[18]

The penumbra zone is recruited into the infarction in the absence of intervention. This led to the idea of a therapeutic window; that is, a window of opportunity during which the tissue may be salvaged through appropriate physiological or pharmacological intervention.[40] If DWI could identify ischemic tissue before irreversible damage occurred, it would serve as an invaluable technique to assess therapy. To this end, comparisons have been made between the sizes of DWI hyperintense regions and final lesion size, as determined by subsequent histology. Without pharmacological intervention or reperfusion, the area of hyperintensity recorded within the first few hours of ischemia in the rodent brain clearly correlates with the ultimate infarct size measured via triphenyl tetrazolium chloride (TTC) or histology.[41,42] However, in a rat MCAO model, DW hyperintensity returned to control level as early as 2 hours following 30 minutes of ischemia with reperfusion. This supports the idea that acute reversal of DWI hyperintensity is indicative of tissue salvage.[43] Verheul et al.[39] convincingly demonstrated the reversibility of DWI correlation with tissue viability. They showed that DWI hyperintensity resulting from the intrastriatal injection of NMDA could be completely reversed if MK-801 antagonist was administered within 30 minutes. This reversal was consistent with neuronal protection as determined from subsequent histology. Delayed treatment (1 to 6 hours) resulted in incomplete reversal of the hyperintensity and eventual tissue necrosis.

These early studies together with more recent clinical data indicated that reversal of DWI hyperintensity was an early predictor of tissue salvage and thus a marker of therapeutic efficacy. This has important implications for drug discovery and can streamline clinical trials designed to evaluate neuroprotectant activity. More recent studies have, however, shown that the acute reversal of DWI hyperintensity alone is not an indicator of tissue salvage since delayed pathology that occurs relatively late in the ischemic cascade can produce a secondary decline in ADC in the ischemic brain.[44] This responsive to transient ischemia is illustrated in Figure 3.6. The apparent discrepancy reflects the nature of the experimental protocol and the model. The acute pathophysiological consequences resulting from a brief cessation of blood flow can be reversed readily with reperfusion. The ischemic episode will, however, trigger events that ultimately lead to cell death. The exact cellular processes responsible for the secondary ADC decline appear to require increased protein synthesis but remain unknown. They may include apoptosis, inflammation, and secondary energy failure. Nevertheless, a reversal of ADC is clearly indicative of potentially viable tissue since regions with persistent hyperintensity become infarcted.

While the acute pathophysiology of ischemia causes a decrease in ADC and therefore hyperintensity on the DWI, tissue necrosis will occur as ischemic damage evolves. Cellular degradation and the onset of tissue necrosis are associated with morphological changes that remove the barrier to free diffusion. As a result, regions within the subacute ischemic lesion exhibit high ADC and reduced diffusion anisotropy[45] most likely associated with necrotic tissue. The ability to delineate regions of tissue necrosis can also be valuable in assessing severity of ischemia damage and time course. This approach has found many applications in cancer therapy and will be discussed in more detail below.

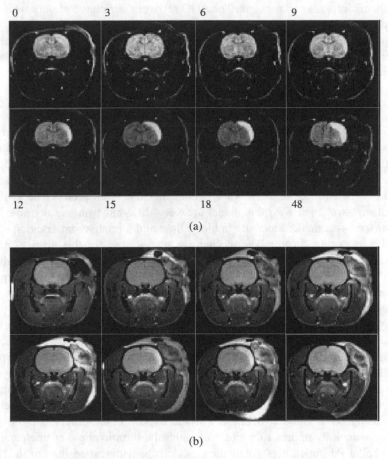

FIGURE 3.6 (a) Biphasic response in hyperintensity seen in the ischemic area is evidence from the diffusion-weighted MRI image acquired at the time indicated (hours) following transient occlusion of the middle cerebral artery in the rat. Equivalent T_2 weighted MRI images are shown in (b) for comparison. Note the DWI clearly highlights the ischemic area during the occlusion (time point 0) and is completely reversed when the tissue is reperfused. A secondary diffusion-weighted imaging change is seen at 9 hours following onset of ischemia and becomes more dramatic 15 to 18 hours later. This secondary response is accompanied by a change in T_2 (b) consistent with reperfusion injury or secondary energy failure.

It is provocative to think that the ADC value can be used to characterize the pathophysiological state of tissue. Several studies have intended to establish an ADC threshold below which irreversible ischemia damage occurs. For example, Hasegawa et al.[46] showed that ADC recovery occurred only in ischemic regions where ADC decreased by less than 0.25×10^{-5} mm^2/second. It should be noted, however, that the ADC obtained depends on the experimental conditions and animal models used; the values published by different laboratories are not necessarily comparable.

Hossmann et al.[37] reported that the recovery of the ADC in cats following resuscitation after complete cerebrocirculatory arrest for 1 hour depended on the postischemic reperfusion pressure. The ADC recovery correlated closely with tissue pH and metabolic recovery in animals that demonstrated no ADC recovery, global depletion of ATP and glucose, and severe lactic acidosis. Conversely, animals that recovered ADC exhibited replenishment of ATP and glucose and substantial reversal of lactic acidosis.

3.5.2 EPILEPSY RESEARCH

Diffusion weighted MRI has been used to investigate seizure activity in rodent models. Bicuculline, an antagonist of γ-aminobutyric acid (GABA), induced status epilepticus when administered intraperitoneally in experimental animals and was used to model some aspects of acute epilepsy in humans. Immediately after administration of bicuculline, a 14 to 18% decline in ADC was seen.[47] The CBF and metabolism associated with this model are very different from results noted with focal strokes — a marked increase in blood flow and a relative preservation of ATP levels occur during seizure. The mechanism responsible for this change in DWI signal intensity is not clear. While it is not possible to identify unequivocally the underlying pathology responsible for the DWI changes seen during status epilepticus, it is likely that a disruption of ion homeostasis and changes in cell volume are again involved.

DWI was used to demonstrate the pathology resulting from chronic exposure to vigabatrin, an inhibitor of GABA-transaminase that raises cerebral GABA. Vigabatrin has been proven clinically effective in treating intractable complex partial seizures, but animal experiments involving prolonged exposure led to intramyelinic edema and the formation of microvacuoles in cerebral white matter.[48] Animal models of chronic exposure to vigabatrin demonstrated that this pathology can be detected *in vivo* using DWI. Upon cessation of chronic exposure, the observed DWI hyperintensity eventually returns to normal, although the intramyelinic edema persists in the cerebellar Purkinje fibers. Again the exact mechanism responsible for the hyperintensity seen with DWI has not been fully explained, but these data serve to illustrate the diversity and scope for DWI in the study of cerebral pathology.

3.5.3 DIFFUSION WEIGHTED MRI IN ONCOLOGY

DWI has altered our understanding of pathology and evolution of ischemic damage in animal models of stroke. The ability to assess acute damage influenced treatment protocols and enhanced our understanding of the modes of action of putative stroke therapies. The initial observations of experimental models rapidly translated to clinial practice. DWI remains an established diagnostic technique for evaluation of stroke patients and recently received FDA approval for clinical diagnostic use.

The utility of DWI in studying CNS tumors is less compelling and its diagnostic value remains controversial.[49] Animal models of intracranial tumors showing that diffusion MRI can be used as an early surrogate marker for therapeutic intervention failed to compare DWI with other MRI modalities.[50,51] Nevertheless, a number of interesting studies indicate that, while DWI may not be sensitive to acute pathology, it provides unique insight into tumor tissue heterogeneity and assessment of tissue necrosis.

Peritumor edema is common and pronounced in experimental and clinical brain tumors. Accurate delineation of the tumor mass is not possible with conventional T_2-weighted MRI because hyperintensity from the edema will dominate the image. T_1-weighted MRI and contrast-enhanced MRI with Gd-based agents are often used to depict regional disruption of the blood–brain barrier (see Chapter 1). Since DWI is sensitive to cellular events including swelling and lysis, it was postulated that DWI may be sensitive to the pathology of CNS tumors. The hope was that DWI could serve as an early predictor of response to therapy and provide an accurate demarcation of tumor mass. Unfortunately, results of early studies using DWI to evaluate CNS tumors in experimental models were equivocal.[52,53]

Diffusion weighted MRI performed on a number of intracranial tumors derived from different cell lines inoculated in the brains of rats failed to distinguish peritumor edema from the tumor mass and showed no differences between tumor types. Accurate demarcation was only possible with contrast-enhanced T_1-weighted scans. These initial animal studies and some clinical experience suggest that a diffusion protocol offers little advantage over conventional MRI approaches and that DWI will have only limited utility in experimental neurooncology.

More recent studies have, however, shown that DW is sensitive to the heterogeneity within a tumor mass. DW scans were able to distinguish solid tumor masses from regions of coagulative necrosis.[50] As stated earlier, tissue necrosis is associated with increased water mobility and a consequent increase in ADC. Mapping ADC values provides an estimate of degree of tissue necrosis. The diffusivity of water and change in signal intensity measured in MR experiments depend on diffusion time. Structural information about pore size and cell shape can be deduced even with very short diffusion times.[54]

Hardware limitations prohibit performance of these types of experiments with conventional MRI scanners. Most diffusion experiments in practice involved relatively long diffusion times and the ADC reflected average properties of the medium including measures of tortuosity, volume fraction, and cellular permeability. It appears that as the barrier to free diffusion became disrupted, ADC values increased with the onset of tissue necrosis. A good correlation between time-dependent diffusion in experimental tumors and tissue necrosis defined by histology was indicated.[55,56] Longer diffusion times provided greater contrast between the necrotic and surrounding tissue within signal-to-noise limits.

3.5.4 PHYSIOLOGICAL BASES FOR TISSUE CHANGES

Many studies attempted to account for the dramatic changes in ADC and underlying pathology following interruption of the blood supply to the brain. While a precise description of the altered physiochemical properties causing the decrease in the apparent diffusion coefficient of water remains controversial, a qualitative description of the nature of the process emerged from biological experimentation. The following section describes the consensus on the basis of diffusion changes during ischemia, although research continues in this evolving area.

While it is generally assumed that acute cell swelling is the *physiological* process underlying the acute ADC decrease during ischemia, the *physical* mechanism by

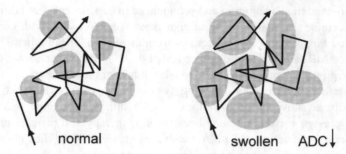

FIGURE 3.7 The ADC decrease in acute stroke occurs with cytotoxic edema, long before vasogenic edema becomes apparent on T_2-weighted images. Upon cellular energy failure, the intracellular space increases rapidly from ~80 to ~90% and water molecules spend relatively more time diffusing within the cell membranes than in the extracellular spaces.

which the swelling results in decreased water diffusion is much less clear. The initial hypothesis was that water diffusion was slower inside cells than in the extracellular space.[57] Cell swelling following cellular energy failure means that water molecules spend more time diffusing within cells (Figure 3.7), thus decreasing average diffusion coefficient.

Recent data show that *both* intracellular and extracellular water diffusion decreases during ischemia.[58,59] Szafer proposes that changes in cell membrane permeability may play a role. Computer modelling suggests that permeability changes alone are not sufficient to explain all the diffusion changes during ischemia.[60,61] Increased extracellular tortuosity during cell swelling may cause reduced extracellular ADC. Since 80 to 90% of tissue water is intracellular, it is reasonable to expect that intracellular processes primarily affect the measured ADC. A loss in active intracellular water transport (cytoplasmic streaming) with energy failure may be another cause of decreased intracellular diffusion. However, the observation that ADC decreases (similar to those accompanying ischemia) occur without energy failure in status epilepticus[47] and SD[29] argues against a mechanism directly dependent on cell energy status.

Beyond the acute phase of stroke, the initially decreased ADC value has been observed to recover and subsequently increase above normal, both in animal models[62] and humans.[63] In the long term (several weeks) it is believed that cell lysis and subsequent cell membrane breakdown result in reduced hindrance to water motion and hence faster diffusion. In the intermediate term, however, normalized or pseudo-normalized ADC values have been detected in highly abnormal (histologically) tissue. This suggests that perhaps a balance of abnormal cellular processes such as localized necrosis and cytotoxic and vasogenic edema in different cell populations within a voxel may also produce normal ADC values. This clearly implies that ADC values must be interpreted with care in the context of an evolving disease process.

3.6 DIFFUSION TENSOR IMAGING AND ANISOTROPY

A large number of studies employing diffusion imaging to investigate cerebral pathology have been qualitative in nature and relied on the visual appearance of the

DWI or used the Stejskal–Tanner equation to determine the ADC of water. They assumed isotropic diffusion — diffusion that exhibits no directionality. It is important to remember that diffusion is a three-dimensional process. In biological systems, it is likely to have directional dependence, i.e., exhibit anisotropy.

3.6.1 THEORY

The microstructures of specific biological media including certain muscle fibers and axonal tracts exhibit diffusion restriction that has directional dependence. The diffusion of water is less restricted along the long axis of the group or bundle of aligned tissue fibers than it is perpendicular to the long axis. The anisotropic diffusion that arises when displacement along one direction occurs more readily than in another direction is defined by a *tensor*. As indicated in Figure 3.1, if the free diffusion of water molecules is restricted in one dimension due to the presence of semipermeable or impermeable membranes, the diffusion coefficient of water perpendicular to these boundaries can be significantly reduced.

Diffusion anisotropy in the brain occurs primarily in white matter tracts. The myelin sheaths and other structures surrounding the nerve fibers hinder water diffusion. As a result, water diffusion across nerve fibers is about four times slower than diffusion along the fibers, and thus is anisotropic.[64] In general, diffusion in three dimensions is characterized by a mathematical *tensor* quantity. In the case of axial symmetry (as in nerve fibers), the diffusion coefficient plotted in three dimensions is an ellipsoid.[65]

3.6.1.1 Diffusion Tensor

Diffusion tensor imaging (DTI) is the term used to describe the extension of DWI to three spatial directions where the full diffusion tensor is measured. The measured diffusion properties of anisotropic tissues will differ when the diffusion gradients are applied along different directions. The complete characterization of the diffusion properties of an anisotropic structure requires that the full effective diffusion tensor be measured.[66,67]

$$\mathbf{D} = \begin{bmatrix} D_{xx} & D_{xy} & D_{xz} \\ D_{yx} & D_{yy} & D_{yz} \\ D_{zx} & D_{zy} & D_{zz} \end{bmatrix}$$

The tensor equation for diffusion attenuation is:

$$\ln\left(\frac{A(b)}{A(0)}\right) = -\sum_{i=1}^{3}\sum_{j=1}^{3} b_{ij}D_{ij} = -\mathbf{b}:\mathbf{D}$$

where **:** is the generalized dot product A(b) is the signal intensity for b, A(0) is the signal intensity for b equal to 0, and **b** is a 3×3 matrix that describes the orientation,

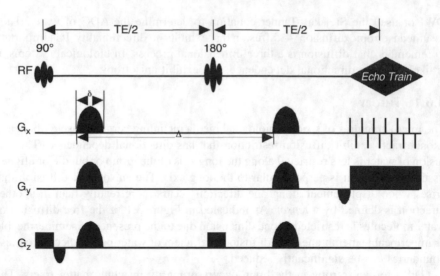

FIGURE 3.8 Stejskal–Tanner PGSE-NMR EPI sequence for diffusion tensor imaging. The appropriate gradient amplitude and direction are applied to obtain the desired diffusion orientation and weighting. For example, to obtain D_{xx}, only G_x is employed. For D_{xy}, $0.707G_x$ and $0.707G_y$ are employed.

strength, duration, and separation of the applied magnetic field gradients. Due to symmetry, the diffusion tensor can be determined by applying the gradients in a minimum of six different directions at varying amplitudes. Figure 3.8 is an example of Stejskal–Tanner PGSE (pulsed gradient spin echo)-NMR EPI sequence for diffusion tensor imaging. The use of rapid imaging such as EPI makes diffusion tensor imaging reasonable where measurement of the full diffusion tensor can be completed in several minutes.

The appropriate gradient amplitude and direction are applied to obtain the desired diffusion orientation and weighting. For example, to obtain D_{xx}, only G_x is employed. For D_{xy}, 0.707Gx and 0.707Gy are employed.

The principal diffusivities or eigenvalues of the diffusion tensor (λ_i) provide the rate of diffusion along three mutually perpendicular directions (principal axes or eigenvectors) where molecular translations are uncorrelated. For a diffusion metric to be truly quantitative, it must be rotationally invariant. The measured value must be independent of the orientation of the sample relative to the directions of the gradients. A rotationally invariant measure of isotropic diffusion is the mean of the principal diffusivity (D), which is equivalent to the average of the diagonal elements of the diffusion tensor $(\mathbf{D})$:[66,68]

$$\langle D \rangle = \frac{\text{Trace}(\mathbf{D})}{3} = \frac{D_{xx} + D_{yy} + D_{zz}}{3} = \frac{\lambda_1 + \lambda_2 + \lambda_3}{3}$$

Measurement time can be reduced by measuring diagonal elements of the diffusion tensor that will provide a rotationally invariant measure of isotropic diffusion.

3.6.1.2 Diffusion Tensor Metrics

The diffusion tensor, $\mathbf{D}$, can be separated into an isotropic component, $\langle D \rangle \mathbf{I}$, where $\mathbf{I}$ is the identity tensor, and a anisotropic component, $\boldsymbol{D}$,[69] termed the diffusion deviation tensor or diffusion deviatoric:

$$\mathbf{D} = \langle D \rangle \mathbf{I} + \boldsymbol{D}$$

Several quantitative scalar measures of anisotropy in which indices are constructed from rotationally invariant components of the diffusion tensor (eigenvalues and eigenvectors) have been developed. These measures of anisotropy can be divided into two groups: intravoxel and intervoxel. Intravoxel measures are constructed from the diffusion tensor of the voxel of interest. Intervoxel techniques assume that neighboring voxels in the same anisotropic tissue will have similar principal axes (eigenvectors) due to their similar orientations. Thus, intervoxel metrics employ similarity measures between the eigenvectors of the voxel of interest and its neighbors.

A simple intravoxel metric of anisotropy is the ratio of the first and third eigenvalues (principal diffusivities) of the diffusion tensor. The eigenvalues are sorted with the largest receiving the assignment as the first eigenvalue. The ratio provides a measure of the relative magnitude of the diffusivity along the direction of maximum diffusion compared to the orthogonal direction. In addition, the effects of sorting eigenvalues can be reduced by employing the average of the orthogonal diffusivities (second and third eigenvalues) in the denominator:

$$\text{ratio} = \frac{\lambda_1}{\lambda_3}$$

$$\text{or} \quad = \frac{\lambda_1}{\frac{1}{2}\left(\lambda_2 + \lambda_3\right)}.$$

Sorting eigenvalues is prone to variations due to noise. The relative anisotropy (RA) and fractional anisotropy (FA) indices are two metrics proposed by Basser and Pierpaoli[69] that do not require sorting. These metrics are constructed from the isotropic and anisotropic parts of the diffusion tensor. The magnitude of a tensor is given by the square root of the tensor dot product with itself. RA is the ratio of the magnitude of anisotropic and isotropic components of the diffusion tensor:

$$\text{RA} = \frac{\sqrt{\boldsymbol{D} . \boldsymbol{D}}}{\sqrt{\langle D \rangle \mathbf{I} : \langle D \rangle \mathbf{I}}} = \frac{\sqrt{\left(\lambda_1 - \langle D \rangle\right)^2 + \left(\lambda_2 - \langle D \rangle\right)^2 + \left(\lambda_3 - \langle D \rangle\right)^2}}{\langle D \rangle \sqrt{\mathbf{I} : \mathbf{I}}}$$

$$\text{RA} = \frac{\sqrt{3 Var(\lambda)}}{\sqrt{3}\langle D \rangle} = \frac{SD(\lambda)}{E(\lambda)}$$

The RA index equals the ratio of the standard deviation of the principal diffusivities to the mean of the principal diffusivities. The FA index is the scaled ratio of the magnitudes of the diffusion deviatoric to the diffusion tensor:[69]

$$FA = \sqrt{\frac{3}{2}} \frac{\sqrt{\boldsymbol{D.D}}}{\sqrt{\boldsymbol{D:D}}} = \frac{3}{\sqrt{2}} \frac{SD(\lambda)}{\sqrt{\lambda_1^2 + \lambda_2^2 + \lambda_3^2}}$$

The principal axes of the diffusion tensor for adjacent voxels should be correlated when they contain the same anisotropic tissue. Whereas for truly isotropic tissues, the principal axes of adjacent voxels will be randomly oriented and, thus, uncorrelated. Intervoxel methods determine the degree of similarity between principal axes of adjacent diffusion tensors. The tensor dot product between neighboring tensors provides a measure of their similarity and is the basic operation employed by intervoxel metrics. The tensor dot product between the diffusion deviatorics of neighboring pixels is a measure of similarity of anisotropic parts of neighboring diffusion tensors.

Basser and Pierpaoli[69] proposed the use of the tensor dot products between deviatorics as a measure of fiber–tract organization. Pierpaoli and Basser[70] incorporated these metrics into an intervoxel measure of anisotropy called the lattice anisotropy (LI) index. The LI intervoxel metric is defined as:

$$LI_N = \frac{\sqrt{3}}{\sqrt{8}} \frac{\sqrt{\boldsymbol{D}_{ref} : \boldsymbol{D}'_N}}{\sqrt{\boldsymbol{D}_{ref} : \boldsymbol{D}'_N}} + \frac{3}{4} \frac{\boldsymbol{D}_{ref} : \boldsymbol{D}'_N}{\sqrt{\boldsymbol{D}_{ref} : \boldsymbol{D}_{ref}} \sqrt{\boldsymbol{D}'_N : \boldsymbol{D}'_N}}$$

$$LI_{ref} = \frac{\sum_{N=1}^{8} a_N LI_N}{\sum_{N=1}^{8} a_N}$$

where a weighted average is formed from the lattice index between the neighboring voxels (N) and the reference voxel. The lattice index is weighted according to the distance from the reference pixel, where a_N is the weighting factor and is equal to 1.0 for horizontal and vertical voxels relative to the reference voxel and 0.707 is for voxels diagonal to the reference voxel. Pierpaoli and Basser[70] found that the lattice measure demonstrated low error variance and was less susceptible to bias than other rotationally invariant indices.

3.6.1.3 Displaying Diffusion Tensor Data

FA, RA, and LI are scalar quantities derived from the diffusion tensor, from which spatial maps can be constructed. They provide tremendous contrast that can be exploited to identify and quantify anisotropic tissue structures *in vivo* (Figure 3.9). While the eigenvalues of the diffusion tensor represent rates of diffusion along the principal axes, the eigenvectors provide the direction to the axes and allow insight

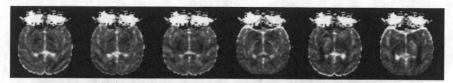

ADC maps using 6 non-collinear diffusion gradients

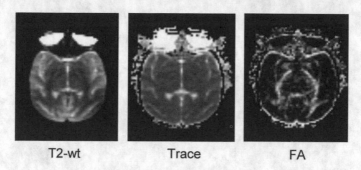

T2-wt   Trace   FA

FIGURE 3.9 ADC maps of normal macaque brain acquired using diffusion gradients oriented in six noncollinear directions, showing differing contrasts in white matter tracts. The data can be used to calculate the full diffusion tensor at each pixel position. From the diffusion tensor, various scalar invariant quantities can be calculated. For example, the trace removes diffusion anisotropy effects (presenting an average diffusion image) or the fractional anisotropy (FA)-accentuating regions of anisotropic diffusion while showing more isotropic regions (e.g., gray matter) as dark.

into the orientations of anisotropic structures. The first or principal eigenvector provides the direction of maximum diffusion. For white matter tracts, this is the axis parallel to fiber tract orientation.[66]

A number of color encoding and graphic techniques have been proposed to display fiber tract orientation within a single image.[66,71,72] Pierpaoli and Basser[70] represented fiber orientation by mapping the three vector components of the principal eigenvector to the primary colors (red, green, and blue) of a color image and scaled the brightness by the lattice anisotropy index. Figure 3.10 shows an example of this method where the brightness was scaled by the FA index. The integrity of a patient's white matter tracts was evaluated 2 weeks after onset of stroke symptoms. The maps of fiber orientation show reduced connectivity (bottom row) in the regions corresponding to the lesion in the T_2 maps (top row). The diffusion tensor data was collected by a rapid imaging technique. Whole brain coverage was achieved with isotropic voxels in about 15 minutes.[74]

Another common method for displaying fiber tract orientation is generating a graphical representation of a three-dimensional geometric shape such as an ellipsoid,[66,70] octahedral,[74] or vector;[75] where the long axis of the object is aligned along the principal axis of diffusion. This method is best suited for close looks at small structures, where orientation of the graphical object is easily visible. The main problem is that a three-dimensional object must be represented in a two-dimensional image. As an example, fiber tract orientation perpendicular to the plane of the image

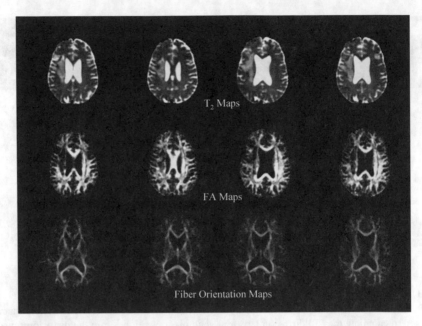

FIGURE 3.10 T_2, fractional anisotropy (FA), and color-coded direction maps of the brain acquired 2 weeks after a stroke. The maps of fiber orientation (bottom row) and FA (middle row) show reduced connectivity in regions that correspond to the lesion visible in the T_2 maps (top row). (Courtesy of Fernando Zelaya, Ph.D. and Derek Jones, Ph.D., Institute of Psychiatry, London.) See Color Figure 3.10 following page 210.

will appear as a sphere when an ellipsoid is employed to provide orientation. In this case, a highly anisotropic structure will appear isotropic.

Graphical and color-coded maps of fiber tract direction provide a qualitative, visual view of axonal connectivity. Another area of research associated with fiber tract orientation is developing a quantitative assessment of connectivity.[76–81] The algorithms focus on linking voxels whose characteristics indicate that they belong to the same fiber tract. These features include estimates of diffusion anisotropy, principal eigenvector, and the heuristic knowledge of white matter tract contours and orientation.

Jones et al.[78] employed FA thresholds to identify white matter voxels and then, based on an assumption that fiber tracts form circular arcs, neighboring white matter voxels were linked when their principal eigenvectors satisfied a model of expected curvature. Figure 3.11 shows an example of fiber tractography; individual white matter tracts were extracted from DTI data of a human brain. Basser et al.[79] modelled the trajectory of white matter tracts as a three-dimensional space curve. The local tangent vector was identified as the principal eigenvector. Curvature and torsion (twisting) were calculated from the white matter trajectory. They also employed continuous representations of the principal eigenvectors by fitting the discrete voxel data with a B-spline function. This smoothing of the data improved the performance of the tract-following algorithm compared with the performance achieved with interpolated data.

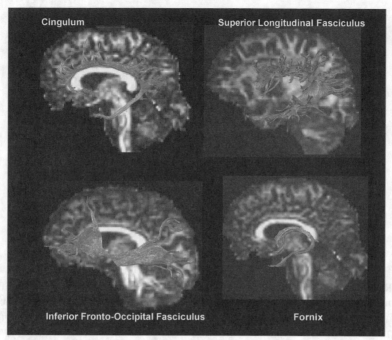

Cingulum

Superior Longitudinal Fasciculus

Inferior Fronto-Occipital Fasciculus   Fornix

FIGURE 3.11 Example of fiber tractography applied to the human brain. Individual white matter tracts were extracted from DTI data with the use of a fiber tractography algorithm. (Courtesy of Derek Jones, Ph.D., Institute of Psychiatry, London.) See Color Figure 3.11 following page 210.

3.6.2 IN VIVO APPLICATIONS OF DIFFUSION TENSOR IMAGING

The measurement of diffusion in many biological tissues varies with the measurement direction because the structural organizations of many tissues create preferred directions for diffusion. Figure 3.12 illustrates how the effects of structural organization greatly affect the measurement of water diffusion in a highly anisotropic structure — a celery stalk. Filaments run parallel to the long axis. They are visible in the diffusion maps when the diffusion gradients are applied perpendicular to the long axes of the filaments (Figures 3.12A and 3.12B). This is due to the restriction of diffusion provided by filament walls that hinders the movements of water molecules along the perpendicular axes and leads to a reduction in the rate of diffusion within the filaments. Diffusion appears homogeneous when the rate of diffusion is measured along the long (z) axis of the celery stalk (Figure 3.12C). The filaments are not visible in this measurement direction.

It is now generally accepted that diffusion can only fully be quantified in biological systems by measuring the complete diffusion tensor.[66] The filaments are easily visible in the spatial map of mean diffusivity, $\langle D \rangle$, where the measured ADC is independent of the direction of the applied diffusion gradients and the orientation of the tissue within the voxel (Figure 3.12D). The anisotropic nature of the celery stalk is most dramatically characterized in the fractional anisotropy map (Figure 3.12E) which is constructed from the diffusion tensor. DWI of rat brain

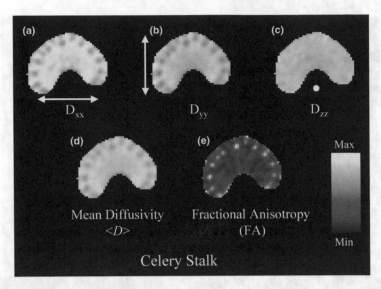

FIGURE 3.12 Diffusion tensor imaging of a celery stalk. Spatial maps of the rate of diffusion were measured perpendicular (a and b) and parallel (c) to the long axis of the stalk. The mean diffusivity (d) and fractional anisotropy (e) maps are rotationally invariant measures of isotropic and ansiotropic diffusion, respectively. See Color Figure 3.12 following page 210.

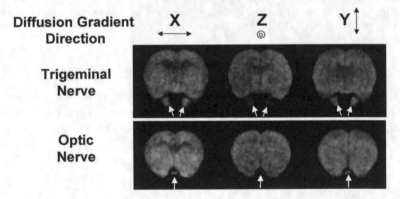

FIGURE 3.13 Diffusion-weighted imaging of rat brain showing trigeminal and optic nerves (arrows). The rate of water diffusion is faster along the nerve direction than perpendicular to it. This results in greater signal attenuation when the diffusion gradients are oriented parallel to the nerve bundles (Z direction). (Courtesy of Christian Beaulieu Ph.D., University of Alberta, Edmonton.)

(Figure 3.13) also shows a directional dependency associated with the trigeminal and optic nerves (arrows). The rate of water diffusion is faster along the nerve direction perpendicular to it, which results in greater signal attenuation when the diffusion gradients are oriented parallel to the nerve bundles (Z direction).

Brain tissues exhibit a wide range of diffusion anisotropy. White matter tracts exhibit a high degree of diffusion anisotropy; gray matter shows less anisotropy and cerebral spinal fluid is isotropic. Many neurological disorders produce structural changes in gray and/or white matter. Although disease processes differ, neurological disorders such as multiple sclerosis, Alzheimer's disease, and stroke exhibit tissue structure losses that can be monitored by DTI.

3.6.2.1 Axonal Maturation

White matter tracts exhibit high degrees of diffusion anisotropy. Myelin sheets cover the nerve axons that comprise these tracts. Myelin is a hydrophobic layer of lipids and proteins. It provides a high degree of electrical insulation and increases the speed of electrical conduction down the axons. The hydrophobic nature of myelin hinders the diffusion of water along paths perpendicular to the tracts. The measured rate of diffusion is higher when diffusion gradients are applied parallel to the directions of white matter tracts as compared to a perpendicular orientation.[81–83]

Wimberger et al.[84] showed that changes in diffusion anisotropy provided indicators of premyelination of maturing white matter in rat pups. The ratio of corresponding pixels within different DWIs served as a measure of anisotropy; the images were acquired with the diffusion gradients applied in perpendicular directions. The study showed an increase in anisotropy in white matter as the pups matured. The increase in anisotropy began before myelin was detectable via histological examination. Anisotropy rapidly increased as the amount of detected myelin increased.

The increase in diffusion anisotropy preceded changes in T_2-weighted images. The initial rise in diffusion anisotropy was attributed to premyelination changes in the axons, which included thickening of the cell membranes. Further increases in anisotropy were attributed to the increased presence of myelin.

DTI was also used to study mouse brain development, and it should prove to be a valuable to tool to study brain development in knockout and transgenic models of neurological disease.[85] Figure 3.14 shows characterization of mouse brain development by DTI. White matter tract development can easily be seen comparing weeks E14 with E16 and E18.

Neil et al.[87] employed DTI to characterize diffusion in human newborns. They employed the RA index (scaled by 0.707), a rotationally invariant measure of anisotropy, to quantify the relationship of diffusion anisotropy and gestation age. Isotropic diffusion quantified the relationship and was significantly higher in white and gray matter in the brains of newborns as compared to adults. It was also inversely correlated with gestational age; it decreased with increasing gestational age. Diffusion anisotropy of white matter was found to be lower in newborns. Only diffusion anisotropy measured in the centrum semiovale was correlated with gestational age.

3.6.2.2 Fiber Orientation Mapping

Scalar indices of anisotropy such as FA, RA, and LI provide outstanding contrast that allows easy identification of anisotropic structures. White matter tracts in the brain represent areas of high diffusion anisotropy relative to the neighboring gray matter and CSF. Graphic representations[66,69,74,75] and color-coded maps[66,71,88] of fiber tract direction provide a qualitative view of axonal connectivity. Connectivity

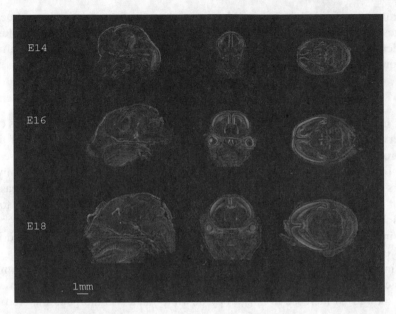

FIGURE 3.14 Diffusion tensor imaging of mouse brain development. *Ex vivo* imaging of a mouse brain at 14, 16, and 18 weeks of embryonic development. Brain samples were fixed by paraformaldehyde. RGB direction color coding: red = superior–inferior, green = right–left, and blue = anterior–posterior. Images were acquired at isotropic resolution of approximately 80 μm. (Courtesy of Susumu Mori, Ph.D., Johns Hopkins University, Baltimore.) See Color Figure 3.14 following page 210.

algorithms[76–81,89] provide the means to quantify these structures and confirm connections among different regions of the brain.

The application of fiber mapping and connectivity allows us to determine neuronal connectivities of different regions of the brain. White matter integrity is of particular interest in studies of many medical disorders. Lim et al.[90] found that the white matter of patients suffering from schizophrenia exhibited lower anisotropy than white matter of age-matched controls. They noted no differences in white matter volume or gray matter anisotropy. The schizophrenic patients exhibited reduced gray matter volume consistent with the disease.

Chronic alcohol abuse has been associated with the loss of white matter integrity. DTI was employed to quantify white matter changes associated with chronic alcoholism.[91] Alcoholics exhibited lower regional values of FA, when compared to normal controls. In addition, splenium FA was correlated with working memory. Attention correlated positively with intervoxel coherence of the genu. Function MRI (fMRI) is another area where neuronal connectivity is of particular interest. DTI was combined with fMRI[92] to determine whether sites of functional activation are linked.

3.6.2.3 CNS Diseases

Many neurodegenerative disorders affect humans, including multiple sclerosis (MS), Alzheimer's disease (AD), Krabbe's disease, Alexander's disease, and Wallerian degeneration. MS, Krabbe's disease, and Alexander's disease are demyelination disorders. MS is an immune-mediated disease of the white matter in which myelin is attacked by the immune system. In diseases such as Alzheimer's disease and Wallerian degeneration, demyelination occurs after cell injury. The ability to estimate the degree of neurodegeneration *in vivo* can provide valuable information in diagnosis of these disorders and planning treatment and evaluating potential therapies *in vivo*.

A disease that alters the microstructure of a tissue will likely alter its anisotropic diffusion properties. Consequently, neurodegenerative diseases can potentially be studied using diffusion anisotropy measures. Demyelination of axons in MS results in a reduction in the restrictions to water diffusion. Ono et al.[93] employed rotationally variant measure of anisotropy to show that diffusion anisotropy can provide differentiation of a demyelination disorder (Krabbe's disease) and a dysmyelination (abnormal myelin development) disorder (Pelizaeus–Merzbacher disease) of cerebral white matter. Both disorders showed high intensity lesions in T_2-weighted images. The demyelination disorder (Krabbe's disease) lost its diffusion anisotropy, while the dysmyelination disorder demonstrated high diffusion anisotropy. This study demonstrates the diagnostic potential of diffusion anisotropy.

Bammer et al.[101] employed an interleaved-EPI DTI sequence to characterize MS lesions. They found a decrease in FA in NAWM relative to healthy controls and FA was also decreased in lesions that exhibited T_1-hypointensity. In this study, contrast-enhancing lesions did not exhibit reduced anisotropy, which had been observed in other studies.[92,100] These contradictory results were attributed to diffusion differences that may be associated with an early phase of inflammation.

Several clinical studies have shown elevated diffusion in MS lesions, which has been attributed to an increase in the extracellular space due to demyelination and edema.[92,94–98] These studies have shown that normal-appearing white matter (NAWM) in MS patients exhibit elevated rates of diffusion. In addition, serial MRI studies have shown that increases in diffusion occur in normal-appearing white matter prior to detection of Gd-enhancing lesions.[92,98] Diffusion imaging has also been shown to be able to differentiate between hypo- and isointense, nonenhancing T_1 lesions.[99]

Several groups have employed DTI to investigate the anisotropic nature of multiple sclerosis lesions. Diffusion anisotropy was found to be reduced in several categories of MS lesions[92,100–103] and NAWM.[92,101–103] Diffusion and fractional anisotropy measures have been found to correlate with clinical measures of disability.[102,103] Tievsky et al.[100] employed rotationally invariant anisotropy measures (FA and RA) to confirm a reduction in anisotropy in the center of acute MS lesions and to differentiate between varying degrees of demyelination and remyelination. They concluded that a peripheral rim of restricted diffusion, which exhibited low ADC values and intermediate values of anisotropy, characterizes acute MS lesions. These values for ADC and anisotropy were attributed to acute demyelination. Chronic lesions were isotropic with high ADC values, while remyelinated plaques exhibited intermediate levels of anisotropy.

Alzheimer's disease is a neurodegenerative disorder associated with the deposition of amyloid plaques, neuron death, and demyelination. Hanyu et al.[104] employed a rotationally variant measure of diffusion anisotropy to evaluate white matter integrity in AD patients. They found reduced diffusion anisotropy in the white matter of patients who did not exhibit lesions in T_2-weighted images. The reduction was attributed to the loss of myelin. Isotropic diffusion has also been shown to be elevated in the white matter of AD patients.[104–106]

Diffusion tensor imaging has been applied to the study of AD. Rose et al.[107] used a color-encoding scheme to evaluate the integrity of association fiber WMTs in patients with AD. In patients with probable AD, WMTs related to association (splenium of the corpus callosum, superior longitudinal fasciculus, and cingulum) exhibited reduced anisotropy, while WMTs related to motor control (pyramidal tract) were normal. In addition, the LI index of the splenium of the corpus callosum correlated with cognitive ability (Mini-Mental State Exam, MMSE).

The progression of the cerebral ischemia results in cytotoxic edema, cell death, axon demyelination, cell lysis and eventual removal of cellular debris by glial cells and macrophages. These events will reduce barriers to diffusion and result in a reduction in anisotropy. Kajima et al.[108] evaluated diffusion anisotropy in a rat model of focal ischemia at acute and chronic time points. Anisotropy was greatly reduced 24 to 48 hours after occlusion. Their study was hindered because the investigator did not employ a rotational invariant measure of anisotropy; only differences between the ADCs measured along three orthogonal gradient axes were related as measures of anisotropy.

DTI was employed to characterize the temporal course of FA and LI during acute and subacute cerebral ischemia in a rat stroke model.[45] The evolution of the parameters was compared with other MR parameters already characterized in rat models of cerebral ischemia. FA and LI were dramatically reduced during the subacute phase, 24 to120 hours after middle cerebral artery occlusion (MCAO) in rat models of transient ischemia (60 minutes; see Figure 3.15). Figure 3.16 shows parametric maps obtained at acute and subacute time points (3 and 48 hours post MCAO, respectively). The temporal evolutions of proton density, T_2, CBF_i and mean diffusivity were compared with FA and LI during the acute and subacute stages for subcortical (Figure 3.15a) and cortical (Figure 3.15b) regions within the ischemic lesions. The parametric values were normalized by their respective control values. The control values for acute data were the preocclusion values. The corresponding contralateral values provided controls for subacute time points.

The temporal evolution of $<D>$, T_2 and proton density (M0) within the ischemic lesions exhibited a well characterized pattern for a rat model of cerebral ischemia.[62] Diffusion was dramatically reduced during the acute period and T_2 and M0 peaked 24 to 48 hours post MCAO. Carano et al.[45] showed that the diffusion anisotropy indices were reduced to approximately 30% of control values during the subacute period and remained depressed for the remaining subacute time points. This suggests that diffusion anisotropy may provide a more stable parameter for generating subacute lesion contrast than T_2 or M0, since the contrast for these parameters peaked 24 to 48 hours post MCAO and then declined.

Knight et al.[62] described the breakdown of the cytoarchitecture within subacute ischemic lesions in rat brains. This disruption of the cytoarchitecture is consistent with the observed reduction in diffusion anisotropy. In addition, the renormalization

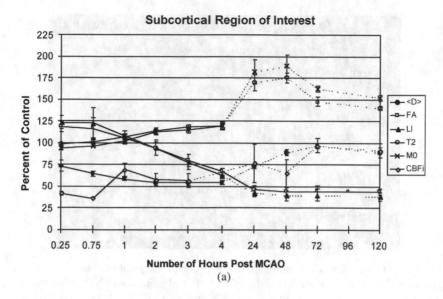

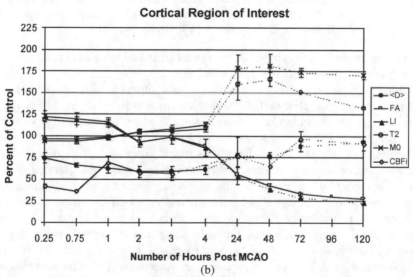

FIGURE 3.15 Temporal evolution of the following parameters is shown for a rat model of transient cerebral ischemia: mean diffusivity ($<D>$), T_2, proton density (M0), cerebral blood flow index (CBF_i), fractional anisotropy (FA), and lattice anisotropy index (LI). Region of interest (ROI) measurements were made within the subcortical (a) and cortical (b) regions of the rat brain during and after 60 minutes of temporary middle cerebral artery occlusion. ROI data shown as the ratio of the parameter with the corresponding control value. Preocclusion data were employed as control values for acute data (0 to 4 hrs) except for CBF_i. The contralateral ROI was employed as the control for acute CBF_i (0 to 3 hours) and all subacute parameters (24 to 120 hrs after occlusion). Seven animals were evaluated during the acute period. A total 16 animals were studied at subacute time points (24 (n = 7), 48 (n = 3), 72 (n = 4), or 120 (n = 2) hours after occlusion).

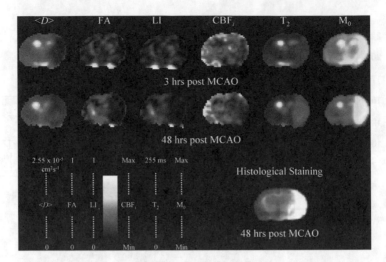

FIGURE 3.16 Spatial maps of mean diffusivity (<D>), fractional anisotropy (FA), lattice anisotropy (LI), cerebral blood flow index (CBF_i), T_2 and proton density (M_0) are shown for a cerebral ischemic lesion imaged at 3 and 48 hours after middle cerebral artery occlusion in a rat model of 60 minutes of transient ischemia. The corresponding postmortem TTC-stained slice is also shown. See Color Figure 3.16 following page 210.

or hypernormalization of isotropic diffusion was attributed to a loss of cell membrane integrity consistent with the observed histology.

Clinical studies of diffusion anisotropy have observed similar trends during cerebral ischemia. A decline in diffusion anisotropy was found during late acute and chronic stages of human stroke by Maier et al.,[109] where the standard deviation of three orthogonal ADC values was used as an anisotropy metric (rotationally variant).

Several clinical DTI studies have shown that isotropic diffusion and FA are reduced in acute ischemic lesions.[110,111] Isotropic diffusion was elevated and FA reduced in chronic white matter lesions relative to normal white matter characteristics.[78] Yang et al.[112] observed a heterogeneous temporal evolution of diffusion anisotropy characteristics within acute and subacute ischemic lesions. Regions of reduced diffusion anisotropy were found in acute and subacute ischemic lesions. Figure 3.15 shows an apparent trend toward increases in hyperacute diffusion anisotropy. No statistical difference was apparent between the region of interest measurements of diffusion anisotropy in the ipslateral and contralateral hemispheres. Increases in FA and LI after MCAO were seen in both hemispheres. They may have resulted from an increase in respiratory noise due to hyperventilation after in-bore occlusion since diffusion anisotropy metrics are sensitive to noise.[45]

Diffusion and DTI have also been applied to studies of normal and diseased spinal cords. The spinal cord is a highly anisotropic structure that serves as a novel target for diffusion imaging and DTI. It exhibits a high degree of diffusion anisotropy.[82,113–116] Due to a fairly consistent orientation of its fibers, diffusion symmetries may be exploited with the use of rotationally variant measures of anisotropy as a means to reduce imaging time, although the field of view will be restricted due to curvature of the spine.

Diffusion imaging of the spine is prone to artefacts associated with susceptibility effects arising from neighboring vertebrae, motion due to CSF movement, arterial flow and respiration, and partial volume averaging with neighboring CSF. Despite these difficulties, diffusion imaging offers a promising technique for early detection and evaluation of spinal cord injuries. As with white matter disorders, diffusion imaging of spinal cord injuries detects changes in isotropic and anisotropic diffusion associated with a reduction in the barriers of diffusion, such as demyelination.

Ex vivo spinal cord measurements of the ADC have shown anisotropic changes in a rat spinal injury model. Ford et al.[113] reported a reduction in diffusion measured along the longitudinal axis of the spinal cord and an increase in diffusion measured along the transverse axis after injury. A reduction in anisotropy was seen by construction of a rotationally variant measure of anisotropy from the ratio of the ADC values.

Ex vivo DTI has been shown to detect a reduction in diffusion anisotropy of spinal cord due to demyelination in an experimental allergic encephalomyelitis mouse model.[116] *In vivo* estimates of diffusion anisotropy via DTI confirmed high levels of anisotropy of white and gray matter within the rat spinal cord, with higher anisotropy found within the white matter tracts.[117] The application of diffusion anisotropy to the study of the spinal cord was shown to be feasible in clinical practice. DTI was used to study corticospinal tract damage associated with amyotrophic lateral sclerosis (ALS).[118] Elevated rates of diffusion and reduced anisotropy were found within the ALS lesions. Elevated diffusion was also found within spinal cord lesions of MS patients.[97]

3.7 CONCLUSIONS

Diffusion weighted MRI offers a unique technology that can provide insight into CNS pathology and morphologies as diverse as spreading depression. ischemia, and axonal connectivity and maturation. DWI is noninvasive, offers high spatial and temporal resolution, and is equally applicable to neuroscience research in animal models and in clinical investigation and diagnosis. It provides physiological and anatomical information that is not available from other imaging modalities or from invasive methods. Despite the lack of complete understanding of the mechanisms underlying the changes seen with DWI, its role in neuroimaging is established.

REFERENCES

1. Tanner, J.E. and E.O. Stejskal, Restricted and self-diffusion of protons in colloidal systems by the pulsed-gradient, spin-echo method. *J. Chem. Phys.*, 49, 1768, 1968.
2. Stejskal, E.O. and J.E. Tanner, Spin diffusion measurements: spin-echoes in the presence of a time-dependent field gradient. *J. Chem. Phys.*, 42, 288, 1965.
3. Le Bihan, D., E. Breton, and D. Lallemand, Separation of diffusion and perfusion in intravoxel incoherent motion (IVIM) MR imaging. *Radiology*, 168, 497, 1988.

4. Le Bihan, D. et al., MR imaging of intravoxel incoherent motions: application to diffusion and perfusion in neurologic disorders. *Radiology*, 161, 401, 1986.
5. Le Bihan, D., Intravoxel incoherent motion imaging using steady-state free precession. *Mag. Res. Med.*, 7, 346, 1988.
6. Ahn, C.D. et al., Effects of random directional distributed flow in nuclear magnetic resonance imaging. *Med. Phys.*, 14, 43, 1987.
7. Turner, R., Angiography and perfusion measurements by NMR. *Prog. Nucl. Mag. Res. Spectrosc.*, 23, 93, 1987.
8. King, M.D. et al., Perfusion and diffusion MR imaging. *Mag. Res. Med.*, 24, 288, 1992.
9. Pekar, J., C.T. Moonen, and P.C. van Zijl, On the precision of diffusion/perfusion imaging by gradient sensitization. *Mag. Res. Med.*, 23, 122, 1992.
10. Moseley, M.E., M.F. Wendland, and J. Kucharczyk, Magnetic resonance imaging of diffusion and perfusion, *Top. Mag. Res. Imaging*, 3, 50, 1991.
11. Anderson, A. and J. Gore, Analysis and correction of motion artifacts in diffusion-weighted imaging, *Mag. Res. Med.*, 32, 379, 1994.
12. de Crespigny, A. et al., Navigated diffusion imaging of normal and ischemic human brain, *Mag. Res. Med.*, 33, 720, 1995.
13. Mansfield, P., Multiplanar image formation using NMR spin-echoes, *J. Phys. Chem. Solid State Phys.*, 10, L55, 1977.
14. Turner, R. and D. Le Bihan, Single-shot diffusion imaging at 2.0 tesla, *J. Mag. Res.*, 86, 445, 1990.
15. Butts, K. et al., Diffusion-weighted interleaved echo-planar imaging with a pair of orthogonal navigator echoes, *Mag. Res. Med.*, 35, 763, 1996.
16. Does, M.D., J. Zhong, and J.C. Gore, *In vivo* measurement of ADC change due to intravascular susceptibility variation, *Mag. Res. Med.*, 41, 236, 1999.
17. Moseley, M.E. et al., Early detection of regional cerebral ischemia in cats: comparison of diffusion- and T_2-weighted MRI and spectroscopy, *Mag. Res. Med.*, 14, 330, 1990.
18. Astrup, J., B.K. Siesjo, and L. Symon, Thresholds in cerebral ischemia: the ischemic penumbra, *Stroke*, 12, 723, 1981.
19. Hansen, A.J., Effect of anoxia on ion distribution in the brain, *Physiol. Rev.*, 65, 101, 1985.
20. Busza, A.L. et al., Diffusion-weighted imaging studies of cerebral ischemia in gerbils: potential relevance to energy failure, *Stroke*, 23, 1602, 1992.
21. Allen, K. et al., Acute cerebral ischaemia: concurrent changes in cerebral blood flow, energy metabolites, pH, and lactate measured with hydrogen clearance and 31P and 1H nuclear magnetic resonance spectroscopy III. Changes following ischaemia, *J. Cereb. Blood Flow Metabol.*, 8, 816, 1988.
22. de Crespigny, A.J. et al., Rapid monitoring of diffusion, DC potential, and blood oxygenation changes during global ischemia: effects of hypoglycemia, hyperglycemia, and TTX, *Stroke*, 30, 2212, 1999.
23. Decanniere, C. et al., Correlation of rapid changes in the average water diffusion constant and the concentrations of lactate and ATP breakdown products during global ischemia in cat brain, *Mag. Res. Med.*, 34, 343, 1995.
24. Hansen, A.J. and C.E. Olsen, Brain extracellular space during spreading depression and ischemia, *Acta Physiol. Scand.*, 4, 355, 1980.
25. Benveniste, H., L.W. Hedlund, and G.A. Johnson, Mechanism of detection of acute cerebral ischemia in rats by diffusion-weighted magnetic resonance microscopy, *Stroke*, 23, 746, 1992.
26. Leao, A.A.P., Spreading depression of activity in the verebral cortex, *J. Neurophysiol.*, 7, 359, 1944.

27. Back, T., K. Kohno, and K.A. Hossmann, Cortical negative DC deflections following middle cerebral artery occlusion and KCl-induced spreading depression: effect on blood flow, tissue oxygenation, and electroencephalogram, *J. Cereb. Blood Flow Metabol.*, 14, 12, 1994.

28. de Crespigny, A. et al., Magnetic resonance imaging assessment of cerebral hemodynamics during spreading depression in rats, *J. Cereb. Blood Flow Metabol.*, 18, 1008 1998.

29. Latour, L. et al., Spreading waves of decreased diffusion coefficient after cortical stimulation in the rat brain, *Mag. Res. Med.*, 32, 189, 1994.

30. Hossmann, K.A., Peri-infarct depolarizations, *Cerebrovasc. Brain Metabol. Rev.*, 8, 195, 1996.

31. Takano, K. et al., The role of spreading depression in focal ischemia evaluated by diffusion mapping, *Ann. Neurol.*, 39, 308, 1996.

32. Yenari, M.A. et al., Diffusion- and perfusion-weighted magnetic resonance imaging of focal cerebral ischemia and cortical spreading depression under conditions of mild hypothermia, *Brain Res.*, 88, 208, 2000.

33. Sotak, C.H., New NMR measurements in epilepsy: diffusion-weighted magnetic resonance imaging of spreading depression, *Adv. Neurol.*, 79, 925, 1999.

34. Rother, J. et al., Recovery of apparent diffusion coefficient after ischemia-induced spreading depression relates to cerebral perfusion gradient, *Stroke,* 27, 980, 1996.

35. Kastrup, A. et al., High speed diffusion magnetic resonance imaging of ischemia and spontaneous peri-infarct spreading depression after thromboembolic stroke in the rat, *J. Cereb. Blood Flow Metabol.*, 20, 1636, 2000.

36. Hoehn-Berlage, M. et al., Evolution of regional changes in apparent diffusion coefficient during focal ischemia of rat brain: the relationship of quantitative diffusion NMR imaging to reduction in cerebral blood flow and metabolic disturbances, *J. Cereb. Blood Flow Metabol.*, 15, 1002, 1995.

37. Hossmann, K.A. et al., NMR imaging of the apparent diffusion coefficient (ADC) for the evaluation of metabolic suppression and recovery after prolonged cerebral ischemia, *J. Cereb. Blood Flow Metabol.*, 14, 723, 1994.

38. Back, T. et al., Penumbral tissue alkalosis in focal cerebral ischemia: relationship to energy metabolism, blood flow, and steady potential, *Ann. Neurol.*, 47, 485, 2000.

39. Verheul, H.B. et al., Comparison of diffusion-weighted MRI with changes in cell volume in a rat model of brain injury, *Nucl. Mag. Res. Biomed.*, 1994. 7(1–2), 96–100.

40. Heiss, W.D., M. Forsting, and H.C. Diener, Imaging in cerebrovascular disease, *Curr. Opin. Neurol.*, 14, 67, 2001.

41. Minematsu, K. et al., Reversible focal ischemic injury demonstrated by diffusion-weighted magnetic resonance imaging in rats, *Stroke*, 23, 1304, 1992.

42. van Bruggen, N., T.P. Roberts, and J.E. Cremer, The application of magnetic resonance imaging to the study of experimental cerebral ischaemia, *Cerebrovasc. Brain Metabol. Rev.,* 1994. 6(2): p. 180–210.

43. Mintorovitch, J. et al., Comparison of diffusion- and T2-weighted MRI for the early detection of cerebral ischemia and reperfusion in rats. *Mag. Res. Med.*, 18, 39. 1991.

44. van Lookeren-Campagne, M. et al., Secondary reduction in the apparent diffusion coefficient of water, increase in cerebral blood volume, and delayed neuronal death after middle cerebral artery occlusion and early reperfusion in the rat, *J. Cereb. Blood Flow Metabol.*, 19, 1354, 1999.

45. Carano, R.A. et al., Multispectral analysis of the temporal evolution of cerebral ischemia in the rat brain, *J. Mag. Res. Imaging*, 12, 842, 2000.

46. Hasegawa, Y. et al., MRI diffusion mapping of reversible and irreversible ischemic injury in focal brain ischemia, *Neurology*, 44, 1484, 1994.
47. Zhong, J. et al., Changes in water diffusion and relaxation properties of rat cerebrum during status epilepticus, *Mag. Res. Med.*, 30, 241, 1993.
48. Jackson, G.D. et al., Vigabatrin-induced lesions in the rat brain demonstrated by quantitative magnetic resonance imaging, *Epilepsy Res.*, 18, 57, 1994.
49. Zimmerman, R.D., Is there a role for diffusion-weighted imaging in patients with brain tumors or is the "bloom off the rose"? *Am. J. Neuroradiol.*, 22, 1013, 2001.
50. Chenevert, T.L., P.E. McKeever, and B.D. Ross, Monitoring early response of experimental brain tumors to therapy using diffusion magnetic resonance imaging, *Clin. Cancer Res.*, 3, 1457, 1997.
51. Chenevert, T.L. et al., Diffusion magnetic resonance imaging: an early surrogate marker of therapeutic efficacy in brain tumors, *J. Natl. Cancer Inst.*, 92, 2029, 2000.
52. Eis, M. et al., Quantitative diffusion MR imaging of cerebral tumor and edema, *Acta Neurochir. Suppl.* (Wien), 60, 344, 1994.
53. Els, T. et al., Diffusion-weighted MR imaging of experimental brain tumors in rats, *Magma*, 3, 13, 1995.
54. King, M.D. et al., q-Space imaging of the brain, *Mag. Res. Med.*, 32, 707, 1994.
55. Helmer, K.G., B.J. Dardzinski, and C.H. Sotak, The application of porous media theory to the investigation of time-dependent diffusion in *in vivo* systems, *Nucl. Mag. Res. Biomed.*, 8, 297, 1995.
56. Helmer, K.G., S. Han, and C.H. Sotak, On the correlation between the water diffusion coefficient and oxygen tension in RIF-1 tumors, *Nucl. Mag. Res. Biomed.*, 11, 120, 1998.
57. Moseley, M.E. et al., Diffusion-weighted MR imaging of acute stroke: correlation with T_2-weighted and magnetic susceptibility-enhanced MR imaging in cats, *Am. J. Neuroradiol.*, 11, 423, 1990.
58. Stanisz, G.J. et al., An analytical model of restricted diffusion in bovine optic nerve, *Mag. Res. Med.*, 37, 103, 1997.
59. O'Shea, J.M. et al., Apparent diffusion coefficient and MR relaxation during osmotic manipulation in isolated turtle cerebellum, *Mag. Res. Med.*, 44, 427, 2000.
60. Szafer, A. et al., Diffusion-weighted imaging in tissues: theoretical models, *Nucl. Mag. Res. Biomed.*, 8, 289, 1995.
61. Szafer, A., J. Zhong, and J.C. Gore, Theoretical model for water diffusion in tissues, *Mag. Res. Med.*, 33, 697, 1995.
62. Knight, R. et al., Magnetic resonance imaging assessment of evolving focal cerebral ischemia, *Stroke*, 25, 1252, 1994.
63. Marks, M.P. et al., Acute and chronic stroke: navigated spin-echo diffusion-weighted MR imaging [erratum in *Radiology* 200, 289, 1996], *Radiology*, 199, 403, 1996.
64. Moseley, M., Y. Cohen, and J. Kucharczyk, Anisotropy in diffusion-weighted MRI, *Mag. Res. Med.*, 14, 330, 1990.
65. Basser, P.J., Inferring microstructural features and the physiological state of tissues from diffusion-weighted images, *Nucl. Mag. Res. Biomed.*, 8, 333, 1995.
66. Basser, P.J., J. Mattiello, and D. Le Bihan, Estimation of the effective self-diffusion tensor from the NMR spin echo, *J. Mag. Res. Biomed.*, 103, 247, 1994.
67. Basser, P.J., J. Mattiello, and D. Le Bihan, MR diffusion tensor spectroscopy and imaging, *Biophys. J.*, 66, 259, 1994.
68. van Gelderen, P. et al., Water diffusion and acute stroke, *Mag. Res. Med.*, 31, 154, 1994.

69. Basser, P.J. and C. Pierpaoli, Microstructural and physiological features of tissues elucidated by quantitative-diffusion-tensor, *J. Mag. Res. Biomed.*, 111, 209, 1996.

70. Pierpaoli, C. and P.J. Basser, Toward a quantitative assessment of diffusion anisotropy, *Mag. Res. Med.*, 36, 893, 1996.

71. Douek, P. et al., MR color mapping of myelin fiber orientation, *J. Comput. Assist. Tomogr.*, 15, 923, 1991.

72. Pajevic, S. and C. Pierpaoli, Color schemes to represent the orientation of anisotropic tissues from diffusion tensor data: application to white matter fiber tract mapping in the human brain, *Mag. Res. Med.*, 42, 526, 1999.

73. Gilbert, R.J. et al., Determination of lingual myoarchitecture in whole tissue by NMR imaging of anisotropic water diffusion, *Am. J. Physiol.*, 275, 363, 1998.

74. Jones, D.K. et al., Isotropic resolution diffusion tensor imaging with whole brain acquisition in a clinically acceptable time, *Hum. Brain Mapping*, 15, 216, 2002.

75. Makris, N. et al., Morphometry of *in vivo* human white matter association pathways with diffusion-weighted magnetic resonance imaging, *Ann. Neurol.*, 42, 951, 1997.

76. Conturo, T.E. et al., Tracking neuronal fiber pathways in the living human brain, *Proc. Natl. Acad. Sci. U.S.A.*, 96, 10422, 1999.

77. Xue, R. et al., *In vivo* three-dimensional reconstruction of rat brain axonal projections by diffusion tensor imaging, *Mag. Res. Med.*, 42, 1123, 1999.

78. Jones, D.K. et al., Non-invasive assessment of axonal fiber connectivity in the human brain via diffusion tensor MRI, *Mag. Res. Med.*, 42, 37, 1999.

79. Mori, S. et al., Three-dimensional tracking of axonal projections in the brain by magnetic resonance imaging, *Ann. Neurol.*, 45, 265, 1999.

80. Basser, P.J. et al., *In vivo* fiber tractography using DT-MRI data, *Mag. Res. Med.*, 44, 625, 2000.

81. Poupon, C. et al., Towards inference of human brain connectivity from MR diffusion tensor data, *Med. Image Anal.*, 5, 1, 2001.

82. Moseley, M.E. et al., Anisotropy in diffusion-weighted MRI, *Mag. Res. Med.*, 19, 321, 1991.

83. Chenevert, T.L., J.A. Brunberg, and J.G. Pipe, Anisotropic diffusion in human white matter: demonstration with MR techniques *in vivo*, *Radiology,* 177, 401, 1990.

84. Doran, M. et al., Normal and abnormal white matter tracts shown by MR imaging using directional diffusion weighted sequences, *J. Comput. Assist. Tomogr.,* 14, 865, 1990.

85. Wimberger, D.M. et al., Identification of "premyelination" by diffusion-weighted MRI, *J. Comput. Assist. Tomogr.*, 19, 28, 1995.

86. Mori, S. et al., Diffusion tensor imaging of the developing mouse brain, *Mag. Res. Med.,* 46, 18, 2001.

87. Neil, J.J. et al., Normal brain in human newborns: apparent diffusion coefficient and diffusion anisotropy measured by using diffusion tensor MR imaging, *Radiology,* 209, 57, 1998.

88. Pierpaoli, C., Oh no! One more method for color mapping of fiber tract direction using diffusion MR imaging data, *Proc. ISMRM 5th Annl. Mtg.*, Vancouver, B.C., 1997.

89. Jones, D.K. et al., Characterization of white matter damage in ischemic leukoaraiosis with diffusion tensor MRI, *Stroke*, 30, 393, 1999.

90. Lim, K.O. et al., Compromised white matter tract integrity in schizophrenia inferred from diffusion tensor imaging, *Arch. Gen. Psychiatr.*, 56, 367, 1999.

91. Pfefferbaum, A. et al., *In vivo* detection and functional correlates of white matter microstructural disruption in chronic alcoholism, *Alcohol Clin. Exp. Res.*, 24, 1214, 2000.

92. Werring, D.J. et al., A direct demonstration of both structure and function in the visual system: combining diffusion tensor imaging with functional magnetic resonance imaging. *Neuroimage*, 9, 352, 1999.

93. Ono, J. et al., Differentiation of dys- and demyelination using diffusional anisotropy, *Pediatr. Neurol.*, 16, 63, 1997.

94. Christiansen, P. et al., Increased water self-diffusion in chronic plaques and in apparently normal white matter in patients with multiple sclerosis, *Acta Neurol. Scand.*, 87, 195, 1993.

95. Horsfield, M.A. et al., Apparent diffusion coefficients in benign and secondary progressive multiple sclerosis by nuclear magnetic resonance, *Mag. Res. Med.*, 36, 393, 1996.

96. Droogan, A.G. et al., Comparison of multiple sclerosis clinical subgroups using navigated spin echo diffusion-weighted imaging, *Mag. Res. Imaging*, 17, 653, 1999.

97. Werring, D.J. et al., The pathogenesis of lesions and normal-appearing white matter changes in multiple sclerosis: a serial diffusion MRI study, *Brain*, 123, 1667, 2000.

98. Rocca, M.A. et al., Weekly diffusion-weighted imaging of normal-appearing white matter in MS, *Neurology*, 55, 882, 2000.

99. Nusbaum, A.O. et al., Quantitative diffusion measurements in focal multiple sclerosis lesions: correlations with appearance on TI-weighted MR images, *Am. J. Roentgenol.*, 175, 821, 2000.

100. Tievsky, A.L., T. Ptak, and J. Farkas, Investigation of apparent diffusion coefficient and diffusion tensor anisotrophy in acute and chronic multiple sclerosis lesions, *Am. J. Neuroradiol.*, 20, 1491, 1999.

101. Bammer, R. et al., Magnetic resonance diffusion tensor imaging for characterizing diffuse and focal white matter abnormalities in multiple sclerosis, *Mag. Res. Med.*, 44, 583, 2000.

102. Filippi, M. et al., Diffusion tensor magnetic resonance imaging in multiple sclerosis, *Neurology*, 56, 304, 2001.

103. Ciccarelli, O. et al., Investigation of MS normal-appearing brain using diffusion tensor MRI with clinical correlations, *Neurology*, 56, 926, 2001.

104. Hanyu, H., et al., Increased water diffusion in cerebral white matter in Alzheimer's disease, *Gerontology*, 43, 343, 1997.

105. Hanyu, H. et al., Regional differences in diffusion abnormality in cerebral white matter lesions in patients with vascular dementia of the Binswanger type and Alzheimer's disease, *Eur. J. Neurol.*, 6, 195, 1999.

106. Kantarci, K. et al., Mild cognitive impairment and Alzheimer's disease: regional diffusivity of water, *Radiology*, 219, 101, 2001.

107. Rose, S.E. et al., Loss of connectivity in Alzheimer's disease: an evaluation of white matter tract integrity with colour coded MR diffusion tensor imaging, *J. Neurol. Neurosurg. Psychiatr.*, 69, 528, 2000.

108. Kajima, T. et al., Diffusion anisotropy of cerebral ischaemia, *Acta Neurochir. Suppl.* (Wien), 60, 216, 1994.

109. Maier, S.E. et al. Diffusion anisotropy imaging of stroke, *Proc. ISMRM 5th Annl. Mtg.*, Vancouver, B.C., 1997.

110. Zelaya, F. et al., An evaluation of the time dependence of the anisotropy of the water diffusion tensor in acute human ischemia, *Mag. Res. Imaging*, 17, 331, 1999.

111. Sorensen, A.G. et al., Human acute cerebral ischemia: detection of changes in water diffusion anisotropy by using MR imaging, *Radiology*, 212, 785, 1999.

112. Yang, Q. et al., Serial study of apparent diffusion coefficient and anisotropy in patients with acute stroke, *Stroke*, 30, 2382, 1999.

113. Ford, J.C. et al., MRI characterization of diffusion coefficients in a rat spinal cord injury model, *Mag. Res. Med.,* 31, 488, 1994.

114. Nakada, T., H. Matsuzawa, and I.L. Kwee, Magnetic resonance axonography of the rat spinal cord, *Neuroreport*, 5, 2053, 1994.

115. Matsuzawa, H., I.L. Kwee, and T. Nakada, Magnetic resonance axonography of the rat spinal cord: postmortem effects, *J. Neurosurg.*, 83, 1023, 1995.

116. Ahrens, E.T. et al., MR microscopy of transgenic mice that spontaneously acquire experimental allergic encephalomyelitis, *Mag. Res. Med.*, 40, 19, 1998.

117. Fenyes, D.A. and P.A. Narayana, *In vivo* diffusion characteristics of rat spinal cord, *Mag. Res. Imaging*, 17, 717, 1999.

118. Ellis, C.M. et al., Diffusion tensor MRI assesses corticospinal tract damage in ALS, *Neurology*, 53, 1051, 1999.

119. Ries, M. et al., Diffusion tensor MRI of the spinal cord, *Mag. Res. Med.*, 44, 884, 2000.

4 Functional Magnetic Resonance Imaging

Mathias Hoehn

CONTENTS

0-8493-0122-X/03/$0.00+$1.50

4.1 INTRODUCTION

The discovery of a close coupling of functional brain activity, metabolism, and blood flow under normal physiological conditions was cited in the literature as early as 1890.[1] The potential of this relationship, however, was not exploited until the late 20th century when various imaging modalities permitted the regional evaluation of blood flow and metabolism. Using the xenon clearance technique, Lassen et al. demonstrated the coupling of brain function and highly localized increases of blood flow in corresponding brain regions.[2]

In parallel, Sokoloff et al.[3] developed the autoradiographic deoxyglucose technique that provided spatially resolved data on glucose consumption during brain activation. Their technique was soon adapted for noninvasive use in humans when Phelps[4] applied ^{18}F-deoxyglucose, a positron-emitting tracer. The real breakthrough for functional brain imaging was the first application of nuclear magnetic resonance (NMR) imaging for functional activation studies. In the first investigation by Belliveau et al.,[5] increases in blood flow and volume were recorded in the visual cortex during visual stimulation with the NMR contrast agent GdDTPA in 1990. The most common functional magnetic resonance imaging (fMRI) technique, blood oxygen level-dependent (BOLD) magnetic resonance imaging (MRI) followed in 1991[6] and led to an astounding evolution and expansion of cognitive science.

Despite this rapid development, we must remember that many functional imaging methods are only indirect indicators of the brain activity, i.e., recording the hemodynamic response to a stimulus. Their correct interpretation depends on the intact coupling of brain activity and the induced metabolic or hemodynamic change. The situation is even more complex with the BOLD technique because the BOLD signal change is based on an increase in blood flow that is overproportional compared to the increase of oxygen consumption during functional activation. It must be emphasized, therefore, that the conclusions drawn from BOLD fMRI data are valid only when and if the coupling mechanisms are kept intact.

The large amount of data acquired by different imaging modalities confirms the robustness of this coupling of electrical activity and blood flow response in the healthy brain. However, the situation may be different in disease states. Coupling is achieved by the interaction of a complex system of biochemical and neurogenic mediators that are subject to pathological interference and may modulate both the effect of functional activation on metabolism and the response of blood flow to the change in metabolic activity. Knowledge of such disturbances is vital to understanding the coupling mechanisms and interpreting activation studies under clinical conditions.

In recent years, a number of laboratories turned to investigation of the somatosensory activation of the rat cortex as the most established model. For this reason,
most of this chapter is dedicated to the discussion of results obtained with this model
and species.

4.2   CHOICE OF ANESTHETIC

A major factor to keep in mind for fMRI studies in animals is the requirement to
anesthetize the animals unless time-consuming and challenging training periods are
allowed to accustom the animals to exposure to the magnet environment and scanner
noise during study periods.

The coupling of functional activity of the cerebral cortex with blood flow and
metabolism is very sensitive to anesthetics.[7] Many anesthetics reduce or suppress
the coupling of functional activation and metabolic and blood flow response.[7,8] For
this reason, most activation studies in experimental animals were done with animals
in the awake state. However, this limits such investigations to autoradiographic
studies of freely moving or minimally restrained animals because the only invasive
intervention required is the insertion of intravascular catheters that can be done under
light inhalation anesthesia prior to the experiment. More sophisticated techniques,
in particular the opening of the skull for electrophysiological or continuous blood
flow recordings, require surgical anesthesia. This also applies to most MR investigations because the animals must be immobilized to prevent movement artefacts.

Several anesthetics have been tested for compatibility with functional activation.[9–11] The best suited anesthetic is α-chloralose,[12] a compound used extensively
in neurophysiological research for tracing multisynaptic pathways. When administered intravenously at 80 mg/kg, α-chloralose produces surgical anesthesia that can
be maintained for many hours when supplemented intermittently by small additional
doses. Successful functional activation of the somatosensory cortex was demonstrated after whisker movement or electrical stimulation of the paws in mice, rats,
and cats. For more intense functional activation, as induced by electrical stimulation
of the cortex or spreading depression, halothane or barbiturate anesthesia can also
be used[13] but the coupling mechanism may be different from the one that operates
during more physiological activation procedures.

Recently, the same animal model of somatosensory stimulation of the rat paw
was used to investigate the feasibility of new anesthetics for fMRI studies. Several
authors[14,15] were able to show that propofol also permitted the detection of the
activated somatosensory cortex, but the intensity of the BOLD-activated signal was
clearly lower than that usually reported for α-chloralose. This was confirmed in a
study comparing fMRI signals in propofol-anesthetized and awake restrained animals.[16] Due to the investigative limits imposed by anesthesia, several authors investigated the possibility of performing fMRI studies on awake animals. However, data
obtained from awake animals were found rather unreliable and weak compared to
data from animals in the anesthetized state.[16–18] In other studies, extensive measures
were taken to train the animals to accustom them to the magnet environment and
scanner noise. The animals still had to be restrained in straight jackets and their heads
had to be immobilized.[19–21] From the perspectives of animal care and the need to

exclude or minimize stress during functional brain activation, the requirement for restraints and the fact that experimental animal scanners produce noise levels above 115 dB[22] will probably limit fMRI studies to animals anesthetized most preferably with α-chloralose.[12]

4.3 ESTABLISHED STIMULATION PARADIGMS IN RATS

The major stimulation paradigms applied today for experimental fMRI studies in rats focus on the somatosensory system (Figure 4.1). Two different stimuli are used in most laboratories: mechanical whisker stimulation and electrical paw stimulation. The only other well described method for rats is olfactory stimulation. Visual stimulation was reported from one mouse study and several studies in cats (see Section 4.12). Acoustic stimulation appears extremely difficult because the auditory cortex lies too close to the large air-filled ear channels that produce strong susceptibility artefacts resulting in uncontrolled reduction or extinction of the signal in the auditory cortex.

4.3.1 WHISKER STIMULATION

Whiskers are aligned in three rows of individual hairs on both sides of the snout. Each single hair is represented by a cortical structure in the posteriomedial barrel subfield of the somatosensory cortex, containing distinct cylindrical columns of cellular aggregates throughout layer IV of the cortex. The columns are called *barrels* because of their shape. Thus, individual stimulation of a single whisker will result in activation of the corresponding barrel on the contralateral cortex, as extensively characterized by Woolsey and colleagues.[23,24]

Stimulation of all or selected single whiskers can be achieved by applying a focused, pulsed air stream leading to whisker movement of defined strength and frequency (Figure 4.2). Alternatively, whisker movement is achieved by magneto-electrically induced vibration of a thin wire attached to a single whisker and fed by square-shaped electrical pulses from a function generator, with the whole set-up positioned in the static magnetic field of the MRI system.[25] In the case of single whisker stimulation, all whiskers except the selected one are carefully clipped close to the snout surface just before the experiment. Typical stimulation frequencies to achieve strong cortical responses were reported for 8 Hz.[25]

4.3.2 ELECTRICAL PAW STIMULATION

The cortical representation fields of the forepaw and hindpaw are located next to each other and cover a large portion of the primary somatosensory cortex (SI).[26] See Figure 4.1. Stimulation was achieved by insertion of thin needle electrodes under the skin of the paw. Electrical stimulation consisted of square-wave pulses of 0.3-ms duration. Variation of functional response was achieved by varying stimulation frequency; optimal stimulation response was consistently reported for 1.5 to 3 Hz.[27-31]

Response amplitude was shown to increase with increasing current intensity.[29,32] The stimulation current must be adjusted in the range of 0.5 to 2.0 mA to remain

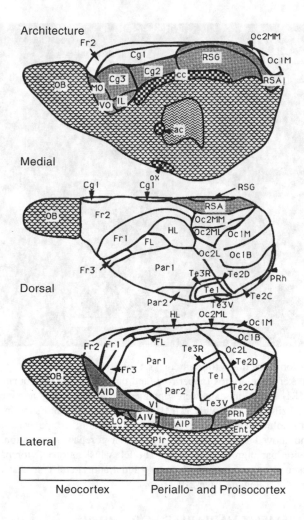

FIGURE 4.1 Axial orientation of the rat brain from dorsal view. (From Paxinos, G., *Rat Brain*, Academic Press, San Diego, 1995. With permission.)

below the threshold of pain (indicated by a rise in blood pressure). Lower current thresholds necessary to induce measurable cortical response were somewhat higher for hindpaw than for forepaw stimulation.[30]

4.3.3 OLFACTORY STIMULATION

The only established nonsomatosensory stimulation paradigm for fMRI investigation in rats is olfactory stimulation with pleasant or obnoxious odors.[33,34] Odor delivery is best achieved through a glass system with a funnel loosely fit over the nose of the spontaneously breathing animal. For quantitative measurements, the flow rate and odorization of the air must be controllable. Duration of odor exposure can be adjusted with a flow valve.[33]

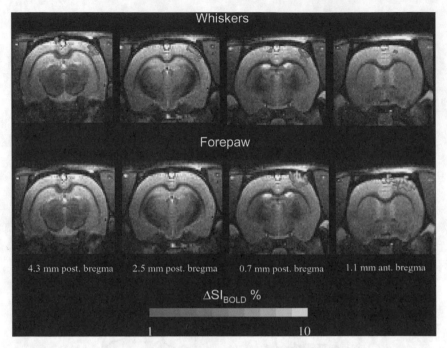

FIGURE 4.2 Coronal sections through the rat brain with the activated representation fields of the whisker barrel cortex (upper row) and the forepaw in the somatosensory cortex demarcated. fMRI activation data were obtained with EPI using a boxcar stimulation protocol and analyzing the data with STIMULATE software,[142] and superimposed on morphological high-resolution images. For whisker stimulation, a tape was stretched across all whiskers and moved by a pulse air stream. For forepaw stimulation, the electrical forepaw stimulation paradigm was applied.[28] The left whiskers or left forepaw were stimulated. The whisker representation area is more caudal and lateral than that of the forepaw. See Color Figure 4.2 following page 210.

4.4 MEASUREMENT VARIABLES FOR fMRI

4.4.1 BOLD MRI

The most common blood oxygenation level-dependent (BOLD) signal increase during functional brain activation is based on Ogawa's investigations in 1990[35,36] and later years.[37] This approach is an indirect measure of hemodynamic response: the overproportionate increase of blood flow as compared to the increase in oxygen consumption leads to an increase in venous blood oxygenation. Since deoxyhemoglobin is paramagnetic, the concentration decrease in paramagnetic material in the vascular bed will lead to a reduction in susceptibility changes, and consequently, a signal increase during functional brain activation.

Using the above-described model of somatosensory forepaw stimulation in rats under α-chloralose anesthesia, Hyder and colleagues performed the first BOLD- based fMRI study on anesthetized animals at 7 T.[27] They reported activation areas extending far beyond the somatosensory cortex SI of the rat. Since they observed blood pressure increases during the stimulation period, these areas of rather unspecific activation are probably due to pain reaction caused by high stimulation currents. However, if physiological conditions are carefully monitored and maintained, the method permits a highly resolved regional assignment of particular stimulation paradigms to cortical representation fields (Figure 4.2).

Bock and colleagues demonstrated a clear separation of the representation fields for the forepaw and hindpaw — two directly adjacent areas within the somatosensory cortex.[30] The hindpaw activation area is more medial and caudal than the corresponding forepaw activation area. Also, hindpaw activation was detected only for stimulation currents of 1.5 mA or higher[30] — a level fully sufficient for most forepaw stimulations. In a similar study using single whisker stimulation, Yang et al. demonstrated the high spatial selectivity of the BOLD method by detecting the corresponding single whisker barrel within the whole barrel field.[25] All such BOLD- based fMRI studies depend on T_2*-weighted imaging; TE values and magnetic field conditions may vary among individual reports. However, the BOLD contrast was maximal for TE = T_2* of the corresponding tissue.

Grüne et al.[38,39] showed in quantitative T_2* measurements of rat brains that the effective T_2* decreases radially toward the upper cortical layers in coronal image sections. Thus, activation areas close to the skull will remain undetected when unsuitably long TE values are chosen. The authors, therefore, concluded that it is necessary to record quantitative T_2* images to obtain reliable information on location and extent of representation fields within the rat cortex. In a recent comparison of gradient echo (GE) and spin echo (SE) BOLD signal behavior at very high fields, Lee and coworkers[40] reported a negligible contribution from intravascular signal to the BOLD signal increase during electrical forepaw stimulation in rats. The authors further concluded that at B_0 fields of 9.4 T or higher, the sensitivities of SE-BOLD experiments will be comparable to those of GE-BOLD studies.

4.4.2 PERFUSION-WEIGHTED MRI

Perfusion-weighted imaging (PWI) is an alternative MRI method first described by Kerskens et al. to observe hemodynamic responses of a functional brain.[41] They used a fast imaging adaptation of the arterial spin tagging technique reported earlier by Detre et al.[42] PWI may be preferable to BOLD imaging because its signal change is interpreted more directly due to the activation-induced cerebral blood flow (CBF) increase. It is also much more sensitive and allows detection of the activated area in the somatosensory cortex from individual images, without reference to statistical analysis of image series under both resting and activated conditions, as is necessary for BOLD-based data. PWI, originally applied at 4.7 T, was later described to gain almost a factor of 3 in sensivity for experiments at 7 T.[43]

Silva and colleagues[32,44] combined BOLD and PWI by implementing the arterial spin labeling (ASL) technique in an echo planar imaging (EPI) sequence. The unlabeled image of the necessary image pair for the PWI served as the T_2*-sensitive (and therefore BOLD-sensitive) image. The subtraction of the image pair yielded perfusion-sensitive data. This technique was applied to study the fast dynamics of hemodynamic response to electrical forepaw stimulus using the activation block design. The authors noted onset of CBF response at 0.6 seconds after stimulation start while the corresponding time for oxygenation changes (BOLD) was 1.1 seconds. Also, no early negative BOLD effect was observed at this high temporal resolution. These findings were interpreted as speaking "against the occurrence of an early loss of hemoglobin oxygenation that precedes the rise in CBF and suggest that CBF and oxygen consumption increases may be dynamically coupled in this animal model of neural activation."[44]

The analysis of the signal behavior of PWI and BOLD under the same activation paradigm was further analyzed by the same authors[32] who showed that the activation centers of both methods colocalize very well while the BOLD activation territory was significantly larger than that of the CBF parameter. By varying stimulation conditions like current intensity or stimulation frequency, they found that the BOLD signal changes follow CBF changes with a very close correlation. Changes in response amplitude between the first activation block and the following blocks were described as functions of intermittent resting periods. For both BOLD and PWI, reduction by approximately 30 to 35% in response amplitude was reported for the second block at a rest period of 1 minute. The first and consecutive blocks were indistinguishable when the resting period was extended to 5 minutes.[32] This observation, confirmed in other studies,[45,46] led to different levels of $CMRO_2$ increase during the first and consecutive blocks of activation.[45]

A technique of combined BOLD and PWI data recording, similar to that reported by Silva et al.[32] but with a lower temporal resolution, described by Hyder et al., permitted calculation of quantitative maps of R_2^*, R_2, and CBF at a temporal resolution of approximately 30 seconds.[47]

4.4.3 CEREBRAL BLOOD VOLUME MRI

A third variable for the detection of brain activation is the change of cerebral blood volume (CBV) recorded with intravascular contrast agents, in particular magnetic iron oxide nanoparticles (MIONs). This highly sensitive technique is based on the observation that the concentration of paramagnetic agent in voxels increases during increases of CBV and leads to increased susceptibility differences between vessels and surrounding tissue. In consequence, this results in a blood volume-proportional decrease in T_2^*-sensitive signal intensity.

Since this method produces a signal change running opposite to the BOLD effect, it is the preferable technique at low fields at which the opposing BOLD contribution is weak and difficult to detect. Successful application of this approach to delineate the activation area in the somatosensory cortices of rats was first reported by van Bruggen et al.[48] and Mandeville et al.[49] The former group showed the spatial agreement of activation areas found by BOLD and consecutive CBV maps.[48] They were able to produce CBV activation maps of high spatial resolution at a less than 6-second temporal resolution due to the high sensitivity to T_2^* changes at high magnetic field.[50]

Mandeville and Marota[51] performed a detailed analysis of BOLD signal behavior and CBV changes during stimulation of the rat brain. They concluded that the existing gradient of CBV from the inner to the outer cortical layers led to distinctly different signal behaviors of BOLD and CBV, resulting in a dorsal shift of the BOLD activation area in respect to that of CBV, in obvious contradiction to van Bruggen's report[48] of spatial agreement of the activation areas of BOLD and CBV.

CBV as a sensitive MRI parameter for detection of functional brain activation was then applied in several studies including analyses of the dynamics of the hemodynamic response[49,52,53] (Section 4.6) and for determination of $CMRO_2$ changes[45,46,54] (Section 4.7). Detailed analysis of signal contributions from CBV-dependent susceptibility and from blood oxygenation-dependent susceptibility changes was performed by Kennan et al.[15] and expanded by Zhong et al.[55]

4.5 STRUCTURE AND FUNCTION RELATIONSHIPS OF ESTABLISHED STIMULATION PARADIGMS

4.5.1 WHISKER STIMULATION

The whiskers have a one-to-one relationship with the barrel structure on the contralateral somatosensory cortex.[23,24] The approximate diameters of these barrels range from 300 to 500 μm. A rat's whiskers are its most sensitive tactile sensors and are indispensable for spatial orientation and movement. These properties make the whisker barrel field of the rat an ideal model for studying functional brain activation. This stimulation is well established and used widely with other techniques, especially autoradiography and laser-Doppler flowmetry, to investigate physiological parameters during functional brain activation.[56]

Another important application for whisker stimulation has been the study of learning-induced plasticity and the role of glutamate receptors.[57,58] Yang et al. reported the detection of a single whisker barrel by stimulation of a single whisker after clipping all others.[25] The high spatial image resolution in their fMRI experiments permitted them to distinguish the locations of barrels assigned to whiskers D1 and D4, i.e., barrels within one row, with representation of two other whiskers (D2 and D3) lying between the detected activation areas. The same authors[59] compared the localization and spatial extent of the activation area recorded during single whisker stimulation with electrophysiological data reported in the literature.[60]

Defining two thresholds in the BOLD activation maps, Yang and colleagues found good agreement with the earlier reported electrical activity. The area encompassing all positive BOLD pixels was closely similar to the extent that more than 0.5 spikes/stimulus were recorded using microelectrophysiology. The focal response area (>2 spikes/stimulus) correlated well with the BOLD activation area if a cut-off threshold at 75% of the maximal BOLD signal was applied. Although the result that the indirect BOLD signal reflects the center of electrical activity is encouraging, it is necessary as a note of caution to point out that the BOLD signal behavior is strongly dependent on the experimental conditions, as clearly shown by Grüne et al.[38] Therefore, such threshold determinations are simply arbitrary in an effort to obtain spatial agreement with the independent variable (electrical activity in this case) and lack physiological justification for such choices.

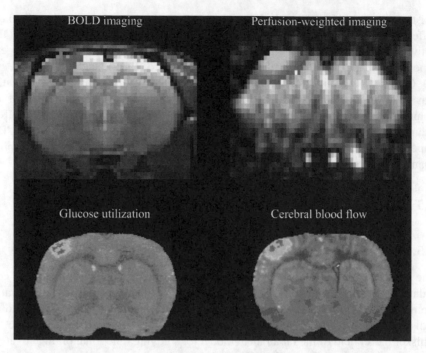

FIGURE 4.3 Coronal sections highlighting the activation of somatsosensory cortex by fMRI (upper) and autoradiographic (lower) techniques, respectively. fMRI data were obtained with BOLD and a perfusion-weighted sequence. Autoradiographic images reflect recording of the cerebral metabolic rate of glucose and cerebral blood flow. Note good spatial correspondence of activated areas of the four different techniques. (From Brinker, G. et al., *Mag. Res. Med.*, 41, 469, 1999. With permission.) See Color Figure 4.3 following page 210.

4.5.2 PAW STIMULATION

This stimulation paradigm is the most widely applied one for fMRI studies on anesthetized animals due to its robustness and reproducibility. The forepaw representation area recorded with BOLD and PWI was demonstrated to be in full agreement[61] with the areas of increased blood flow and increased glucose consumption revealed by autoradiographic experiments (Figure 4.3).[62] Confirming that no pain reaction due to noxious stimulation current intensity occurred, several authors showed the BOLD activation to be very stable and reproducible in both localization and spatial extent.[22,28,29,38,50,54,63–65]

The paradigm of electrical paw stimulation can be further extended to distinguish the directly adjacent representation fields of forepaw and hindpaw within the somatosensory cortex SI.[30] The technique of fMRI-based detection of somatosensory cortex activation has been shown convincingly to provide high spatial resolution and sensitivity to distinguish directly neighboring representation fields[30] and separate barrel fields of rather minute spatial extent.[25]

Although most investigations exclusively focused on the cortex, brain activity can also be registered in the cerebellum. Peeters and colleagues[66] studied cerebellar activity during electrical forepaw and hindpaw stimulation in rats. Their main observation was the rather patchy appearance of the activation areas. Although they noted some interindividual variation in patterns, they found a clear and unexpected horizontal organization. The activation was bilateral, mainly patchy, and expressed a mediolateral band organization that was more pronounced ipsilateral to the paw stimulation. No overlap was observed between forepaw and hindpaw representations. The patchy appearance was tentatively attributed to the afferent input components of the mossy fibers.[66] The cerebellum receives afferent inputs from both mossy fibers and climbing fibers.[67] The organization of climbing fibers is well defined; the mossy fibers, originating from spinal cord and corticopontine projections, have patchy and fractured somatotopy in the cerebellum.[68]

4.5.3 OLFACTORY STIMULATION

The olfactory bulb (OB) of the mammal has different areas and activation patterns within its glomerular layers, depending on particular stimuli. The axons of the olfactory sensory neurons terminate in these glomerular layers. Yang et al.[33] and Xu et al.[34] applied odors of iso-amyl acetate (IAA) solution and limonene. While typical BOLD activation levels of whisker or forepaw stimulation are in the range of a 4 to 10% signal increase, the authors observed a 20 to 30% BOLD increase during olfactory stimulation.

The highest activity was observed in the glomerular layers, composed of axon terminals and presynaptic and postsynaptic dendrites. Since they have the highest synaptic density in the OB, the authors inferred that synaptic activity gave rise to the BOLD signal.[33] They also noted that for sustained odor stimulation, the BOLD signal was reduced after several minutes. A slow and delayed decline of the BOLD signal after termination of the odor stimulus was interpreted as most likely due to slow clearance of the odor molecules from the olfactory receptors and the relatively high concentration of the odor stimulus. Investigations of variation of odor stimulus or intensity[34] showed that for IAA and limonene, overlapping but significantly different activation areas were observed. BOLD activity was found to increase with odorant concentration.[34]

4.6 fMRI: NORMAL PHYSIOLOGICAL CONDITIONS

4.6.1 TEMPORAL RESPONSES

Mandeville and coworkers reported several studies dealing with the temporal behavior of CBF, CBV, and BOLD signals in response to electrical forepaw stimulation in rats.[49,52] They measured BOLD and CBV responses sequentially; CBF response was determined in a separate group of animals using laser-Doppler flowmetry (LDF).[52]

Comparison of SE- and GE-dependent CBV measurements resulted in equivalent CBV changes, a result interpreted to indicate proportional CBV changes for capillaries and small vessels. At a 3-Hz stimulation rate, a CBV increase of $24 \pm 4\%$

was found for a stimulation duration of 30 seconds,[49] while the CBV increase was only 10% during a 6-second stimulation period.[52]

The CBV response to the stimulation was clearly delayed when compared to the much faster responses of BOLD and CBF. The latter two parameters reached the new stimulation-induced steady state almost instantaneously (BOLD was delayed by approx. 1 second relative to CBF). CBV exhibited a two-phase behavior: a fast component followed by a slow increase. When fitting this signal curve to a monoexponential function, the authors obtained a time constant of approximately 14 seconds. A similar procedure applied to the CBF data resulted in a time constant of 2.4 ± 0.8 seconds.[69]

This temporal mismatch of three hemodynamic variables in response to the stimulus led the authors to formulate a modified Windkessel model. They described the temporal evolution of the CBV changes as a rapid elastic response of capillaries and veins followed by slow venous relaxation of stress. Delayed venous compliance was suggested as the mechanism for the observed poststimulus undershoot in the BOLD signal curve.[69] All three variables were measured separately: BOLD and CBV changes were recorded sequentially on the same animals so that some fluctuations in response intensity and size of activation must always be considered between the individual stimulation periods. CBF was determined in a different group of animals, using LDF which lacks spatial resolution. Nevertheless, the qualitative description of the temporal behavior of these variables is in good agreement with more recent investigations by Burke and colleagues[45,46] who recorded all three variables using only MRI technology. The latter approach permitted the authors to register CBF and BOLD changes simultaneously using the EPI-based version of arterial spin tagging perfusion imaging.[32,44]

4.6.2 PHYSIOLOGICAL MECHANISMS CONTRIBUTING TO FUNCTIONAL BRAIN ACTIVATION

The issue of the contributions of various factors to neuronal excitability and the coupling of neuronal activity to blood flow is a very broad topic that can be touched upon only slightly in this chapter in the direct connection to presently available fMRI data dealing with this complex field.

Kennan and coworkers[70] addressed the influence of hypoglycemia on the functional activation signal in medial nerve stimulation in rats. Under mildly hypoglycemic conditions (blood glucose level reduced from 6.6 ± 0.3 to 2.8 ± 0.2 mmol/L) they observed a reduction of BOLD signal amplitude by 40% during stimulation (Figure 4.4). However, no global BOLD signal effect was noted during resting conditions. Because the authors registered only BOLD signals and recorded no CBF changes during stimulation under euglycemic and hypoglycemic conditions, the interpretation of the observations remains unclear. The question remains whether a hemodynamic, metabolic, or even electrical adaptation to decreased glucose availability exists. Future studies should combine such investigations with CBF recording and measurement of electrical activity via somatosensory-evoked potentials (SEPs).

Following a CO_2-induced challenge, Bock et al.[29] noted an increase in CBF response amplitude by 100% relative to normal conditions during electrical forepaw

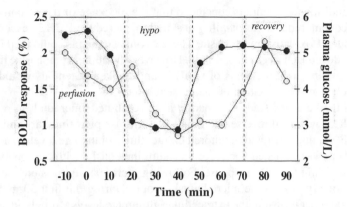

FIGURE 4.4 BOLD fMRI response to median nerve stimulation as a function of blood glucose level. BOLD signal response decreases in parallel with induction of hypoglycemia and follows the recovery of normoglycemia. The full circles and right vertical axis indicate the time course for plasma glucose. Open circles and the left vertical axis indicate the BOLD fMRI signal change. (From Kennan, R.P. et al., *J. Cereb. Blood Flow Metabol.*, 20, 1352, 2000. With permission.)

stimulation. In contrast, BOLD response amplitude increased only marginally from 6 to 7%. This hypercapnic up-regulation was registered after the CO_2 challenge at a time when blood gases had already returned to normocapnic conditions so that a direct influence of the CO_2 challenge was excluded. This enhanced CBF response was transient and leveled off again about 3 hours after the CO_2 challenge, but could be elicited repetitively by further CO_2 challenge. This condition of doubled CBF response amplitude to the same stimulus was considered a welcome, nontoxic sensitivity enhancement of CBF-based fMRI studies. However, in a later study by Schwarzbauer and Hoehn on awake humans, presence of this hypercapnic up-regulation of the CBF response to stimulation could not be confirmed.[71]

These authors interpreted the absence of this effect in awake humans and its presence in anesthetized rats as a modulatory effect of the α-chloralose anesthesia on the cholinergic systems of rats. Earlier investigations by Scremin et al.[72,73] showed that the cholinergic system is involved in the CO_2 effect on cerebrovascular resistance, and that this effect is anesthesia-dependent.[74]

Two recent investigations were dedicated to the role of the glutamatergic system in brain activation and its coupling to cerebral blood flow increase. Under normal physiological conditions, neurotransmitters are released from vesicles after an influx of Na^+ ions through presynaptic voltage-dependent Na^+ channels. Inhibitors of these channels and the Na^+ current they modulate suppress neuronal excitability and neurotransmitter release. Kida et al.[75] applied such a neuronal voltage-dependent Na^+ channel blocker and glutamate release inhibitor, lamotrigine, to rats during electrical forepaw stimulation. Lamotrigine application reduced the BOLD response by more than 50% (from 6.7 to 3.0% BOLD amplitude) while the CBF response was decreased by approximately one order of magnitude. Based on earlier independent studies with lamotrigine that showed reduced cortical excitability, also under clinical conditions, the authors concluded that the blockage of the glutamate release and consequent reduced excitability resulted in a reduced CBF response and a lowered rate of oxidative metabolism. These two mechanisms could then lead to the strongly reduced BOLD effect observed. However, the authors emphasize that further studies including measurements of $CMRO_2$ and evoked potentials would permit a more conclusive interpretation of the present data.

In another elegant study, Forman et al.[76] combined microdialysis with CBF-based fMRI. They used reverse microdialysis to infuse picrotinin, a γ-amino butyric acid (GABA) antagonist and monitored extracellular glutamate levels. The microdialysis set-up was adjusted for recording simultaneously with the ongoing fMRI studies, providing the CBF response. Following picrotoxinin infusion, the CBF was increased locally around the microdialysis probe. During the first 30 minutes after GABA antagonist infusion, the extracellular glutamate levels strongly increased and were linearly proportional to the CBF increase. This was interpreted as showing that the picrotoxinin-induced CBF increase was tightly coupled to increased neuronal activity as reflected by increased extracellular glutamate levels. However, after picrotoxinin infusion glutamate levels fell again while the CBF increase persisted. This may have been due to a depletion of the releasable glutamate pools in local neurons. Furthermore, after long exposure to picrotoxinin, the CBF increase may be driven by other endogenous stimuli.

4.6.3 CORRELATION OF fMRI WITH ELECTROPHYSIOLOGICAL SIGNALS

As discussed earlier, it is highly desirable to have electrophysiological data complementary to data on the hemodynamic response to the stimulus available. Often, only this combination will allow unambiguous interpretation of fMRI data, particularly under pathophysiological conditions or when the mechanisms coupling electrical activity to hemodynamic response are investigated. However, several problems are connected with such a complex experimental set-up.

The major issue is selection of electrode materials that will avoid susceptibility and thus image artefacts, particularly in the strongly T_2^*-weighted image sequences usually applied for fMRI studies. If this is not successful, then artefact-free images can only be recorded in planes shifted away from the plane of the electrode positions. This may compromise the desired correlation between electrophysiological signals and fMRI results. The other major problem arises from artefacts on the EEG traces induced by switching of the magnetic field gradient during imaging. The fast gradient switching may induce currents stronger than the EEG signal in the EEG leads. The strong interferences between imaging requirements and electrophysiological needs have prevented most laboratories from making strong efforts to resolve the problem. Sijbers et al.[77] described a method of restoring MR-induced artefacts in simultaneously recorded EEG data. Although apparently successful, their approach needs to extract and eliminate the induced EEG artefacts. Since they used Ag/AgCl electrodes that will produce susceptibility artefacts in their neighborhood, the colocalization of MRI and EEG data registration is not assured.

However, a set-up for artefact-free EEG and even DC potential recording has been described by Kohno et al.[78] and Busch et al.[79] for application to animal studies in high field experimental systems. Although developed and applied to investigations of experimental cerebral ischemia, the technique of Busch et al. was later adapted by Brinker et al.[31] for fMRI studies using strongly T_2*-sensitive MRI sequences. They used calomel electrodes to record EEG and SEPs simultaneously with fMRI data registration during electrical forepaw stimulation in rats. Their set-up did not require data postprocessing for artefact correction and did not produce image artefacts because of the choice of electrode material. They were able to demonstrate a close correlation between amplitude of SEP and BOLD signal amplitude during forepaw stimulation (Figure 4.5).

These results show that the indirect BOLD activation level can serve as a surrogate for true brain activation. However, a note of caution at this point is to emphasize that this correlation was only shown to hold under normal physiological conditions. When pathophysiological conditions or situations of functional recovery (see Section 4.11)[80] are studied, an uncoupling of both variables, the electrophysiological signal and the BOLD amplitude, cannot be excluded.

In situations where a break or disturbance of coupling between electrical brain activity and hemodynamic response may exist, the meaning of the BOLD signal must be interpreted with caution. Ogawa et al.[81] applied a technical solution similar to the one described by Brinker et al.[31] to study the interaction of closely following stimuli and their effects on both SEP and BOLD signals (see Section 4.8).

The only other correlation between BOLD and electrophysiological data is the literature comparison of Yang et al.[59] concerning the activation area of single stimulated whiskers and the size of the field with electrical activity (see Section 4.4). However, electrophysiological data were not recorded. They were taken from the literature for the animal model with the stimulation paradigm.

4.7 FUNCTION-RELATED CHANGES IN METABOLISM

To cover the increased metabolic demand during functional brain activation, two sources are principally available: glucose and oxygen. The cerebral metabolic rate of glucose (CMRglc) has been shown by quantitative autoradiography to increase over 50% during somatosensory stimulation of rats.[62] The study of the cerebral metabolic rate of oxygen ($CMRO_2$) increase, mainly investigated by PET imaging, provided a wide range of values and a trend of smaller $CMRO_2$ increases than CMRglc increases, thus indicating stimulation of anaerobic glycolysis.[82]

Several authors discussed the reason for glucose utilization. Sokoloff[83] suggested that the ion flux associated with functional activation stimulates energy-dependent Na^+-, K^+-ATPase to transport Na^+ and K^+ ions back into the cells for restoration of ionic gradients. Pellerin and Magistretti[84] formulated an alternative hypothesis that glucose is mainly used to provide energy for the back-transport of glutamate released during functional activation into astrocytes.

To investigate further the source of glucose consumption and determine whether glucose is oxidatively consumed, Hyder and colleagues reviewed a series

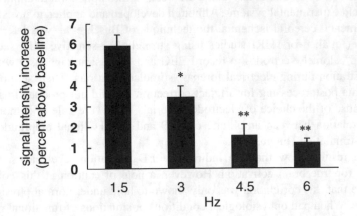

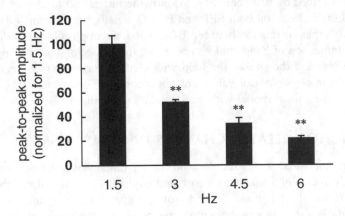

FIGURE 4.5 Increase of signal intensity in T_2*-weighted images (top) and normalized SEP amplitudes (bottom) at increasing stimulation frequencies. SEP amplitudes were normalized to a 1.5-Hz value. Note the corresponding frequency behavior of BOLD fMRI and SEP amplitudes (* = $p < 0.05$; ** = <0.01; statistically different from data at 1.5 Hz). (From Brinker, G. et al., *Mag. Res. Med.*, 41, 469, 1999. With permission.)

of publications discussing glutamate turnover during various brain activation states and calculated glucose and oxygen consumption.[85–88] Glucose was labeled in the C1 or C1 and C6 positions with a ^{13}C isotope and infused. The NMR spectroscopy technique known as proton-observed carbon edit (POCE) was used to record the flux of this label from glucose into the C4 position of the glutamate molecule.

Using earlier models,[89] the authors calculated tricarboxylic acid flux values (V_{TCA}).[85-88] and converted them to cerebral metabolic rates of glucose oxidation (oxidative CMR_{glc}) and oxygen consumption ($CMRO_2$). The main conclusion was that oxidative glycolysis is the main source of energy for increased brain activity.[86]

These experiments permitted Sibson et al.[87] to calculate the glutamate-neurotransmitter cycling between neurons and astrocytes, which reflects a quantitative measure of glutamatergic neuronal activity. By measuring V_{TCA} and glutamine synthesis, an almost 1:1 stoichometry between oxidative glucose metabolism and glutamate-neurotransmitter cycling in the cortex was determined. The authors interpreted this finding to indicate that most cortical energy production supports functional (synaptic) glutamatergic neuronal activity. Sibson et al. also concluded that these data indicate that mapping of cortical oxidative glucose metabolism reflects a quantitative measure of synaptic glutamate release. The results, strongly in support of the hypothesis expressed by Pellerin and Magistretti[84] must be seen in relation to certain arguments. The applied POCE spectra do not provide a signal-to-noise ratio for robust fits to the models. The spectroscopy studies, with the exception of one investigation using spectroscopic imaging,[88] did not permit spatial resolution; data were averaged across the somatosensory cortex, leading to severe partial volume effects. This aspect of partial volume dilution may be especially serious in the case of bilateral activation because of the medial parts of the cortex selected by the authors.[85,86]

Hyder et al.[90,91] and Kida et al.[64] combined NMR spectroscopy data for CMR_{glc} determinations with CBF and BOLD recording during various states of brain activation globally induced by variation of the state of anesthesia or by electrical forepaw stimulation under α-chloralose anesthesia. These data were used to extend the models of oxygen delivery (relationship between CBF increase and $CMRO_2$ increase) by introducing a new parameter Ω describing the O_2 diffusivity of the capillary bed. The model results led to the authors' supposition that the effective oxygen diffusivity of the capillary bed is not constant; it presumably varies to meet local requirements in oxygen demands.

Because current methods sensitive to changes of oxygen consumption (positron emission tomography, intrinsic optical imaging, microelectrodes) lack spatial/temporal resolution or are invasive, efforts have been made during the last few years to establish MRI-based mapping of $\Delta\ CMRO_2$.[45, 46, 54, 92-95] In some cases, these strategies require measurements in addition to MRI, e.g., laser-Doppler flowmetry (LDF)[54] or need to assume a relationship between CBV and CBF changes or apply calibration procedures based on hypercapnia.[93,94] The latter calibration by CO_2-induced CBF increase was recently challenged by Hyder et al.[96] who showed that CBV changes are different during functional activation and during CO_2 challenge. Only a few studies were based on or applied to experimental animal work,[45,46,54] but they are based on the basic relationship between BOLD signal intensity change and changes of $CMRO_2$, CBF and CBV, as originally described by Ogawa et al.[37] and represented by Equation 4.1:

$$\frac{\Delta CMRO_2}{CMRO_{2rest}} = \left(1 + \frac{\Delta CBF}{CBF_{rest}}\right)\left(1 - \left(\frac{\Delta SI_{BOLD}}{SI_{BOLDrest}} \frac{1.32}{2\pi B_0 TE\left(Y_a - Yv_{rest}\right)CBV_{rest}\,\Delta\chi} + \frac{\Delta CBV}{CBV_{rest}}\right)\right) - 1$$

(4.1)

The $_{rest}$ indices indicate values under resting conditions, TE is echo time, B_0 is the static magnetic field strength, $\Delta\chi$ is the susceptibility difference between fully oxygenated and deoxygenated blood, and 1.32 is an experimentally determined numerical factor. The calculation of changes in $CMRO_2$ thus requires three parameters, i.e., $\Delta CBF/CBF_{rest}$, $\Delta CBV/CBV_{rest}$, and $\Delta SI_{BOLD}/SI_{BOLD,rest}$, all of which must be measured during activation.

The BOLD signal change was measured with a T_2^*-sensitive imaging sequence. CBV was determined by using MIONs as an intravascular contrast agent (see Section 4.4). CBF was recorded using laser-Doppler flowmetry in the report by Mandeville et al.[54] (Figure 4.6) and measured via arterial spin tagging PWI by Burke[45] and Schwindt et al.[46] All three investigations used the electrical forepaw stimulation paradigm in rats.

Results of $CMRO_2$ changes were in very good agreement — varying between $19 \pm 17\%$[54] and $20 \pm 12\%$.[45,46] The increase in $CMRO_2$ in anesthetized rats was in concordance with most studies in awake humans. Those investigations using the above-described MRI technique[92,94,95] or positron emission tomography[97,98] revealed values ranging from 16 to 25%, independent of techniques applied. However, using the ^{13}C NMR spectroscopic approach to determine glutamate flux through the TCA cycle, Hyder et al.[85,86] reported $CMRO_2$ increases of 100 to 400%. These values are in striking contrast to other reported values that led Mandeville and colleagues[54] to challenge the validity of the basic assumptions of the models[89] and corrections used by Hyder et al.[86]

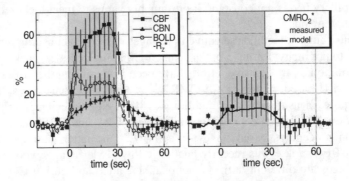

FIGURE 4.6 Time course of cerebral blood flow (crosses), cerebral blood volume (closed circles), and negative BOLD relaxation rate (open circles) during electrical forepaw stimulation (left). The cerebral metabolic rate of oxygen ($CMRO_2$) is calculated from these parameters at each time point. The gray shaded area demarcates the activation period. (From Mandeville, J.B. et al., *Mag. Res. Med.*, 42, 944, 1999. With permission.)

Interestingly, both Mandeville et al.[54] and Schwindt et al.[46] report that the centers of activation do not colocalize for the different variables. Mandeville et al. had only regional information for CBV and BOLD changes and interpreted the activation mismatch as due to the gradient of resting state CBV across the cortex. Schwindt et al. also found the mismatch with the center of activation for CBF, with best concordance between changes of CBF and CMRO$_2$ calculated from CBF, CBV, and BOLD (Figure 4.7). BOLD-based fMRI alone may give misleading results about the exact localization of areas of increased neuronal activity (reflected by increased metabolism). In the opinion of Schwindt et al.[46] areas of brain activation may be more reliably represented by PWI (which best colocalizes with CMRO$_2$ maps).

CMRO$_2$ is principally accessible with another MRI technique. Inhalation of the $^{17}O_2$ isotope becomes visible with ^{17}O-NMR only after its conversion to $H_2{}^{17}O$. Thus, it can be used as a tracer for NMR-based quantification of metabolism. Two approaches exploit this phenomenon. The first is direct detection of ^{17}O, which is feasible for *in vivo* studies only at high fields due to the low sensitivity of ^{17}O-NMR. The other strategy takes advantage of the fact that the ^{17}O isotope

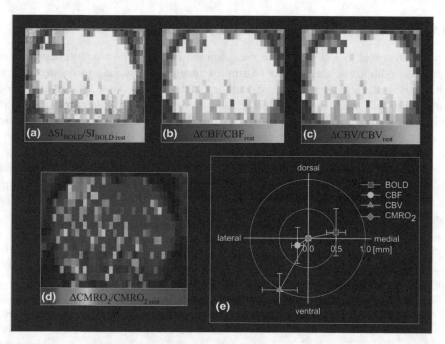

FIGURE 4.7 Coronal activation maps for BOLD (left), cerebral blood flow (center), and cerebral blood volume (right) for electrical forepaw stimulation of rats. Below is the CMRO$_2$ map, calculated pixelwise for pixels showing activation in individual parameter activation maps and following the algorithm appearing in Equation 4.1 in the text. Also shown are the average centers of mass for the three parameters, relative to the center of mass of the calculated CMRO$_2$ activation map. Note that the largest mismatch is observed for cerebral blood volume and BOLD changes. Cerebral blood flow changes are closest to the ΔCMRO$_2$. (From Schwindt, W. et al., *Proceedings of Symposium on Brain Activation and CBF Control*, Tokyo, 2001. With permission.) See Color Figure 4.7 following page 210.

incorporated into a water molecule will influence water proton relaxation behavior. This indirect method has been proposed to overcome the low sensitivity of direct ^{17}O detection.[99,100]

Recent conference contributions revealed the first *in vivo* examples for both approaches. For direct ^{17}O detection, a three-dimensional NMR spectroscopic imaging sequence was implemented to record the conversion of 68.2% enriched $^{17}O_2$ to $H_2^{17}O$.[101] The authors reported a linear increase of the ^{17}O signal of $H_2^{17}O$ water with time. Using a simplified model calculation,[102,103] the signal change was converted to $CMRO_2$ so that spatially resolved $CMRO_2$ maps could be produced.[101] In the case of indirect detection, a $T_{1\rho}$ imaging sequence was used.[104] The authors also observed a rapid increase in ^{17}O water concentration.[105] The method was capable of detecting approximately 2% signal change in the $T_{1\rho}$ image per 2 mM increase in $H_2^{17}O$. The authors[104] were reluctant to estimate $CMRO_2$ data without knowledge of arterial input function. However, both techniques appear promising for fast and spatially resolved determination of $CMRO_2$. It remains to be seen whether the approaches will be validated with independent techniques to assure their reliability.

4.8 FACILITATION/INHIBITION OF ACTIVATION

The brain reacts to a stimulus in a well-defined manner. The reaction depends on certain conditions of the stimulus. Stimulus repetition may lead to habituation or alternatively to learning situations; variations of the stimulus (e.g., frequency or amplitude) will result in facilitation or inhibition of response. Many modifications involve synaptic changes, i.e., changes in the effectiveness of specific synaptic connections. Investigation of these mechanisms under controlled experimental animal conditions is appealing because interesting new information may be gained.

In an early application of fMRI to anesthetized animals, Gyngell et al.[28] studied the response of the somatosensory cortex as a function of stimulus frequency. Using the electrical forepaw stimulation paradigm in rats, they described a dependence of neuronal response on the repetition rate of the sensory stimulus. However, in contrast to the results obtained in awake human volunteers, the BOLD response in anesthetized rats decreased significantly after increase of forepaw stimulus frequency from 1.5 to 7.5 Hz (less than 20% of the BOLD amplitude observed at 1.5 Hz). At 9 Hz, the BOLD signal was completely lost.

This response reduction with increasing frequency, which begins at frequencies above 1.5 to 3 Hz, was described in cats.[12] CBF and SEP measurements were used. Response reduction was related to postexcitatory inhibition, i.e., occlusion of evoked potentials at increasing frequencies. In a later investigation, Brinker et al.[31] confirmed the results of Gyngell et al.[28] in their report on simultaneous recording of BOLD response and SEPs in forepaw stimulation rat models. In a consecutive study by Silva and others,[32] frequency dependence was further extended combining BOLD and CBF measurements during electrical forepaw stimulation.

The authors described a close correlation between BOLD and CBF responses with a matched intensity increase with increasing stimulation intensity (Figure 4.8). Their observation of frequency dependence of the response intensity for BOLD and CBF was in full agreement with the results of Gyngell et al.[28] for BOLD and Brinker

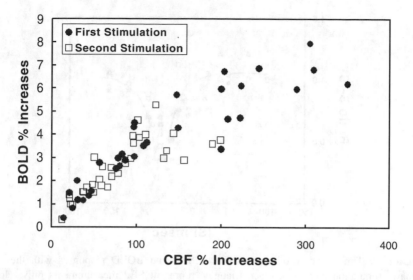

FIGURE 4.8 Correlation of relative BOLD changes and relative cerebral blood flow changes from individual measurements. The data obtained from the second stimulation block (open circles) showed weaker response compared to the first stimulation block (closed circles). Excellent correlation was obtained independent of stimulation block. (From Silva, A.C. et al., *J. Cereb. Blood Flow Metabol.*, 19, 871, 1999. With permission.)

et al.[31] for BOLD and SEPs, i.e., decreases in signal amplitude with increasing stimulus frequency. Although Silva and colleagues do not discuss this, their data indicate that couplings of electrical activity, metabolic increase, and hemodynamic response remain tight, at least qualitatively. If the coupling was disturbed due to postexcitatory inhibition, CBF would not decrease with increasing stimulus rate. At the same time, if the metabolism remained at a higher level, oxygen extraction would increase. In consequence. the BOLD signal would decrease much faster than the CBF signal. On the other hand, a stronger decrease in metabolism would produce a less noticeable change of the BOLD signal as a function of stimulus frequency.

In a recent report by Ogawa et al.,[81] the refractory processes of neural origin were investigated further. The authors developed an approach for measuring temporal resolution of evoked neural events on a millisecond time scale. They extended the paradigm of Brinker et al.[31] by recording SEPs and BOLD signal behavior for individual short periods of activation. At interstimulus intervals of approximately 600 ms (1.5 Hz), they observed a decrease of the second SEP and second BOLD intensity, normalized to the first event. At around 300 ms, the second response was completely suppressed, thus explaining the earlier reported decrease of averaged SEP amplitude during change from 1.5- to 3-Hz stimulation frequency.[31]

Ogawa et al.[81] also examined the interaction of stimuli originating at two different sites using stimulation of the left and right forepaws of rat models with a varying interval between left and right stimuli. The evoked potential that appeared at 25 ms after the stimulus pulse at the left forepaw was highly suppressed at an interstimulus interval (ISI) of 30 to 40 ms (Figure 4.9). The suppressive interaction at one site by

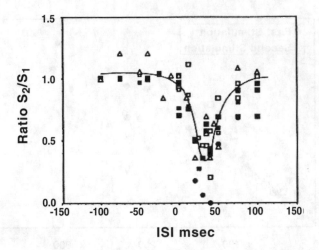

FIGURE 4.9 Time window of suppression of SEP and BOLD responses with the two-forepaw stimulation paradigm. Open triangles represent SEP measurements only; closed circles represent fMRI data only. Squares represent simultaneous measurements of SEPs (open squares) and fMRI (closed squares). All responses were normalized to respective values at interstimulation intervals of –100 ms. (From Ogawa, S. et al., *Proc. Natl. Acad. Sci. U.S.A.*, 97, 11026, 2000. With permission.)

the preceding stimulus at the other paw occurred at a well-defined short range of ISI values. In the absence of known contralateral projections of thalamocortical sites, this suppression was likely to come through the callosal (cross-hemisphere) projection with disynaptic connections.[106] Most interestingly, Ogawa et al. pointed out that the first stimulus alone did not lead to metabolic or hemodynamic activation on the ipsilateral hemisphere — a finding in full agreement with autoradiographic data obtained for single paw stimulation.[62]

When a defined stimulus is to be studied by fMRI, care must be taken to ensure that this stimulus is not disturbed or influenced by other sensory inputs because of possible interactions. During fMRI studies, a strong background noise level due to fast gradient switching for the space encoding the fMRI signal is always present. This led to investigations by Burke et al.[22] that extended the concept of stimulus interactions to polysensory stimuli interactions.

The rat electrical forepaw stimulation paradigm was used; acoustic stimulation was provided by strong MRI gradient noise. Reducing the noise level significantly (approximately 30 dB) allowed somatosensory activation to cover a smaller area with smaller maximum signal amplitude in the BOLD activation images. To ensure the difference was not due to secondary causes like gradient-induced mechanical vibrational stimuli, the animals were cochleotomized after the first series of experiments. In the second series, the activation response was independent of noise level and in full agreement with the results from the first series obtained with reduced noise levels. The authors observed facilitating interaction of an acoustic stimulus on somatosensory activation. The two sensory representation fields were not adjacent and thus did not share polysensory fields, in contrast to experiments performed with electrophysiological[107] and optical imaging techniques[108] in which interactions between two adjacent representation fields were investigated and activation of shared polysensory fields was observed.

4.9 CALCIUM-DEPENDENT SYNAPTIC ACTIVITY AND NEURONAL TRACT TRACING: Mn^{2+}-BASED fMRI

4.9.1 Mn^{2+}-CONTROLLED SIGNAL CHANGE DURING CALCIUM-DEPENDENT SYNAPTIC ACTIVITY

A clever and interesting MRI technique takes advantage of the similarities of para-magnetic Mn^{2+} and Ca^{2+} ions. The influx of Ca into cells is required for the release of neurotransmitters during functional activation. Mn^{2+} ions have van der Waals radii similar to those of Ca^{2+} ions, and can therefore enter cells through voltage-gated Ca channels. Such accumulation of Mn^{2+} ions was first shown by Lin and Koretsky[109] to decrease T_1 water relaxation time in rat brain. By using continuous intravenous infusion of Mn ions and parallel breakage of the blood–brain barrier by mannitol injection, the authors introduced an imaging technique to record a parameter directly related to neuronal activation. They showed a strong signal increase across the brain hemisphere after glutamate injection through a catheter in the common carotid artery. Glutamate is an excitatory neurotransmitter inducing Ca^{2+} influx in postsynaptic and presynaptic sites that in turn causes release of neurotransmitters. Manganese also enters cells along with the Ca^{2+} influx. The authors also showed that electrical stimulation of the forepaw led to a well-circumscribed signal increase in the soma-tosensory cortices of rats in T_1-weighted images (Figure 4.10). The authors claim that this technique will also be applicable to detecting activation in awake rats by performing MRI after the stimulation. This is feasible because the half-life of manganese in the brain was set between 54 and 260 days due to its low clearance rate from the brain.

Shortly after this first report, Duong et al.[110] extended the study of Mn^{2+}-based recording of synaptic activity during electrical forepaw stimulation and compared the data with BOLD and CBF activation maps recorded directly before Mn^{2+} admin-istration. The mannitol, needed for transient breakage of the blood–brain barrier for delivery of Mn^{2+}, was applied through a catheter in the external carotid artery (ECA) to provide direct access to the internal carotid artery (ICA) without interrupting blood flow to the brain. This surgical procedure is very similar to that used for intraluminal thread occlusion of the middle cerebral artery (MCA) in the rat stroke model.[78] The strongest Mn^{2+}-induced T_1 reduction reflecting the highest Ca activity occurred in cortical layer IV. Direct inputs into cortical layer IV are projected from the thalamus. This layer has the highest neuron density and exhibits the highest level of synaptic activity relative to the other cortical layers. Based on *in vitro* calibration systems of the Mn^{2+}-dependent T_1 relaxation time decrease, the authors estimated the manganese concentration in the cells to be around 100 μM.

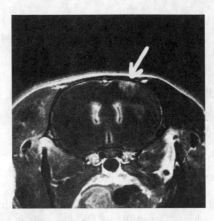

FIGURE 4.10 Electrical stimulation of the left forepaw led to the activation area in the somatosensory cortex obtained after Mn^{2+} administration and recording the signal change with a T_1-weighted sequence. The $MnCl_2$ infusion pump was turned on 30 seconds before electrical stimulation; hypertonic mannitol solution was injected through the right carotid artery to open the blood–brain barrier 30 seconds after start of electrical stimulation. (From Lin, Y.J. and Koretsky, A.P., *Mag. Res. Med.*, 38, 378, 1997. With permission.)

Comparison of the activation map of synaptic activity (Mn^{2+}-dependent T_1 decrease) with those of BOLD and CBF showed complete agreement of the center of mass (COM) of the activation areas in all three parameters. The COM offsets between any two activation maps were less than 200 μm for all three imaging modalities. The authors concluded that hemodynamic changes during functional brain activation such as BOLD and CBF reflect the neuronal activity very well at high fields, where the signal contributions from large vessels are negligible.

4.9.2 NEURONAL TRACT TRACING BASED ON Mn^{2+} INFUSION

Tract tracing techniques contributed large amounts of information to our current understanding of neuronal connections. However, all established methods to date are invasive. This prevents repetitive studies under varying physiological conditions.

Pautler et al.[111] exploited the calcium-mimicking properties of manganese ions to monitor anterograde tract tracing with T_1-weighted MRI. They investigated the olfactory and visual pathways in mice. They administered Mn^{2+} topically to the nares or injected it into the vitreous humor, producing readily detectable highlighting of the associated neuronal pathways of live mice by MRI. In the olfactory pathways, the transport of Mn^{2+} was observed from the olfactory bulb to the primary olfactory cortex. For the visual pathway, the transport was recorded from the eye through the optic nerve to the superior colliculus. From this latter data, the authors estimated the transport speed to be approximately 2 mm/hour.

This technique of tract tracing by Mn^{2+}-induced MRI contrast was used by Watanabe et al.[112] to investigate the visual pathway in rats by injecting Mn^{2+} intra-ocularly. They were able to follow with high resolution MRI the contrast agent from the retina through the optic nerve to the chiasm, then through the contralateral optic

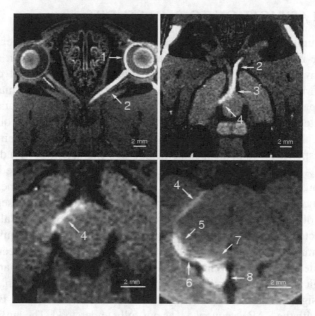

FIGURE 4.11 Signal enhancement of the visual pathway in the rat 24 hours after Mn^{2+} administration into the left eye, presented in oblique planes relative to the coronal imaging plane. The following structures are enhanced: (1) left retina; (2) left optic nerve; (3) optic chiasm; (4) right optic tract; (5) right lateral geniculate nucleus; (6) right brachium of the superior colliculus; (7) right pretectal region; (8) right superior colliculus. (From Watanabe, T. et al., *Mag. Res. Med.*, 46, 424, 2001. With permission.)

tract to the dorsal and ventral lateral geniculate nucleus. The parallel pathway was followed to the superior colliculus (Figure 4.11). At 24 hours, the contrast was strongest in the optic tract. At 48 hours, the contrast was fading. From the time after injection when the contrast enhancement was observed in the superior colliculus, the velocity of Mn^{2+} enhancement along the projection fibers was estimated at 2.8 mm/hour, in close agreement with the earlier estimate of Pautler et al.[111] In contrast, Watanabe et al. saw no evidence of transsynaptic crossing of Mn.$^{2+}$ and no enhancement was reported for the visual cortex areas.

Van Meir et al.[113] reported an elegant application of this Mn^{2+}-based tract tracing technique to the analysis of singing bird brains. A complex system involving several nuclei in the brain is responsible for singing. The most caudal nuclei forming the high vocal center (HVC) and the robust nucleus of the archistriatum (RA), are essential for song production. The more rostral nuclei, Area X, and the lateral portion of the magnocellular nucleus of the neostriatum (IMAN) are involved in song learning. All these nuclei are completely indiscernible in native MRIs; they provide no contrast with the surrounding tissues. Van Meir and colleagues injected Mn^{2+} directly into the HVC. After transport of the contrast agent to the other nuclei, the nuclei lit up in the strongly T$_1$-weighted images, thus allowing for volume determination — a topic of great interest as these nuclei change in volume during mating season and also during development of the young to adult birds.

4.10 fMRI APPLICATION TO PAIN STUDIES

The investigation of pain and hyperalgesia is of great interest. Application of MRI as a sensitive imaging modality has already been assessed in human studies. In a systematic investigation using experimental animals, Porszasz and colleagues[114] reported on fMRI signal changes in the rat spinal cord following formalin injection into the hindpaw. They injected 50 μl of a 5% formalin solution subcutaneously and the signal intensity change was recorded with a RARE (Rapid Acquisition with Relaxation Enhancement) sequence at the L1 to L6 level of the spinal cord. An immediate response noted in the ipsilateral side was characterized by a drop in signal intensity at L4 and L5. A maximum signal change of 12.7% occurred 10 minutes after injection, after which the intensity slowly returned to baseline. The major formalin-induced signal changes were observed in the L4 and L5 segments with involvement of the corresponding dorsal root ganglia. The more caudal L6 segment was less affected. When pretreatment by lidocaine was performed 4 minutes before formalin administration, the development of the signal intensity decrease on the ipsilateral side was fully prevented. This indicates the approach is applicable for pharmacological evaluation and provides a basis for the study of analgesics. The unexpected signal decrease — contrary to the commonly observed BOLD signal increase — with the RARE sequence was not fully understood. The authors' putative explanations include signal dephasing by increased blood flow and/or increased oxygen metabolism leading to a negative BOLD effect.

Tuor et al.[115] used the formalin-induced pain stimulus alternatively with electrical forepaw stimulation at high currents (15V, 9mA) to investigate CNS processing of pain and its modification by analgesics in animals. Several cortical areas besides the primary somatosensory cortex SI are highlighted upon pain stimulation. The forma-lin-induced BOLD effect was reduced after morphine administration. The same treatment for the electrical forepaw-induced pain led to suppression of all activation with the exception of the somatosensory cortex.

In a similar study from the same laboratory, Malisza et al.[116] induced pain in rats by subcutaneous administration of capsaicin into forepaws. Capsaicin is the active ingredient of hot peppers and produces an intense pain reaction following activation of the vanilloid receptors. In agreement with the report by Tuor et al.,[115] BOLD activation was observed in various cortical regions, followed by a slight negative BOLD effect, called deactivation, and claimed to be in agreement with observations in human pain studies. Morphine application reduced the extents of activation and deactivation.

The field of experimental pain investigation using fMRI techniques is still in its infancy. However, the experimental data are encouraging and allow us to speculate that this research field will become very important and fMRI will make essential contributions to the area of pain studies in experimental animals under controlled conditions. This is ultimately expected to provide new insights into the pharmacology of analgesics.

4.11 ACTIVATION UNDER PATHOPHYSIOLOGICAL CONDITIONS/BRAIN PLASTICITY

fMRI applications to various aspects of physiological brain activation have been presented in this chapter. However, the method is certainly of equal importance and interest for the investigation of pathophysiological alterations of brain activation, including aspects of recovery of functional activation after cerebral lesions. This technique will in principle provide information about activation areas and thus suggest reorganizational processes.

A quantitative approach should provide data on gradual recovery processes. As with the investigations into pain mechanisms, the field is still rather young, partly due to the fact that only few laboratories can combine expertise with pathophysio-logical animal models with animal fMRI. The early applications are encouraging and illuminate the potential of the methodological approach for the understanding of functional restitution processes.

4.11.1 FUNCTIONAL ACTIVATION AFTER CEREBRAL ISCHEMIA

Reese et al.[117] studied the functional brain activities of rats with focal cerebral ischemia induced by permanent occlusion of the middle cerebral artery (MCA). The functional activation was studied 24 hours after onset of ischemia using simultaneous electrical stimulation of both forepaws. The CBV response was monitored in both hemispheres applying a T_2*-sensitive imaging sequence in conjunction with an intravascular NMR contrast agent. The authors described normal activation of the contralateral nonischemic hemisphere. No response was observed on the ischemic somatosensory cortex. Treatment of some animals with isradipine, a calcium antagonist, led to smaller infarct size on the diffusion-weighted images and normal appearing somatosensory cortex without functional response to the stimulus.

To sort out the possibility of subcortical irreversible lesions in relay nuclei (e.g., thalamus) as reasons for response suppression, the authors studied the response to systemically applied bicuculline. Although blood flow appeared unchanged in the isradipine-treated animals, no response to bicuculline was observed on the ipsilateral side. The authors took that as an indication that the absence of cortical response was not due to damaged subcortical structures including afferent tracts. They argued in favor of functional impairment of the cortical areas, due to inhibition of neurons to become activated or disturbance of neurovascular coupling. Future experiments including electrophysiology to test electrical activity will hopefully clarify the functional state and excitability of the neurons in response to the chosen stimulation paradigm.

Dijkhuizen et al.[118] extended this protocol by investigating functional recovery during chronic periods after onset of stroke, i.e., after 2 days and after 2 weeks. A CBV increase in response to electrical forepaw stimulation was recorded using intravascular contrast agents. At day 2 after stroke induction, no functional activity was seen in the ischemic hemisphere. However, vascular reactivity using CO_2 was preserved. Baseline CBV was not elevated, indicating no severe vasodilation that would prohibit further stimulation-induced vasodilation. After 2 weeks, behavioral tests showed a significant, almost complete, improvement of the formerly impaired limb via a forelimb placing test. Signs of activation were evident in the infarction border zone in and adjacent to the sensorimotor cortex. The authors interpreted this as indicative of extension of forelimb representation fields into adjacent cortical areas and conclude that restoration of sensorimotor function may be associated with recruitment of perilesional and contralesional functional fields in the brain.

Using a permanent MCA occlusion model, Abo et al.[119] described extensive plastic changes 2 weeks after the induction of ischemic insult. Behavioral studies indicated complete functional recovery in the beam walking test within 10 days after ischemia induction. fMRI experiments showed that during electrical stimulation of the previously paretic hind limb, two normally inactive brain regions were activated. One region was the undamaged contralateral sensorimotor cortex and the other was located lateral to the lesion. The results indicated that behavioral recovery can be explained by functional reorganization and neuromodulation of the brain. The authors also hypothesized that during recovery, a neuromodulatory mechanism enables the activation of previously inhibited but existing and preserved pathways.

4.11.2 RESTITUTION OF FUNCTIONAL ACTIVITY AFTER RESUSCITATION

After a period of global ischemia, the cerebral vasculature is transiently paralyzed, mainly because of extracellular acidosis that acts as a potent vasodilator.[120] As a consequence, CBF increases above normal (postischemic hyperemia) and remains elevated for a period that roughly corresponds to the duration of the preceding ischemia.[121] Only under conditions of microcirculatory impairment — possibly resulting from increased blood viscosity and edema-induced narrowing of the capillary lumen — blood recirculation may remain below normal until blood stagnation is resolved.[122]

During postischemic hyperemia, autoregulation and CO_2 reactivity of blood flow were abolished. As a consequence, the flow rate passively followed blood pressure but did not respond to mediators of flow coupling, such as potassium or hydrogen ions.[123] After hyperemia ceased, cerebral vessels constricted and blood flow declined as much as 50% below control (postischemic hypoperfusion) level. During this phase, autoregulation recovered and CO_2 reactivity remained suppressed. This led to a peculiar pathophysiological situation in which blood flow did not respond to alterations in blood pressure or metabolic activity. The duration of the phase depended on the duration of ischemia. After 15 minutes of cardiac arrest, CO_2 reactivity returned to control level within 5 hours.[124] After 1 hour of cerebral ischemia, CO_2 reactivity remained reduced as long as 1 year.[125]

A direct consequence of postischemic hypoperfusion is uncoupling between metabolism and blood flow. This may produce relative hypoxia because the oxygen consumption of the brain gradually increases after ischemia in parallel with the restoration of spontaneous electrocortical activity.[126] The dissociation of oxygen supply and consumption is reflected by a gradual increase of oxygen extraction that may rise as high as 80%. When oxygen extraction exceeds a critical value of about 50%, anaerobic glycolysis is stimulated, resulting in secondary lactacidosis and energy depletion. Restoration of the coupling between metabolism and blood flow is, therefore, an important therapeutical goal for improving postischemic resuscitation.

The question whether impaired functional coupling reflects disturbances of functional integrity of the brain or impaired cerebrovascular reactivity was addressed by studies of reanimation after 10 minutes of cardiac arrest in rats for up to 7 days.[124] MRI measurements of apparent diffusion coefficient (ADC) showed complete normalization of ADC within 45 minutes after resuscitation, indicating fast recovery of water and ion homeostasis upon organ reperfusion. As demonstrated in an earlier investigation, normalization of ADC after global cerebral ischemia is a reliable indicator of metabolic recovery of the brain.[127] Neurological performance scoring during this period demonstrated gradual recovery with ongoing recirculation.

After 7 days, animals showed only slightly retarded reaction to visual stimulation and pinching of tail or hind leg and no overt neurological deficits. SEP amplitude recovered slowly and reached approximately 40% of control amplitude at the end of the observation period. While CO_2 reactivity normalized within 5 hours after reanimation, stimulus-induced increase of CBF (LDF measurement) as a functional response to forepaw stimulation recovered only to about 40% of control level within a week.

The slower recovery of the CBF response to functional activation is therefore not limited by reduced cerebrovascular sensitivity.[124] LDF-derived data are in full agreement with those obtained with PWI, indicating slow and ongoing improvement of the stimulus-induced signal intensity increase, reaching a value about half as high as under control conditions. In contrast, T_2^*-weighted imaging recovered much faster and showed a stimulus-induced signal intensity increase 1 day after reanimation comparable to that under control conditions (Figure 4.12).[80,128]

The apparent decoupling of the T_2^*-WI behavior and CBF (measured by perfusion-weighted MRI) is due to the different physiological variables behind the NMR parameters. The BOLD signal is inversely proportional to tissue oxygen extraction i.e., oxygen consumption. From T_2^*-WI data alone, one would have concluded full functional recovery 1 day after resuscitation. However, blood flow response to the stimulus was reduced to approximately 40% of control level then. Thus, with the same oxygen extraction at reduced blood flow, the BOLD signal should have been smaller due to relatively high deoxyhemoglobin content. This was not observed. Therefore, the data are interpreted to indicate reduced oxygen extraction upon activation at 24 hours despite full and fast normalization of basal metabolism of the brain after a short period of cardiac arrest. The partial recovery of neuronal activity was in full agreement with reduced SEP amplitudes 1 day after resuscitation.[129]

4.11.3 LESION-INDUCED PLASTICITY

Therapeutic strategies aimed at preservation of lesioned tissue, e.g., after stroke, have not demonstrated the desired success. Although animal studies have shown positive and encouraging results of drug treatment,[130] clinical trials with beneficial effects are the exceptions. Two potential approaches may allow functional restitution

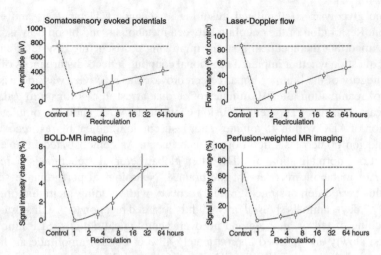

FIGURE 4.12 Recordings of SEPs and corresponding cortical changes in laser-Doppler flow and signal changes of BOLD and perfusion-weighted MRI during electrical forepaw stimulation. Measurements were performed before (control) and at various recirculation periods after 10 minutes of cardiac arrest. Note severe suppression of the electrical and hemodynamic responses after cardiac arrest, followed by partial and slow recovery to about 50% of control level during the first 24 hours. BOLD response, in contrast, returned to control levels earlier. (From Hossman, K.A. et al., in *Pharmacology of Cerebral Ischemia*, Krieglstein, J., Ed., Medpharm, Stuttgart, 1996, 357. With permission.)

after brain lesion: the new field of regeneration based on (stem) cell implantation and the mechanisms of brain plasticity.

The latter approach deals with the observation that the brain can, in principle, transfer initially lost functions to new, unaffected cortical areas when irreversible lesions prohibit functioning by the original representation areas. This is very pronounced during neonatal development of the brain and is still possible in the mature brain. It is therefore of interest to investigate the conditions for this "plastic" response of the brain to focal lesions. Schwindt et al.[131] studied the concept of neonatal, lesion-induced plasticity. A small, well-circumscribed cortical lesion affecting the somatosensory cortex SI of the right hemisphere was produced in mice 1 day after birth. At adulthood, about 6 months later, animals were investigated using electrical forepaw stimulation while recording responses with SEPs (Figure 4.13). Simultaneous functional MRI studies included BOLD and PWI.

The main finding was reduced N1 amplitude of the SEP over the lesioned hemisphere in parallel with decreased fMRI signal amplitude and reduced activation area, all compared to the contralateral side and to the situation in sham-operated animals. The adult lesioned animals showed no neurological deficits. The expected reorganization was not readily observed. Only in a few cases was simultaneous activation of the unlesioned left hemisphere noted in the secondary somatosensory cortex SII when the left forepaw was stimulated. These observations indicated activation of purely ipsilateral pathways and were similar to the observations of focal ischemia models by Abo et al.[119] and Dijkhuizen et al.[118]

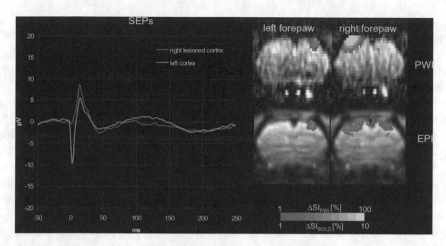

FIGURE 4.13 SEPs and simultaneously recorded EPI-based BOLD and PWI activation maps of adult rats who experienced cortical cold lesions of right hemispheres 1 day after birth. The activation area in the lesioned cortex is clearly reduced relative to cortex of the contralateral healthy hemisphere. In parallel, the corresponding SEP was strongly reduced and distorted. See Color Figure 4.13 following page 210.

4.12 STUDIES OF OTHER SPECIES

4.12.1 fMRI INVESTIGATIONS OF CATS

Few studies have been performed on mammals larger than rodents, apart from the investigations on awake human volunteers and patients. Visual stimulation is the best studied paradigm in humans, but a series of open questions remain. The questions have been approached in cats because cats have highly developed visual systems that resemble human visual systems.

A series of fMRI studies focused on visual stimulation in anesthetized cats. In 1997, Kauppinen et al.[132] investigated the open question whether the tight coupling of glucose and oxygen metabolism in the brain is preserved during visual activation. This question was challenged by early PET studies showing only minor increases in oxygen metabolism in the regions of increased glucose consumption and electrical activity.[82,133] Kauppinen et al. studied lactate production in volume selective ^{1}H-NMR spectroscopy of α-chloralose-anesthetized cats during visual stimulation. Separately recorded visual-evoked potentials (VEPs) were readily observed with a maximal amplitude at 2 Hz. However, no lactate production could be registered even under conditions permitting the detection of lactate levels as low as 0.17 mM. The authors interpreted these results to show that neuronal activation in the cat brain is not associated with aerobic lactate production.

Using high-contrast square-wave drifting gratings for visual stimulation, Jezzard et al.[136] studied BOLD signal changes in isoflurane-anesthetized cats. They clearly observed a BOLD signal increase in area 18 of the visual cortex, with the intensity varying from 0.7 to 2%. They emphasized high interindividual variability but used a small group of animals in the study. Further, the early "dip" before the rise of BOLD signal upon stimulation was not observable.

In two parallel publications, S.G. Kim's group[134,135] reported detailed spatial resolution of iso-orientation columns in visual stimulation data of isoflurane-anesthetized cats. In contrast to Jezzard et al.,[136] they reported a stable and reliable presence of the early "dip" with an amplitude of -0.2 to -0.4% in BOLD data. After a delay of 3 seconds, a positive BOLD signal with a maximal amplitude of 1 to 2% developed. Using the early dip signal behavior instead of the conventionally applied positive and stronger BOLD signal for data analysis, the authors described patchy activation fields for orthogonal orientations of their stimulation patterns. These patchy activation fields occupied territories that were mostly complementary to each other. In contrast to this spatial resolution and specificity, the positive BOLD signal behavior did not show good selectivity. The authors claimed that analysis of the early negative BOLD effect allowed them to detect even pinwheel structures of preferred orientation columns, in good agreement with earlier optical studies.[137,138]

4.12.2 fMRI Investigations of Mice

Mice are increasingly attractive laboratory animals because of the growing availability of genetically altered mouse strains, particularly those suitable for studying neurological diseases. Nevertheless, fewer fMRI investigations focused on mice than on cats. That is probably due, at least in part, to the fact that the model of visual stimulation in the anesthetized cat was established much earlier for optical recording experiments.

While such mouse models were not readily available for use with fMRI, the technique involved additional complications. The mouse brain is much smaller than the rat brain and higher spatial resolution (sensitivity) becomes a necessity. As with rats, it is desirable to keep the animals under physiological control to assure normal physiological blood gases. This is a requirement to maintain stable conditions for recording hemodynamic responses to stimuli.

Huang et al.[139] investigated photic stimulation in spontaneously breathing mice in 1996. The animals were originally anesthetized with pentobarbital. fMRI studies were performed between deep anesthesia and early stages of arousal, after the last application of the anesthetic. The authors observed a BOLD signal increase only in response to stimulus intensity. Also, areas with negative BOLD effect were reported, primarily around major vessels. When the stimulus period was increased stepwise during the fading of the anesthesia, a BOLD increase was observed only at the onset and at turn-off points of the stimulus period but not between them.

The question remains about the physiological origin of this effect, particularly because an animal cannot predict the length of the stimulus period and respond accordingly. It therefore seems worthwhile to further pursue a possible effect like a startle reaction to the changing stimulus condition in the slowly awakening animal. The authors offered a speculative interpretation that the M visual system pathway was recorded. The M channel or luminance pathway provides excitatory signals for increments and decrements in illumination. A major drawback to the interpretation

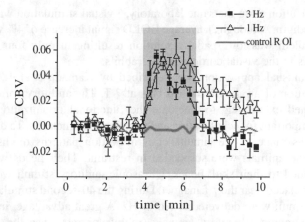

FIGURE 4.14 Time course of cerebral blood volume-based activation in the somatosensory cortices of mice in response to electrical hind paw stimulation. The gray area indicates the stimulation period. (From Mueggler, T. et al., *Proc. Int. Soc. Mag. Res. Med.*, 9, 651, 2001. With permission.)

is that no steady state existed because of the progressive transition from deep anesthesia to awake state. That makes comparison of different sets of data difficult.

Two other mouse fMRI studies focused on the somatosensory cortex, using the electrical hind paw stimulation paradigm in full analogy to the rat model. Both studies may be seen as early reports on the feasibility of fMRI investigations in mice. Mueggler et al.[140] studied isoflorane-anesthetized mice that were artificially ventilated while pCO_2 was monitored by transcutaneous measurement. The authors recorded the CBV increase after administration of iron oxide particles and reported a typical 5% CBV increase in the somatosensory cortex SI during hind paw stimulation (Figure 4.14).

In a report by Ahrens and Dubowitz,[141] α-chloralose-anesthetized, spontaneously breathing mice were studied at 11.7 T. The feasibility of successful recording of fMRI in anesthetized mice was again reported. A drawback, also noted by the authors, was the fact that the system used a vertical bore magnet so that the animals remained in a nonphysiological vertical position for an extended period. Furthermore, no mention was made of monitoring the animals' physiological state.

4.12.3 RABBIT AND BAT STUDIES

In an effort to circumvent the need to anesthetize animals for fMRI studies, Li et al.[19] reported experiments with awake rabbits and use of an established protocol for restraining the animals. The protocol was stereotaxic implantation of headbolts, followed by habituation of the rabbits to the restraining setup for 1 to 2 weeks. The animals were trained to become accustomed to the magnet environment, in particular, to the high noise levels generated during gradient switching. The authors reported good signal stability in awake animals, in good comparison with the situation in anesthetized rabbits.

In an application from the same laboratory,[20] visual stimulation was used as an activation paradigm. Although an average BOLD signal increase of 4% was reported, the major problem was low spatial resolution resulting in only four significantly activated pixels in the visual cortices of the rabbits.

A rather unusual application was described by Kamada et al.[21] They studied auditory activation of awake mustached bats at 7 T. The auditory cortex of the bat has been studied extensively to elucidate the functional organization and neural mechanisms important for echolocation and social communication. To date, no direct observation was made of the simultaneous activation patterns of discrete neural populations. The animals were suspended in restraint. Their heads were fixed by nylon posts glued to their skull bones. Ultrasonic auditory stimuli were delivered from a speaker placed near the 7 T magnet. During the 40-second stimulation periods, the auditory stimuli were delivered at 1 or 4 Hz. A great advantage, in comparison to the more common laboratory animals (rabbits or rats) was the fact that the gradient-generated noise was predominantly at frequencies below the hearing range of the species. The animals were reported to remain calm and completely unaffected by noise during the experimental runs. The regions of BOLD signal elevation during auditory stimulation corresponded to the auditory cortex. Reproducibility was not satisfactory. The authors provided no explanation of the origins of this problem.

4.13 OUTLOOK AND PATHOPHYSIOLOGICAL IMPLICATIONS

Based on the large body of literature available concerning fMRI investigations in laboratory animals, mainly under anesthesia, the perspectives for fast growth of this field are clearly exciting. Although fMRI really had its beginning in human applications, the use of fMRI on anesthetized animals is expanding rapidly, finding more applications, and rightfully claiming its firm place in the range of investigative strategies for understanding functional brain activation. We hope this has been demonstrated by this overview of the breadth of this field.

Mouse fMRI is still in its infancy. More established models and the ability to closely monitor physiological status will allow mouse studies to increase and permit access to studies of various neurodegenerative and other diseases that affect brain functions. Access to transgenic animals will provide information on molecular mechanisms underlying the (patho-)physiology of functional brain activation. The roles of mediators, neurotransmitters, receptors, and ion channels can be studied noninvasively and repetitively *in vivo*.

Larger animals such as cats may be effective for studying paradigms where highly developed mammalian brains are required for comparison with human brains. Studies by Kim's group[134,135] of the spatial resolution of signal encoding and processing of visual stimuli are promising and exciting examples.

Rats (and to an extent, mice) will be used predominantly for pharmacological studies (e.g., pain reaction), studies of cerebral disease models such as stroke, pharmacological modulation of activation mechanisms, and the coupling of neuronal activity and metabolic and hemodynamic response.

Investigations of higher brain functions will require animals in the awake state. Presently, the extremely high gradient-generated noise level forbids most such applications. Even complex training and habituation measures cannot eliminate the reservations about acceptable conditions for the animals when gradient-generated noise levels greatly exceed pain levels. Recent advances in active noise control, particularly progress in noise damping by 30 dB or more, make further studies feasible. If this technical approach can be improved further and used routinely, experimental animal scanners will provide the environment even for studies on awake animals.

The application of functional imaging to the investigation of pathophysiological derangements of the brain is only beginning. The first results appearing in the large body of literature using invasive techniques to study functional brain activation under pathological conditions already indicate that the disturbance of flow regulation is a function of the severity of the lesion impact that can be used to grade the severity of tissue injury. However, it must be emphasized that the absence of functional activation does not necessarily indicate irreversible injury. Full recovery may still occur after considerable time delay relative to metabolic/hemodynamic normalization of the organ. fMRI provides a unique opportunity to evaluate complex brain functions under full surgical anesthesia and will be particularly useful for brain research involving pathological changes in animals under experimental conditions.

ACKNOWLEDGMENT

Support by a grant from NATO (CRG 971053) is gratefully acknowledged.

REFERENCES

1. Roy, C.W. and Sherrington, C.S., On the regulation of the blood supply of the brain, *J. Physiol.* (London), 11, 85, 1890.
2. Lassen, N.A., Ingvar, D.H., and Skinhoj, E., Brain function and blood flow, *Scient. Am.*, 239, 62, 1978.
3. Sokoloff, L. et al., The (^{14}C) deoxyglucose method for the measurement of local cerebral glucose utilization: theory, procedure, and normal values in the conscious and anesthetized albino rat, *J. Neurochem.*, 28, 897, 1977.
4. Phelps, M.E. et al., Tomographic measurement of local cerebral glucose metabolic rate in humans with (F-18)2-fluoro-two-deoxy-D-glucose: validation of method, *Ann. Neurol.*, 6, 371, 1979.
5. Belliveau, J.W. et al., Functional cerebral imaging by susceptibility-contrast NMR, *Mag. Res. Med.*, 14, 538, 1990.
6. Belliveau, J.W. et al., Functional mapping of the human visual cortex by magnetic resonance imaging, *Science*, 254, 716, 1991.
7. Crosby, G. et al., The local metabolic effects of somatosensory stimulation in the central nervous system of rats given pentobarbital or nitrous oxide, *Anesthesiology*, 58, 38, 1983.
8. Meyer, J.S. et al., Effect of stimulation of the brain stem reticular formation on cerebral blood flow and oxygen consumption, *EEG Clin. Neurophysiol.*, 26, 125, 1969.

9. Lindauer, U., Villringer, A., and Dirnagl, U., Characterization of CBF response to somatosensory stimulation: model and influence of anesthetics, *Am. J. Physiol.*, 264, H1223, 1993.

10. Ueki, M., Mies, G., and Hossmann, K.-A., Effect of α-chloralose, halothane, pentobarbital and nitrous oxide anesthesia on metabolic coupling in somatosensory cortex of rat, *Acta Anaesthesiol. Scand.*, 36, 318, 1992.

11. Bonvento, G. et al., Is α-chloralose plus halothane induction a suitable anesthetic regimen for cerebrovascular research?, *Brain Res.*, 665, 213, 1994.

12. Leniger-Follert, E. and Hossmann, K.A., Simultaneous measurement of microflow and evoked potentials in the somatomotor cortex of the cat brain during specific sensory activation, *Pflügers Arch.*, 380, 85, 1979.

13. Kocher, M., Metabolic and hemodynamic activation of postischemic rat brain by cortical spreading depression, *J. Cereb. Blood Flow Metabol.*, 10, 564, 1990.

14 Scanley, B.E. et al., Functional magnetic resonance imgaging of median nerve stimulation in rats at 2.0 T, *Mag. Res. Med.*, 37, 969, 1997.

15. Kennan, R.P. et al., Physiological basis for bold MR signal changes due to neuronal stimulation: separation of blood volume and magnetic susceptibility effects, *Mag. Res. Med.*, 40, 840, 1998.

16. Lahti, K.M. et al., Comparison of evoked cortical activity in conscious and propofol-anesthetized rats using functional MRI, *Mag. Res. Med.*, 41, 412, 1999.

17. Peeters, R. et al., Differences in functional magnetic resonance imaging signal changes between awake and anesthetized condition of rats during forepaw stimulation, *Proc. Int. Soc. Mag. Res. Med.*, 8, 2000.

18. Peeters, R.R. et al., Comparing BOLD fMRI signal changes in the awake and anesthetized rat during electrical forepaw stimulation, *Mag. Res. Imaging*, 19, 821, 2001.

19. Li, L., Chen, N.K., and Wyrwicz, A.M., A conscious animal model for MRI, *Proc. Int. Soc. Mag. Res. Med.*, 7, 969, 1999.

20. Wyrwicz, A.M. et al., Functional MRI of visual system activation in the conscious rabbits, *Proc. Int. Soc. Mag. Res. Med.*, 7, 806, 1999.

21. Kamada, K., Pekar, J.J., and Kanwal, J.S., Anatomical and functional imaging of the auditory cortex in awake mustached bats using magnetic resonance technology, *Brain Res. Protocols*, 4, 351, 1999.

22. Burke, M. et al., Facilitation of electric forepaw stimulation-induced somatosensory activation in rats by additional acoustic stimulation: an fMRI investigation, *Mag. Res. Med.*, 44, 317, 2000.

23. Woolsey, T.A. and Van der Loos, H., The structural organization of layer IV in the somatosensory region (SI) of mouse cerebral cortex: the description of a cortical field composed of discrete cytoarchitectonic units, *Brain Res.*, 17, 205, 1970.

24. Welker, C. and Woolsey, T.A., Structure of layer IV in the somatosensory neocortex of the rat: description and comparison with the mouse, *J. Comp. Neurol.*, 158, 437, 1974.

25. Yang, X., Hyder, F., and Shulman, R.G., Activation of single whisker barrel in rat brain localized by functional magnetic resonance imaging, *Proc. Natl. Acad. Sci. U.S.A.*, 93, 475, 1996.

26. Paxinos, G., *Rat Brain*, Academic Press, San Diego, 1995.

27. Hyder, F. et al., Dynamic magnetic resonance imaging of the rat brain during forepaw stimulation, *J. Cereb. Blood Flow Metabol.*, 14, 649, 1994.

28. Gyngell, M.L. et al., Variation of functional MRI signal in response to frequency of somatosensory stimulation in α-chloralose anesthetized rats, *Mag. Res. Med.,* 36, 13, 1996.
29. Bock, C. et al., Functional MRI of somatosensory activation in rat: effect of hypercapnic up-regulation on perfusion- and BOLD-imaging, *Mag. Res. Med.,* 39, 457, 1998.
30. Bock, C. et al., Brainmapping of α-chloralose anesthetized rats with T_2*-weighted imaging: distinction between the representation of the forepaw and hindpaw in the somatosensory cortex, *NMR Biomed.,* 11, 115, 1998.
31. Brinker, G. et al., Simultaneous recording of evoked potentials and T*$_2$-weighted MR images during somatosensory stimulation of rat, *Mag. Res. Med.,* 41, 469, 1999.
32. Silva, A.C. et al., Simultaneous blood oxygenation level-dependent and cerebral blood flow functional magnetic resonance imaging during forepaw stimulation in the rat, *J. Cereb. Blood Flow Metabol.,* 19, 871, 1999.
33. Yang, X. et al., Dynamic mapping at the laminar level of odor-elicited responses in rat olfactory bulb by functional MRI, *Proc. Natl. Acad. Sci. U.S.A.,* 95, 7715, 1998.
34. Xu, F.Q. et al., Assessment and discrimination of odor stimuli in rat olfactory bulb by dynamic functional MRI, *Proc. Natl. Acad. Sci. U.S.A.,* 97, 10601, 2000.
35. Ogawa, S. et al., Brain magnetic resonance imaging with contrast dependent on blood oxygenation, *Proc. Natl. Acad. Sci. U.S.A.,* 87, 9868, 1990.
36. Ogawa, S. and Lee, T.M., Magnetic resonance iamging of blood vessels at high fields: *in vivo* and *in vitro* measurements and image stimulation, *Mag. Res. Med.,* 16, 9, 1990.
37. Ogawa, S., Lee, T.M., and Barrere, B., The sensitivity of magnetic resonance image signals of a rat brain to changes in the cerebral venous blood oxygenation, *Mag. Res. Med., Medicine,* 29, 205, 1993.
38. Grüne, M. et al., Somatosensory activation in rats detected by quantitative fMRI parameter maps at 7 T: improvement of reliability and separation of BOLD from inflow effects, *J. Cereb. Blood Flow Metabol.,* 19, S402, 1999.
39. Grüne, M. et al., Gradient echo time dependence and quantitative parameter maps for somatosensory activation in rats at 7 T, *Mag. Res. Med.,* 42, 118, 1999.
40. Lee, S.P. et al., Diffusion-weighted spin-echo fMRI at 9.4 T: microvascular/tissue contribution to BOLD signal changes, *Mag. Res. Med.,* 42, 919, 1999.
41. Kerskens, C.M. et al., Ultrafast perfusion-weighted MRI of functional brain activation in rats during forepaw stimulation: comparison with T*$_2$-weighted MRI, *NMR Biomed.,* 9, 20, 1996.
42. Detre, J.A. et al., Perfusion imaging, *Mag. Res. Med.,* 23, 37, 1992.
43. Franke, C. et al., Arterial spin tagging perfusion imaging of rat brain: dependency on magnetic field strength, *Mag. Res. Imaging,* 18, 1109, 2000.
44. Silva, A.C. et al., Early temporal characteristics of cerebral blood flow and deoxy-hemoglobin changes during somatosensory stimulation, *J. Cereb. Blood Flow Metabol.,* 20, 201, 2000.
45. Burke, M., *Die Bestimmung der Änderung des Sauerstoffverbrauchs unter funktioneller Aktivierung mittels Kernspintomographie,* Ph.D. thesis, Technical University of Aachen, 2000. http://sylvester.bth.rwth-aachen.de/dissertationen/2000/63/00 63.pdf

46. Schwindt, W., Burke, M., and Hoehn, M., Activated ares found by BOLD, CBF, CBV and changes in $CMRO_2$ during somatosensory stimulation do not co-localize in rat cortex, *Proceedings of Symposium on Brain Activation and CBF Control,* Tokyo, 2001.

47. Hyder, F. et al., Quantitative multi-modal functional MRI with blood oxygenation level dependent exponential decays adjusted for flow attenuated inversion recovery (BOLDED AFFAIR), *Mag. Res. Imaging,* 18, 227, 2000.

48. van Bruggen, N. et al., High-resolution functional magnetic resonance imaging of the rat brain-mapping changes in cerebral blood volume using iron oxide contrast media, *J. Cereb. Blood Flow Metabol.,* 18, 1178, 1998.

49. Mandeville, J.B. et al., Dynamic functional imaging of relative cerebral blood volume during rat forepaw stimulation, *Mag. Res. Med.,* 39, 615, 1998.

50. Palmer, J.T. et al., High-resolution mapping of discrete representational areas in rat somatosensory cortex using blood volume-dependent functional MRI, *Neuroimage,* 9, 383, 1999.

51. Mandeville, J.B. and Marota, J.J.A., Vascular filters of functional MRI: spatial localization using BOLD and CBV contrast, *Mag. Res. Med.,* 42, 591, 1999.

52. Marota, J.J. A. et al., Investigation of the early response to rat forepaw stimulation, *Mag. Res. Med.,* 41, 247, 1999.

53. Mandeville, J.B. et al., Regional sensitivity and coupling of BOLD and CBV changes during stimulation of rat brain, *Mag. Res. Med.,* 45, 443, 2001.

54. Mandeville, J.B. et al., MRI measurement of the temporal evolution of relative CMR_{O2} during rat forepaw stimulation, *Mag. Res. Med.,* 42, 944, 1999.

55. Zhong, J.H. et al., Quantification of intravascular and extravascular contributions to BOLD effects induced by alteration in oxygenation or intravascular contrast agents, *Mag. Res, Med.,* 40, 526, 1998.

56. Cholet, N. et al., Local injection of antisense oligonucleotides targeted to the glial glutamate transporter GLAST decreases the metabolic response to somatosensory activation, *J. Cereb. Blood Flow Metabol.,* 21, 404, 2001.

57. Polley, D.B., Chen-Bee, C.H., and Frostig, R.D., Two directions of plasticity in the sensory-deprived adult cortex, *Neuron,* 24, 623, 1999.

58. Jablonska, B. et al., Partial blocking of NMDA receptors reduces plastic changes induced by short-lasting classical conditioning in the SI barrel cortex of adult mice, *Cerebral Cortex,* 9, 222, 1999.

59. Yang, X., Hyder, F., and Shulman, R.G., Functional MRI BOLD signal coincides with electrical activity in the rat whisker barrels, *Mag. Res. Med.,* 38, 874, 1997.

60. Armstrong-James, M. and Fox, K., Spatiotemporal convergence and divergence in the rat S1 "barrel" cortex, *J. Comp. Neurol.,* 263, 265, 1987.

61. Hoehn, M. and Hossmann, K.A., Functional activation of the brain under normal and pathological conditions, in *Proceedings, International School of Physics Enrico Fermi, Course 39,* Maraviglia, B., Ed., 1999, 311.

62. Ueki, M., Linn, F., and Hossmann, K.A., Functional activation of cerebral blood flow and metabolism before and after global ischemia of rat brain, *J. Cereb. Blood Flow Metabol.,* 8, 486, 1988.

63. Bock, C. et al., Functional recovery after cardiac arrest and resuscitation in rat: a functional MRI study, *J. Cereb. Blood Flow Metabol.,* 17, S163, 1997.

64. Kida, I. et al., High-resolution CMR_{O2} mapping in rat cortex: a multiparametric approach to calibration of BOLD image contrast at 7 Tesla, *J. Cereb. Blood Flow Metabol.,* 20, 847, 2000.

65 Spenger, C. et al., Functional MRI at 4.7 Tesla of the rat brain during electric stimulation of forepaw, hindpaw, or tail in single- and multislice experiments, *Exp. Neurol.*, 166, 246, 2000.

66. Peeters, R.R. et al., A patchy horizontal organization of the somatosensory activation of the rat cerebellum demonstrated by functional MRI, *Eur. J. Neurosci.*, 11, 2720, 1999.

67. Hawkes, R., An anatomical model of cerebellar modules, *Progr. Brain Res.*, 114, 39, 1997.

68. Shambes, G.M., Gibson, J.M., and Welker, W., Fractured somatotopy in granule cell tactile areas of rat cerebellar hemispheres revealed by micromapping, *Brain Behav. Evol.*, 15, 94, 1978.

69. Mandeville, J.B. et al., Evidence of a cerebrovascular postarteriole Windkessel with delayed compliance, *J. Cereb. Blood Flow Metabol.*, 19, 679, 1999.

70. Kennan, R.P. et al., Effects of hypoglycemia on functional magnetic resonance imaging response to median nerve stimulation in the rat brain, *J. Cereb. Blood Flow Metabol.*, 20, 1352, 2000.

71. Schwarzbauer, C. and Hoehn, M., The effect of transient hypercapnia on task-related changes in cerebral blood flow and blood oxygenation in awake normal humans: a functional magnetic resonance imaging study, *NMR Biomed.*, 13, 415, 2000.

72. Scremin, O.U. et al., Cholinergic control of blood flow in the cerebral cortex of the rat, *Stroke*, 4, 233, 1973.

73. Rovere, A.A. et al., Cholinergic mechanism in the cerebrovascular action of carbon dioxide, *Stroke*, 4, 969, 1973.

74. Scremin, O.U., Rubinstein, E.H., and Schonnenschein, R.R., Cerebrovascular CO_2 reactivity: role of a cholinergic mechanism modulated by anesthesia, *Stroke*, 9, 160, 1978.

75. Kida, I., Hyder, F., and Behar, K.L., Involvement of voltage gated Na^+ channels in the BOLD fMRI response during forepaw somatosensory activation in the rat, *Proc. Int. Soc. Mag. Res. Med.*, 9, 655, 2001.

76. Forman, S.D. et al., Simultaneous glutamate and perfusion fMRI responses to regional brain stimulation, *J. Cereb. Blood Flow Metabol.*, 18, 1064, 1998.

77. Sijbers, J. et al., Restoration of MR-induced artifacts in simultaneously recorded MR/EEG data, *Mag. Res. Imaging*, 17, 1383, 1999.

78. Kohno, K. et al., A modified rat model of middle cerebral artery thread occlusion under electrophysiological control for magnetic resonance investigations, *Mag. Res. Imaging*, 13, 65, 1995.

79. Busch, E. et al., Simultaneous recording of EEG, DC potential and diffusion-weighted NMR imaging during potassium induced cortical spreading depression in rats, *NMR Biomed.*, 8, 59, 1995.

80. Schmitz, B. et al., Recovery of the rodent brain after cardiac arrest: a functional MRI study [erratum: *Mag. Res. Med.*, 40, 340, 1998], *Mag. Res. Med.*, 39, 783, 1998.

81. Ogawa, S. et al., An approach to probe some neural systems interaction by functional MRI at neural time scale down to milliseconds, *Proc. Natl. Acad. Sci. U.S.A.*, 97, 11026, 2000.

82. Fox, P.T. and Raichle, M.E., Focal physiological uncoupling of cerebral blood flow and oxidative metabolism during somatosensory stimulation in human subjects. (PET), *Proc. Natl. Acad. Sci. U.S.A.*, 83, 1140, 1986.

83. Sokoloff, L., Sites and mechanisms of changes in local energy metabolism in neural tissues, *J. Neurochem.*, 61, 241, 1993.

84. Pellerin, L. and Magistretti, P.J., Glutamate uptake into astrocytes stimulates aerobic glycolysis: a mechanism coupling neuronal activity to glucose utilization, *Proc. Natl. Acad. Sci. U.S.A.*, 91, 10625, 1994.

85. Hyder, F. et al., Increased tricarboxylic acid cycle flux in rat brain during forepaw stimulation detected with ^{1}H[^{13}C] NMR, *Proc. Natl. Acad. Sci. U.S.A.*, 93, 7612, 1996.

86. Hyder, F. et al., Oxidative glucose metabolism in rat brain during single forepaw stimulation: a spatially localized ^{1}H[^{13}C] nuclear magnetic resonance study, *J. Cereb. Blood Flow Metabol.*, 17, 1040, 1997.

87. Sibson, N.R. et al., Stoichiometric coupling of brain glucose metabolism and glutamatergic neuronal activity, *Proc. Natl. Acad. Sci. U.S.A.*, 95, 316, 1998.

88. Hyder, F., Renken, R., and Rothman, D.L., *In vivo* carbon-edited detection with proton echo-planar spectroscopic imaging (ICED PEPSI): [3,4-(CH_2)-C_{13}] glutamate/glutamine tomography in rat brain, *Mag. Res. Med.*, 42, 997, 1999.

89. Mason, G.F. et al., NMR determination of the TCA cycle rate and α-ketoglutarate/glutamate exchange rate in rat brain, *J. Cereb. Blood Flow Metabol.*, 12, 434, 1992.

90. Hyder, F., Shulman, R.G., and Rothman, D.L., A model for the regulation of cerebral oxygen delivery, *J. Appl. Physiol.*, 85, 554, 1998.

91. Hyder, F. et al., Dependence of oxygen delivery on blood flow in rat brain: a 7-tesla nuclear magnetic resonance study, *J. Cereb. Blood Flow Metabol.*, 20, 485, 2000.

92. Kim, S.G. and Ugurbil, K., Comparison of blood oxygenation and cerebral blood flow effects in fMRI: estimation of relative oxygen consumption change, *Mag. Res. Med.*, 38, 59, 1997.

93. Davis, T.L. et al., Calibrated functional MRI: mapping the dynamics of oxidative metabolism, *Proc. Natl. Acad. Sci. U.S.A.*, 95, 1834, 1998.

94. Hoge, R.D. et al., Investigation of BOLD signal dependence on cerebral blood flow and oxygen consumption: the deoxyhemoglobin dilution model, *Mag. Res. Med.*, 42, 849, 1999.

95. Kim, S.G. et al., Determination of relative CMR_{O2} from CBF and BOLD changes: significant increase of oxygen consumption rate during visual stimulation, *Mag. Res. Med.*, 41, 1152, 1999.

96. Hyder, F. et al., CBV changes during functional and CO_2 challenges: implications for BOLD calibration, *Proc. Int. Soc. Mag. Res. Med.*, 9, 281, 2001.

97. Marrett, S. and Gjedde, A., Changes of blood flow and oxygen consumption in visual cortex of living humans, *Adv. Exp. Med. Biol.*, 413, 205, 1997.

98. Vafaee, M.S. et al., Frequency-dependent changes in cerebral metabolic rate of oxygen during activation of human visual cortex, *J. Cereb. Blood Flow Metabol.*, 19, 272, 1999.

99. Ronen, I. and Navon, G., A new method for proton detection of $H_2(^{17})O$ with potential applications for functional MRI, *Mag. Res. Med.*, 32, 789, 1994.

100. Reddy, R., Stolpen, A.H., and Leigh, J.S., Detection of ^{17}O by proton $T_1\,\rho$ dispersion imaging, *J. Mag. Res. Series B*, 108, 276, 1995.

101. Zhu, X.H. et al., Feasibility studies of ^{17}O MR imaging for fast and repeatable measurements of three-dimensional $CMRO_2$ image in the rat brain, *Proc. Int. Soc. Mag. Res. Med.*, 9, 649, 2001.

102. Fiat, D. and Kang, S., Determination of the rate of cerebral oxygen consumption and regional cerebral blood flow by non-invasive ^{17}O *in vivo* NMR spectroscopy and magnetic resonance imaging. Part 1: theory and data analysis methods, *Neurol. Res.,* 14, 303, 1992.

103. Fiat, D. and Kang, S., Determination of the rate of cerebral oxygen consumption and regional cerebral blood flow by non-invasive ^{17}O *in vivo* NMR spectroscopy and magnetic resonance imaging. Part 2: determination of CMR_{O2} for the rat by ^{17}O NMR, and CMR_{O2}, rCBF and the partition coefficient for the cat by ^{17}O MRI, *Neurol. Res.,* 15, 7, 1993.

104. Tailor, D.R. et al., Proton MRI detection of metabolically generated $H_2{}^{17}O$ from inhaled $^{17}O_2$, *Proc. Int. Soc. Mag. Res. Med.,* 9, 648, 2001.

105. Pekar, J. et al., *In vivo* measurement of cerebral oxygen consumption and blood flow using ^{17}O magnetic resonance imaging, *Mag. Res. Med.,* 21, 313, 1991.

106. Kandel, A. and Buzsaki, G., Cellular-synaptic generation of sleep spindles, spike-and-wave discharges, and evoked thalamocortical responses in the neocortex of the rat, *J. Neurosci.,* 17, 6783, 1997.

107. Di, S., Brett, B., and Barth, D.S., Polysensory-evoked potentials in rat parieto-temporal cortex: combined auditory and somatosensory responses, *Brain Res.,* 642, 267, 1994.

108. Blood, A.J. and Toga, A.W., Optical intrinsic signal imaging responses are modulated in rodent somatosensory cortex during simultaneous whisker and forelimb stimulation, *J. Cereb. Blood Flow Metabol.,* 18, 968, 1998.

109. Lin, Y.J. and Koretsky, A.P., Manganese ion enhances T_1-weighted MRI during brain activation: an approach to direct imaging of brain function, *Mag. Res. Med.,* 38, 378, 1997.

110. Duong, T.Q. et al., Functional MRI of calcium-dependent synaptic activity: cross correlation with CBF and BOLD measurements, *Mag. Res. Med.,* 43, 383, 2000.

111 Pautler, R.G., Silva, A.C., and Koretsky, A.P., *In vivo* neuronal tract tracing using manganese-enhanced magnetic resonance imaging, *Mag. Res. Med.,* 40, 740, 1998.

112. Watanabe, T., Michaelis, T., and Frahm, J., Mapping of retinal projections in the living rat using high-resolution three-dimensional gradient-echo MRI with Mn^{2+}-induced contrast, *Mag. Res. Med.,* 46, 424, 2001.

113. Van Meir, V. et al., *In vivo* volume measurement of song control nuclei in the brain of European starlings (*Surnus vulgaris*) using manganese-enhanced MRI, *Proc. Inc. Soc. Mag. Res. Med.,* 9, 1470, 2001.

114. Porszasz, R. et al., Signal changes in the spinal cord of the rat after injection of formalin into the hindpaw: characterization using functional magnetic resonance imaging, *Proc. Natl. Acad. Sci. U.S.A.,* 94, 5034, 1997.

115. Tuor, U.I. et al., Functional magnetic resonance imaging in rats subjected to noxious electrical and chemical stimulation of the forepaw, *Proc. Int. Soc. Mag. Res. Med.,* 8, 612, 2000.

116. Malisza, K. et al., Negative functional MRI changes in capsaicin-induced painful stimulation in rats, *Proc. Int. Soc. Mag. Res. Med.,* 9, 657, 2001.

117. Reese, T. et al., Cytoprotection does not preserve brain functionality in rats during the acute post-stroke phase despite evidence of non-infarction provided by MRI, *NMR Biomed.,* 13, 361, 2000.

118. Dijkhuizen, R.M. et al., Temporal pattern of brain reorganization after transient cerebral ischemia in rats: a functional MRI study, *J. Cereb. Blood Flow Metabol.,* 21, S310, 2001.

119. Abo, M. et al., Functional recovery after brain lesion: contralateral neuromodulation: an fMRI study, *NeuroReport*, 12, 1, 2001.

120. Waltz, A.G., Red venous blood: occurrence and significance in ischemic and nonischemic cerebral cortex, *J. Neurosurg.*, 31, 141, 1969.

121. Zimmer, R., Lang, R., and Oberdörster, G., Post-ischemic reactive hyperemia of the isolated perfused brain of the dog, *Pflügers Arch.*, 328, 332, 1971.

122. Hossmann, K.A., Reperfusion of the brain after global ischemia: hemodynamic disturbances, *Shock*, 8, 95, 1997.

123. Waltz, A.G. and Sundt, T.M., Influence of systemic blood pressure on blood flow and microcirculation of ischemic cerebral cortex: a failure of autoregulation, *Progr. Brain Res.*, 30, 107, 1968.

124. Schmitz, B., Böttiger, B.W., and Hossmann, K.A., Functional activation of cerebral blood flow after cardiac arrest in rat, *J. Cereb. Blood Flow Metabol.*, 17, 1202, 1997.

125. Schmidt-Kastner, R., Grosse-Ophoff, B., and Hossmann, K.A., Delayed recovery of CO_2 reactivity after one hour's complete ischaemia of cat brain, *J. Neurol.*, 233, 367, 1986.

126. Hossmann, K.A., Sakaki, S., and Kimoto, K., Cerebral uptake of glucose and oxygen in the cat brain after prolonged ischemia, *Stroke*, 7, 301, 1976.

127. Hossmann, K.A. et al., NMR imaging of the apparent diffusion coefficient (ADC) for the evaluation of metabolic suppression and recovery after prolonged cerebral ischemia., *J. Cereb. Blood Flow Metabol.*, 14, 723, 1994.

128. Hossmann, K.A. et al., Functional magnetic resonance imaging after cardiac arrest in rat, in *Pharmacology of Cerebral Ischemia*, Krieglstein, J., Ed., Medpharm Scientific Publishers, Stuttgart, 1996, 357.

129. Hoehn, M. et al., Validation of arterial spin tagging perfusion MR imaging: correlation with autoradiographic CBF data, *Proc. Int. Soc. Mag. Res. Med.*, 7, 1843, 1999.

130. Hoehn-Berlage, M. et al., Inhibition of non-selective cation channels reduces focal ischemic injury of rat brain, *J. Cereb. Blood Flow Metabol.*, 17, 534, 1997.

131. Schwindt, W. et al., Cortical plasticity after neonatal cold lesions in rats: an fMRI study, in *Proceedings, 30th Annual Scientific Meeting of Society for Neuroscience*, New Orleans, LA, 2000, 861.

132 Kauppinen, R.A. et al., Visual activation in α-chloralose-anaesthetized cats does not cause lactate accumulation in the visual cortex as detected by (^{1}H) NMR difference spectroscopy, *Eur. J. Neurosci.*, 9, 654, 1997.

133 Fox, P.T. et al., Nonoxidative glucose consumption during focal physiologic neural activity, *Science*, 241, 462, 1988.

134. Kim, D.S., Duong, T.Q., and Kim, S.G., High-resolution mapping of iso-orientation columns by fMRI, *Nature Neurosci.*, 3, 164, 2000.

135. Duong, T.Q. et al., Spatiotemporal dynamics of the BOLD fMRI signals: toward mapping submillimeter cortical columns using the early negative response, *Mag. Res. Med.*, 44, 231, 2000.

136 Jezzard, P., Rauschecker, J.P., and Malonek, D., An *in vivo* model for functional MRI in cat visual cortex, *Mag. Res. Med.*, 38, 699, 1997.

137. Bonhoeffer, T. and Grinvald, A., Iso-orientation domains in cat visual cortex are arranged in pinwheel-like pattern, *Nature*, 353, 429, 1991.

138. Shmuel, A. and Grinvald, A., Functional organization for direction of motion and its relationship to orientation maps in cat area 18, *J. Neurosci.*, 16, 6945, 1996.

139. Huang, W. et al., Magnetic resonance imaging (MRI) detection of the murine brain response to light: temporal differentiation and negative functional MRI changes, *Proc. Natl. Acad. Sci. U.S.A.,* 93, 6037, 1996.
140. Mueggler, T., Baumann, D., and Rudin, M., Dynamic CBV imaging of the mouse cortex during electrical stimulation of the hindpaw, *Proc. Int. Soc. Mag. Res. Med.,* 9, 651, 2001.
141. Ahrens, E.T. and Dubowitz, D.J., Peripheral somatosensory fMRI in mouse at 11.7T, *NMR Biomed.,* 14, 318, 2001.
142. Strupp, J.P., Stimulate: a GUI based fMRI Analysis Software Package, *NeuroImage,* 3, S607, 1996.

5 Functional Imaging in Nonhuman Primates

Elizabeth Disbrow

CONTENTS

5.1 INTRODUCTION

The use of functional imaging techniques such as functional magnetic resonance imaging (fMRI), magnetoencephalography (MEG), and positron emission tomography (PET) has grown from a specialized procedure available at a handful of locations to a technology available around the world. While fMRI and MEG are used to study widely divergent phenomena including sensory processing, perception, learning, memory, and cognitive function, our understanding of these techniques has lagged behin d their widespread use. This gap in our knowledge led to the development of an animal model to study the relationship of measured signals obtained from fMRI and MEG and the underlying neural activity that ultimately generates these signals.

Functional imaging in the nonhuman primate in combination with electrophysiological recording techniques will allow us to link the imaging signal and the underlying neural activity and thus bridge the gap between the wealth of data obtained using invasive techniques in nonhuman primates and the rapidly increasing data from human imaging experiments.

Functional imaging techniques such as fMRI and MEG are used to examine stimulus-bound changes in activity in the brain (Figure 5.1). What exactly do they measure? Functional MRI is an indirect estimate of neural activity based on blood

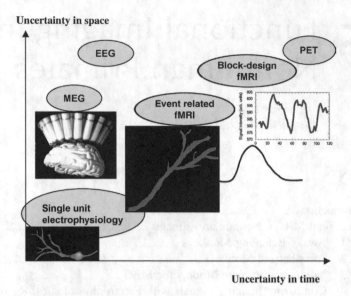

FIGURE 5.1 Spatial and temporal ramifications of indirectness in functional imaging. Techniques have strengths and weaknesses in the spatial and temporal domains. Single unit electrophysiological recording is the "gold standard" with precise spatial and real-time temporal resolution. MEG has submillisecond temporal resolution but reduced spatial resolution due to the ambiguity of the solution of the inverse problem. While EEG has similar temporal resolution, its spatial resolution is considerably reduced due to noise from cerebral fluid and musculature. fMRI and PET have reduced spatial and temporal resolution because the measured signal is based on blood oxygenation level, which indirectly reflects underlying neural activity.

oxygenation levels and called a blood oxygenation level-dependent (BOLD) signal. Active neurons require increased levels of oxygen. Oxygen is carried via hemoglobin, and hemoglobin contains iron. The presence or absence of oxygen on hemoglobin changes the magnetic properties of the iron in hemoglobin, and this difference can be measured externally. In active cortex, the BOLD signal initially dips (1 second poststimulus), reflecting a transient decrease in oxygenated hemoglobin. However, a much larger secondary (2 to 4 seconds poststimulus) increase in local oxygenated hemoglobin dominates the signal. This secondary increase in oxyhemoglobin is the signal commonly measured in fMRI experiments (Ogawa et al., 1990; for review , see Gazzaniga et al., 2002; Posner and Raichle, 1998; Cohen and Bookheimer, 1994) (see Chapter 4).

While this scenario is widely accepted, a host of unanswered questions that are vital to the proper interpretation and use of fMRI data remain. For example, how reliable is the BOLD signal? Is the relationship between the BOLD signal and underlying neural activity linear? How is it regulated? What portion of neural activity does the BOLD signal represent; that is, is it correlated with action potentials, synaptic activity, or postsynaptic potentials? How does the BOLD signal reflect inhibition vs. excitation, and can they be distinguished? Can spatial and temporal resolution be improved? These questions can best be addressed using an animal model in which an examination of the BOLD signal can be combined with direct measures of neural activity such as electrophysiological recording.

MEG has the advantage that it is a more direct measure of neural activity. It measures the magnetic fields associated with neural electrical activity. In theory, the measured magnetic field originates from the current flowing through a large number of parallel dendrites (see Gallen et al., 1995). The dendrites must be tangential to the surface of the head so that the dipolar signal (inflow and outflow of the magnetic field) can be detected. A point source is then calculated based on the solution of the inverse problem (see Hamalainen et al., 1993). It is assumed that the signal originates from the dendrite rather than the axon because the myelination of the axon would disrupt the magnetic field, causing it to cancel itself out.

Data supporting the theory that the MEG signal is derived from large groups of synchronized dendrites comes from an elegant set of studies of the physiological bases of the magnetic signal in the guinea pig hippocampal slice (Wu and Okada, 1998). It was demonstrated that synchronized population spikes and waves of magnetic field occurred when excitatory transmission was blocked. Furthermore, based on source modeling of various temporal components (notably the 20 ms M20 and the 35 ms M35) of evoked responses, speculation has been made as to the cellular mechanisms underlying the temporal profile of electrical activity (Wikstrom et al., 1996). They suggest that the M20 is due to an early excitatory postsynaptic potential while the M35 is due to an inhibitory postsynaptic potential at layer 4. Although the MEG signal is more closely related to neural activity than the BOLD signal, the MEG signal mechanism has been less intensely studied and is still largely theoretical. Thus, a nonhuman primate model for MEG is also necessary for the proper use and interpretation of data.

5.2 FUNCTIONAL MRI IN NONHUMAN PRIMATES

5.2.1 AWAKE BEHAVING MONKEYS

Unlike studying humans, functional imaging in monkeys presents some unique challenges. One of the most important is: how do you maintain the monkey's head in a stable position? There are two schools of thought on this issue. One involves mechanical restraint and the other chemical restraint. Several groups have used a combination of training and head restraint to coerce an awake behaving monkey into the magnet for fMR scanning. In the earliest experiments (Dubowitz et al., 1998; Stephanacci et al., 1998), monkeys were trained to sit in a chair that was gradually tilted to a 90 degree angle. Then in a mock fMRI environment, monkeys were exposed to audio tapes of pulse sequence noise that was gradually increased until it reached levels approximating the actual MR environment. This process took several months.

Head restraint consisted of a plastic head post surgically implanted in the skull of each animal. In one instance (Logothetis et al., 1999), a custom magnet with a vertical bore was designed and built especially to accommodate a monkey in a seated position. Functional imaging in the awake behaving monkey is labor intensive, but results are superior (compared to results from chemically restrained animals) for the

study of behavioral and cognitive issues, and a wealth of data from electrophysiological recording studies of single neurons in behaving macaques exists.

Regional cerebral blood flow has been measured in awake behaving monkeys
using PET. Perlmutter et al. (1991) trained a monkey to sit in a specially designed
chair after surgically implanting an acrylic skullcap for head placement and reposi-
tioning. They were able to measure a significant change in regional cerebral blood
flow in contralateral primary somatosensory cortex following vibratory stimulation
of the hand.

The first fMRI results from nonhuman primates were obtained in awake behaving
monkeys using standard clinical 1.5-T magnets. Stefanacci et al. (1998) showed
activity-dependent signals in the visual cortex in response to passive viewing of a
movie. Dubowitz et al. (1998) performed a more in-depth examination of the BOLD
signal from an awake behaving macaque monkey during passive viewing of a visual
stimulus. They reported activation of primary and extrastriate visual areas and
differences in optimal scan parameters for monkey and human fMR imaging and
similarities in human and monkey fMRI signal amplitude or percent signal change
for the stimulus vs. rest conditions (2 to 4%).

Intravenous contrast agents significantly increased the fMRI contrast-to-noise
ratio (Dubowitz et al., 2001, Vanduffel et al., 2001). Vanduffel and colleagues
examined visual motion areas of macaque cortex using fMRI at 1.5 T. They used a
contrast agent to enhance contrast sensitivity specifically in brain tissue. Monocrystalline iron oxide nanoparticle (MION) was injected intravenously, and awake fix-
ating monkeys were presented with static or coherently moving patterns of dots or
lines. Cortical field boundaries were estimated using sulcal and gyral landmarks
related to existing maps of macaque cortex.

The contrast agent increased fMRI contrast-to-noise ratio by a factor of 5,
increased statistical power, and may have improved spatial localization of activation,
although no direct activity measurements were made. Several motion selective visual
fields were identified including V2, MT, MST, LIP, and VIP. Data were interpreted
in light of the large volume of preexisting data from single unit electrophysiological
recording experiments in nonhuman primates. They compared the relative amplitude
of signal change with the proportion of motion selective cells in a number of cortical
fields. They speculated about the differences in amplitude and proportion at different
levels of the visual motion processing hierarchy, suggesting the influence of attention
as a possible cause. They also compared their data to preexisting human fMRI data
related to the processing of visual motion and found largely similar results.

5.2.2 ANESTHETIZED MONKEYS

The second approach to primate imaging is anesthetizing the monkeys before scanning. The first indication that the BOLD signal could be measured in the anesthetized
preparation involved somatosensory stimuli at the clinical standard 1.5 T (Disbrow
et al., 1999). The medial-lateral organization of primary somatosensory cortex was
examined and showed that the hand and face representations could be discriminated
reliably (Figure 5.2A). Further, the percent signal change for stimulus vs. rest

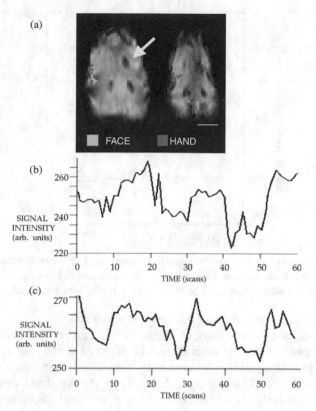

FIGURE 5.2 Cortical activation resulting from stimulation of the hands and face in the anesthetized macaque monkey. (a) Serial axial EPI slices (left = inferior, top = rostral) from stimulation of the hand (red pixels) and the face (green pixels). Arrow indicates the location of fluid-filled probe used for later superposition of anatomical and electrophysiological recording data (Disbrow, E.A. et al., 2000a). (b) Average change in signal intensity over time in voxels active in response to tactile stimulation of the hand (dark pixels in A). (c) Time course of activity in response to identical tactile stimulation in an awake behaving human. Note the similarity in the percent signal change. See Color Figure 5.2 following page 210.

conditions was similar for anesthetized monkeys and awake behaving humans (Figure 5.2(b)(c)).

In a subsequent experiment in anesthetized monkeys (Hayashi et al., 1999), somatotopic organization was demonstrated for both primary and secondary somatosensory cortex. Logothetis et al., (1999) measured the BOLD signal in anesthetized macaque monkeys using a custom-built vertical bore 4.7 T magnet with a voxel size of $1 \times 1 \times 2$ mm. They reported activation of primary and extrastriate cortex and lateral geniculate nucleus in response to reversing checkerboard stimulation. They also measured activation in the superior temporal sulcus, the amygdala, and the caudate and frontal cortex in response to the visual presentation of faces.

Chemical restraint for functional imaging has obvious advantages. Long training periods and surgical implantation of hardware can be avoided, and custom-built

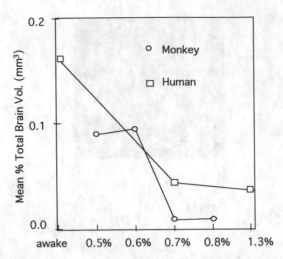

FIGURE 5.3 Human and macaque monkey dose response data for isoflurane general anesthesia. The active brain volume drops off at 0.7% isoflurane in both species. Human data adapted from Antognini, J.F. et al., *Life Sci.,* 61, 349, 1997. With permission.

imaging hardware is unnecessary. However, it requires a significant trade-off. For fMRI, anesthetics exert a variety of effects on the cerebral vasculature, cerebral metabolism, and the link between them. The effects are not entirely understood. Further, the BOLD signal diminishes rapidly with depth of anesthesia (Figure 5.3; Antognini et al., 1997; Disbrow et al., 1999). Thus, the anesthetic window for successful fMRI is small, and it is important to monitor blood gas concentrations and maintain normal levels. Finally, the types of stimuli that can be used with an anesthetized preparation are severely limited, with no options for examining cognitive hypotheses. However, in spite of the limitations, anesthesia is currently the method of choice for researchers interested in combining fMRI and electrophysiological recording techniques in the same monkey (Disbrow et al., 2000; Logothetis et al., 2001).

5.2.3 NONHUMAN PRIMATE MODELS FOR MEG

Development of a nonhuman primate model for MEG has lagged considerably behind development of fMRI. Indeed relatively little work using MEG has been done in any animal. The choice of animals is limited because the neuronal source of the MEG signal must be tangential to the surface of the head in order to be detectable using standard biomagnetometers. Lissencephalic or smooth-brained animals, including readily available new world monkeys, are not appropriate.

The only nonhuman primate study to date (Teale et al., 1994) was performed in an awake behaving *Macaca nemestrina* monkey using auditory stimuli. The monkey was trained to perch in a custom-made chair; the head was restrained using a thin walled plastic helmet. MEG has the advantage of silence, so no noise tolerance training was necessary. Responses were localized to the superior temporal gyrus, probably in the primary auditory cortex, and were similar in morphology to responses seen in humans, although latencies were considerably shorter.

5.2.4 COMPARING IMAGING SIGNALS WITH ELECTROPHYSIOLOGICAL RECORDING DATA: INDIRECT TECHNIQUES (PARAMETRIC STIMULI)

To study the mechanism underlying functional imaging signals, it is ideal to perform both noninvasive and confirmatory invasive techniques in a single animal. However, this process is expensive and labor intensive and requires relatively elaborate facilities. Fortunately, it is possible to shed light on the relationship between the MEG or BOLD signal and underlying neural activity indirectly, based on what we already know about the organization and function of monkey cortex. The underlying assumption is that sensory cortices in the macaque monkey and the human are quite similar. Human imaging data can then be interpreted based on this assumption.

For example, how well do functional imaging signals reflect incremental changes in cortical neural activity? This issue is crucial for the accurate interpretation of functional imaging data. We designed an experiment to examine the issue by drawing on what we know about the organization of the somatosensory cortex of the postcentral gyrus in the monkey. This region contains multiple somatosensory fields (areas 3a, 3b (S1), 1, and 2). Multiunit electrophysiological recording in monkeys revealed that each field contains a complete representation of the body surface, is somatotopically organized, and contains neurons with relatively small receptive fields (see Kaas, 1983). In fact, neurons in this region with receptive fields on digit tips are generally restricted to a single digit (Nelson et al., 1980). Tactile stimulation of one, two, three, and four fingers should result in an incremental increase in the extent of cortical activation in the macaque monkey and presumably in the human as well.

We performed fMRI (1.5 T) and MEG measures of the response to tactile stimulation of one, two, three, and four digits. While fMRI responses were consistently localized to the postcentral gyrus (the presumed location of the hand representation of human primary somatosensory cortex), the data did not accurately reflect the increase in extent of cortical activation with an increase in either percent signal change or extent of fMRI signal at 1.5 T (Figure 5.4). In fact, the number of digits stimulated could not be predicted from the data. On the other hand, increases in extent of cortical activation were correlated with MEG signal intensity (Figure 5.4; Roberts et al., 2000), perhaps reflecting the more direct relationship between instantaneous MEG signal and neuronal activity.

Other comparisons have shown a more reliable relationship between the BOLD signal and preexisting electrophysiological recording data. Rees and colleagues (2000) made a more elaborate comparison of human fMRI and macaque monkey single unit recording data from visual cortical area V5/MT in response to parametric variation in the strength or coherence of the motion stimulus. Six levels of coherence from 0 to 100% were presented to subjects during scanning, and subjects indicated the perceived direction of motion with a button press. Activation in several regions showed a linear relationship with stimulus coherence including V5 bilaterally.

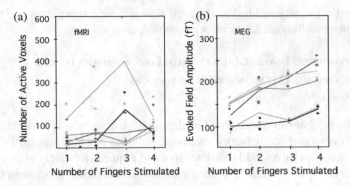

FIGURE 5.4 Extent of cortical activation in response to stimulation of an increasing number of digits. Subjects were scanned three times using fMRI and three times using MEG. (a) fMRI data show considerable within-subject variability (like colored dots) and between-subject variability (different colored lines), with no trend toward increasing area of activation with increasing number of stimulated digits. (b) MEG data indicate significantly less within-subject variability. While between-subject variability was still high, a significant correlation of magnetic field strength and number of digits stimulated was noted. For both (a) and (b), individual subject mean data are shown as solid lines. See Color Figure 5.4 following page 210.

Electrophysiological recording data from a previous study describes a similar correlation between single unit responses and coherence in the preferred direction (Britten et al., 1992). Modeling indicated a simple linear relationship between single unit electrophysiological and fMRI responses with a constant of nine spikes per second per unit percent BOLD contrast.

While these types of studies are useful, they are necessarily based on assumptions that cannot be verified. For example, the observation of an increase in signal amplitude cannot be assumed to result only from an increase in extent of cortical activity. A similar activation pattern may result from an increase in the rate or the synchrony of neural activity. These assumptions are best addressed via direct comparisons.

5.2.5 COMPARING fMRI AND ELECTROPHYSIOLOGICAL RECORDING DATA

Several interesting questions regarding the BOLD signal have been addressed by combining fMRI and electrophysiologcial recording techniques in a single nonhuman primate. One of the simplest questions is how well does fMRI work. Dozens of new fMRI studies appear monthly and most are performed on a standard clinical 1.5 T magnet. While more sophisticated imaging hardware exists, it is not commonly available and the bulk of existing data has been generated at 1.5 T. Thus, it is highly relevant to compare cortical fMRI maps generated using standard clinical equipment with maps derived from electrophysiological recording, and this clearly requres a nonhuman model.

We examined this question by recording responses to simple tactile stimulation using fMRI and comparing these results to maps subsequently obtained with electrophysiological techniques in the same animals using identical stimuli (Disbrow et al., 2000). Somatosensory stimulation was used to determine the location of the

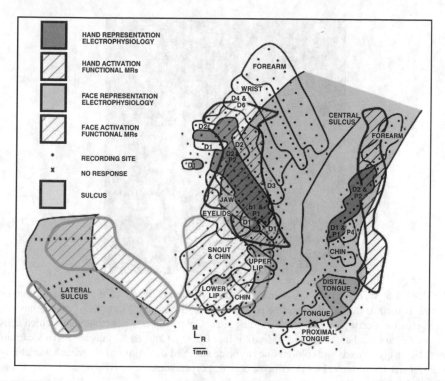

FIGURE 5.5 Correspondence between fMRI and electrophysiological maps obtained from macaque monkey cortex. Identical calibrated tactile stimuli were applied to digits or lips and tongue in both sets of experiments. Resulting maps are displayed on a flattened cortex. Dots represent recording sites in which neurons responded to tactile stimulation, Xs are sites where no response was elicited and black lines indicate borders of body part representations. In some instances, correspondence between the electrophysiological maps (solid red = hand, solid green = face) and the fMRI maps (striped red = hand, striped green = face) was good, e.g., the hand maps and one of the fMRI face maps (right). However, in 45% of the scans, the centroid of the fMRI map did not fall within the electrophysiologically defined map, as in the second face map (left). See Color Figure 5.5 following page 210.

hand and face representations in the primary somatosensory cortices of two anesthetized macaque monkeys. A concordance rate between the two sets of maps was calculated based on the location of the centroid of extended fMRI activation. If it fell within the corresponding electrophysiological map, the fMRI data were considered "concordant." Maps were concordant in 55% of the scans (Figure 5.5). This figure is somewhat lower than anticipated. Errors were predictable and related to the locations of large vessels (Figure 5.6). Thus, while resolution based on hardware capabilities is on the order of 1 to 2 mm, at 1.5 T, the resolution may be as bad as 10 mm, particularly in the planes of multiple parallel large vessels.

The most extensive examination of the relationship between the BOLD signal and the underlying electrophysiology was performed by Logothetis and colleagues (2001). They used a custom-built vertical bore 4.7 T scanner to simultaneously measure BOLD and electrophysiological responses to visual stimuli in anesthetized monkeys. The stimulus consisted of a rotating checkerboard pattern presented at a

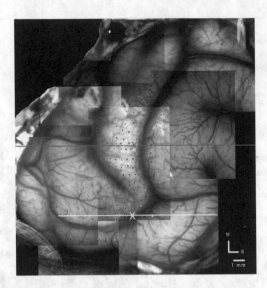

FIGURE 5.6 Variability of fMRI map location. A digital image of the macaque monkey cortex is used to display the anterior-posterior variability in the locations of map centroids. Dots indicate electrophysiological recording sites. Colors indicate penetrations in which cells responded to stimulation of the hand (red) or face (green). Colored Xs indicate mean locations of fMRI map centroids and colored lines indicate standard deviations of the means. Variability was largest in the anterior-posterior direction, perpendicular to major vessels. See Color Figure 5.6 following page 210.

variety of contrasts and a block design at several different durations. Several types of electrophysiological data were collected. They employed single unit and multiple unit recording to measure local spike activity from a population of neurons and local field potentials (LFPs) that reflect synchronized input signals of a population of neurons. The technical difficulties that needed to be overcome to perform simultaneous fMRI and electrophysiological measurements were considerable, including the design of electrophysiological recording equipment, devising a technique for compensating for interference between the two techniques, and construction of a custom vertical bore magnet.

The BOLD signal significantly correlated only with LFP data. Single and multiple unit responses showed adaptation after about 2.5 seconds of stimulus onset, while LFPs showed an increase in activation for the duration of stimulus presentation, much like the BOLD signal. Logothetis et al. concluded that the BOLD signal reflected input and local processing activity rather than output spiking activity. As in previous works (Heeger et al., 1999; Rees et al., 2000), they also found a linear relationship between the BOLD signal and the measured neural contrast response function.

5.2.6 Using Data from Monkeys to Guide Functional Imaging Studies of Cortical Organization

The monkey model is a necessary part of the examination of the relationship of functional imaging signals and underlying electrophysiology. This model can be

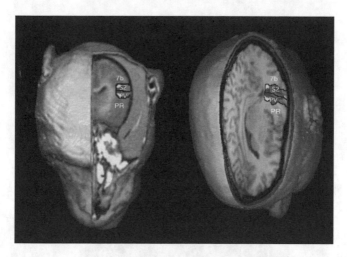

FIGURE 5.7 Schematic of the similarity of organization of higher order somatosensory cortex in the macaque monkey (left) and the human (right). Both species have mirror symmetric S2 and PV and more rostral areas (PR) and more caudal areas (7b) containing cells that respond to tactile stimulation. Macaque monkey data adapted from Krubitzer, L. et al., *J. Neurosci.*, 15, 3821, 1995. Human data adapted from Disbrow, E.A. et al., *J. Comp. Neurol.*, 418, 1, 2000b. With permission. See Color Figure 5.7 following page 210.

used to validate or verify the efficacy of a particular technique and also to guide our exploration of human brain function. Increasingly, fMRI and MEG studies in humans are based on what we learned from the large volume of existing data from monkeys obtained via invasive techniques. Examining different facets of a single question using multiple techniques is a powerful approach to the study of cortical organization and function (Figure 5.7).

A consistent feature of cortical organization is the segregation of sensory information into distinct areas. Determination of cortical areas is based on cytoarchitecture, patterns of connectivity, and neural response properties. Human data on cortical field delineation are sparse; data from monkeys are abundant. The somatosensory cortex of the macaque monkey anterior parietal lobe contains four distinct cortical areas, 3a, 3b, 1, and 2 (Kaas et al., 1979; Nelson et al., 1980; Pons et al., 1985) and each area has a complete somatotopically organized representation of the body surface. Electrophysiological recording data indicate that neurons in 3b and 1 respond to cutaneous stimulation, neurons in area 2 respond to tactile and proprioceptive stimulation, and neurons in 3a respond to proprioceptive stimulation and stimulation of deep receptors (see Kaas, 1983). To examine these regions in humans, Moore and colleagues (2000) took advantage of regional neural stimulus preferences described in monkeys to differentially activate these fields in humans. Using a 3-T scanner, they compared activation from punctate tactile input to activation from performance of a motor task.

Punctate stimulation resulted in activation of two areas of the pre- and postcentral gyri, with a distinct gap of inactivation at the fundus of the central sulcus (Figure 5.8). They concluded that the caudal area of activation on the postcentral gyrus corresponds to areas 3b, 1, and 2, while the activation located on the precentral gyrus was located

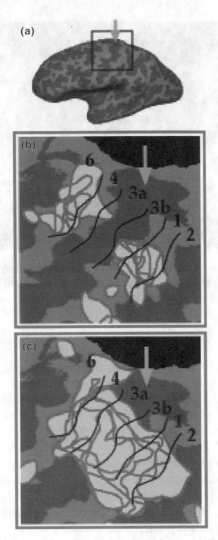

FIGURE 5.8 Activation patterns for tactile and kinesthetic/motor stimulation. (a) The location of activation in (b) and (c) shown on an inflated brain. (b) Average activation pattern from five subjects in response to tactile stimulation displayed on a flattened brain. Note the lack of activation in areas 3a and 2 and the sparse activation in motor area 4. (c) Average activation pattern for kinesthetic/motor stimulation resulting in the stimulation of deep receptors. Significant activation occurred in areas 4, 3a, and 2. See Color Figure 5.8 following page 210.

in premotor area 6. Thus, the gap at the depth of the sulcus indicates the location of area 3a, which was shown in electrophysiological recording experiments to contain neurons that respond to deep stimulation, and motor area 4. This conclusion was supported by the finding that stimulation of deep receptors via performance of a motor task produced a similar pattern of activation, with the exception that significant activation was observed at the depth of the central sulcus, presumably in areas 3a and 4.

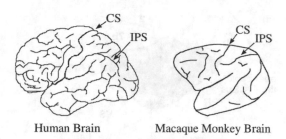

Human Brain   Macaque Monkey Brain

FIGURE 5.9 Line drawings of the human (left) and macaque monkey (right) brain (not to scale). Note the species difference in cortical structures of the central sulcus (CS) and intraparietal sulcus (IPS). The shape and location of the IPS are very different in the human. The human has additional sulci not found in the macaque.

Many similar experiments have been done to subdivide human visual cortex based on data from monkeys. For example, the extrastriate medial temporal area (MT) is well described in monkeys based on its cortical connections (Maunsel and van Essen, 1983; Krubitzer and Kaas, 1990), and direction-selective neural stimulus preferences (Britten et al., 1992). Human MT was identified with fMRI (Tootell et al., 1995) and defined as a region that responded preferentially to moving (as opposed to stationary) stimuli. Human and monkey MT were thought to be analogous. Results from a study by Heeger et al. (1999) strengthen the proposal that human MT is in fact analogous to macaque monkey MT. Their innovative study measured motion opponency in humans and monkeys using fMRI and multiple unit electrophysiological recording techniques, respectively.

Similarities of human and macaque cortical organization are informative because of the wealth of monkey data accumulated over the past 50 years. Also interesting are the differences between the two species. For example, posterior parietal cortex, or the region posterior to somatosensory area 2 and anterior to extrastriate cortex (Figure 5.9), is being studied with increasing intensity in the macaque monkey. This region is generally considered the termination of the dorsal stream for the processing of visual motion and is involved in the integration of visual and somatomotor inputs. It has been subdivided into multiple cortical fields with functions related to saccadic eye movements, attention, visually guided reaching, grasping, and tactile and visual discrimination of shapes (see Culham and Kanwisher, 2001).

While human and monkey visual area MT and somatosensory areas 3a, 3b, 1, and 2 are likely analogous, the relationship between human and monkey posterior parietal cortex is less straightforward. On visual inspection, human and monkey posterior parietal cortices are quite different anatomically. The human brain has additional sulci in this region and a different orientation to the intraparietal sulcus (Figure 5.9). In addition, while human fMRI studies of attention, saccadic eye movements, reaching, grasping, etc. reveal activation in posterior parietal cortex, statements of homology are highly speculative. It seems likely that over the course of evolution, additional cortical fields were added to the human cortex based on increased demands for manual dexterity and visuomotor integration. These species differences are exciting because they provide insight into uniquely human cortical organization and function.

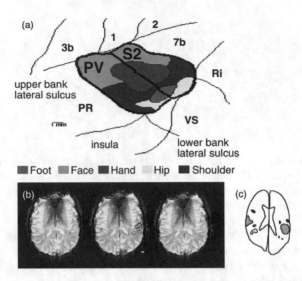

FIGURE 5.10 Somatotopic organization of S2 and PV. (a) Electrophysiological recording data from the upper bank of the lateral sulcus in the macaque monkey. S2 and PV are mirror symmetric, joined at the representations of the face hand and foot, with shoulder and hip representations flanking both sides. Adapted from Krubitzer, L. et al., *J. Neurosci.,* 15, 3821, 1995. With permission. We used this data when examining human cortex, stimulating both distal (hands and feet) and proximal (hip and shoulder) body parts. The upper bank of the Sylvian fissure also contains two fields with similar organization. (b) Three axial slices showing activation from stimulation of the foot (left, red), hand (blue, center), and face (green, right). The positions of the foot and face activation are indicated on the center (hand representation) image, showing the medial-lateral organization of human cortex. The hip and shoulder representations of S2 and PV are located on both sides. (c) Schematic of activation of stimulation of the hand. Three areas of activation were observed, S2/PV in the center (gray), PR (anterior, black) and 7b (posterior, white). Adapted from Disbrow, E.A. et al., 2000b. See Color Figure 5.10 following page 210.

A final example of fMRI studies guided by monkey work is from concurrent monkey and human studies of higher order somatosensory cortex from our laboratory. We used a combination of techniques in humans and monkeys to examine the function of the second somatosensory area (S2). Traditionally this region, located on the upper bank of the Sylvian or lateral sulcus, was thought to contain a single cortical field, S2 (Adrian, 1940; Penfield and Rasmussen, 1968) despite conflicting reports of the orientation and organization of the S2 map in the monkey and the presence of re-representations of some body parts (Whitsel et al., 1969, Robinson and Burton, 1980a and 1980b). In nonhuman primates (Krubitzer et al., 1995) and other mammals (Slutsky et al., 2000; Krubitzer et al., 1993; Krubitzer et al., 1998), extensive explorations of the upper bank of the lateral sulcus using electrophysiological recording techniques revealed two complete body surface representations. The two homunculi were mirror symmetric, joined at the representations of the lips, hands, and feet, and flanked by representations of the shoulder and hip (Figure 5.10A). The second field, in addition to S2, was termed the PV or parietal ventral area.

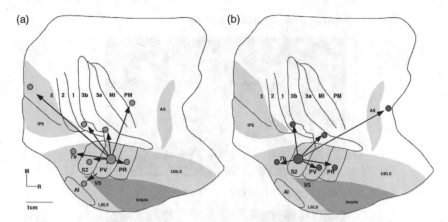

FIGURE 5.11 Schematic of cortico–cortical connections of (A) PV and (B) S2. The connections of S2 are with frontal cortex and predominantly with other somatosensory areas, while the connections of PV are with areas that process inputs from tactile and other systems, such as extrastriate cortex, premotor cortex, and the auditory belt area. Data are displayed on manually flattened macaque monkey cortex. Parts of the occipital and temporal lobes have been removed.

Based on maps of S2 and PV in the monkey, we examined human somatosensory cortex on the upper bank of the Sylvian fissure. We stimulated the lips, hands, feet, as well as the shoulders, and hips to determine whether humans had a similar mirror symmetric organization of two somatosensory cortical fields in this region. Figure 5.10B is an example of fMRI data from these experiments (Disbrow et al., 2000). Humans did indeed have S2 and PV areas with internal organizations similar to those found in monkeys. Two additional fields were observed to be activated by somatosensory stimulation in this region, one rostral and one caudal to S2/PV (Figure 5.10C). The caudal field is in the location designated 7b in the monkey, so we tentatively refer to it as human 7b. The caudal field has not been previously described in detail, and we designated it PR, the parietal rostral ventral area.

We concurrently studied the cortical connections of areas S2 and PV. We mapped these fields using electrophysiological recording techniques. We then injected fluorescent tracers, labeling cell bodies, and axon terminals in fields with connections to S2 and PV (Figure 5.11; Disbrow et al., 1998). Large patches of label were located just rostral and caudal to S2/PV, in a location similar to human PR and 7b, thus confirming the existence of these fields and their role in somatosensory processing.

PV has connections with premotor, extrastriate, and nonprimary auditory cortex, suggesting that it may be involved in sensory motor integration necessary for object exploration and identification. S2 has connections primarily with other somatosensory fields but also with frontal cortex, suggesting that it may be part of a network involved in tactile recognition and memory. Additional evidence from studies of monkeys (see Mishkin, 1979) indicates that S2 may be part of a network including the limbic system involved in tactile learning.

We designed human imaging experiments to test these hypotheses, including studies to examine the role of S2 and surrounding fields in somatomotor integration

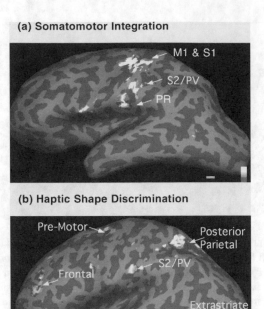

FIGURE 5.12 fMRI data from tasks based on cortico–cortical connections of S2 and PV in macaque monkeys. Because PV has connections with premotor cortex (Figure 5.11), we contrasted activation from somatosensory stimulation with activation from somatomotor stimulation (a). The large area of activation in S2/PV and PR. S2 and PV are also active during haptic shape discrimination as contrasted to a tactile/motor control condition is seen (b). See Color Figure 5.12 following page 210.

(Figure 5.12A), and tactile object identification (Figure 5.12B). We also expanded our electrophysiological and neuroanatomical experiments to include PR, 7b, and surrounding cortex, which will, in turn, help us design further human imaging studies. The interplay of results from invasive and noninvasive techniques provides unique insight into cortical organization and function. Thus, the monkey model is important for the study of the physiological basis of imaging signals and for advancing our understanding of the role of the cortex in sensory processing and cognitive function.

REFERENCES

Adrian, E.D., Double representation of the feet in the sensory cortex of the cat, *J. Physiol.*, 98, 16P, 1940.
Antognini, J.F. et al., Isoflurane anesthesia blunts cerebral responses to noxious and innocuous stimuli: a fMRI study, *Life Sci.*, 61, 349, 1997.

Archer, D.P. et al., Measurement of cerebral blood flow and volume with positron emission tomography during isoflurane administration in the hypnocapnic baboon, *Anesthesiology*, 72, 1031, 1990.

Britten, K.H. et al., The analysis of visual motion: a comparison of neuronal and psychophysical performance, *J. Neurosci.*, 12, 4745, 1992.

Cohen, M.S. and Bookheimer, S.Y., Localization of brain function using magnetic resonance imaging, *Trends Neurosci.*, 17, 268, 1994.

Culham, J.C. and Kanwisher, N.G., Neuroimaging of cognitive functions in human parietal cortex, *Curr. Opin. Neurobiol.*, 11, 163, 2001.

Disbrow, E. et al., The use of fMRI for determining the topographic organization of cortical fields in human and non-human primates, *Brain Res.*, 829, 167, 1999.

Disbrow, E.A. et al., Functional MRI at 1.5 T: a comparison of the blood oxygenation level-dependent signal and electrophysiology, *Proc. Natl. Acad. Sci. U.S.A.*, 97, 9718, 2000a.

Disbrow, E.A., Roberts, T.P.L., and Krubitzer L., Somatotopic organization of cortical fields in the lateral sulcus of *Homo sapiens*: evidence for S2 and PV, *J. Comp. Neurol.*, 418, 1, 2000b.

Disbrow, E., Slutsky, D., and Krubitzer, L., Cortical and thalamic connections of the parietal ventral area (PV) in the macaque monkey, *Soc. Neurosci. Abstr.*, 24, 130, 1998.

Dubowitz, D.J. et al., Functional magnetic resonance imaging in macaque cortex, *Neuroreport*, 9, 2213, 1998.

Dubowitz, D.J. et al., Enhancing fMRI contrast in awake-behaving primates using intravascular magnetite dextran nanoparticles, *Neuroreport*, 12, 2335, 2001.

Gallen, C.C., Hirschkoff, E.C., and Buchanan, D.S., Magnetoencephalography and magnetic source imaging: capabilities and limitations, *Neuroimaging Clin. N. Am.*, 5, 227, 1995.

Gazzaniga, M.S., Ivry, R.B., and Mangun, G.R., *Cognitive Neuroscience: The Biology of the Mind*, W.W. Norton, New York, 2002.

Hamalainen, M. et al., Magnetoencephalography: theory, instrumentation, and applications to noninvasive studies of the working human brain. *Rev. Mod. Physics*, 65, 413, 1993.

Hayashi, T. et al., Mapping of somatosensory cortices with functional magnetic resonance imaging in anaesthetized macaque monkeys, *Eur. J. Neurosci.*, 11, 4451, 1999.

Heeger, D.J. et al., Motion opponency in visual cortex, *J. Neurosci.*, 109, 7162–74, 1999.

Kaas, J.H. et al., Multiple representations of the body within the primary somatosensory cortex of primates, *Science*, 204, 521, 1979.

Kaas, J.H., What, if anything, is S1? Organization of first somatosensory area of cortex, *Physiol. Rev.*, 63, 206, 1983.

Krubitzer, L. et al., Interhemispheric connections of somatosensory cortex in the flying fox, *J. Comp. Neurol.*, 402, 538, 1998.

Krubitzer, L. et al., A redefinition of somatosensory areas in the lateral sulcus of macaque monkeys, *J. Neurosci.*, 15, 3821, 1995.

Krubitzer, L.A. and Kaas, J.H., Cortical connections of MT in four species of primates: areal, modular, and retinotopic patterns, *Vis. Neurosci.*, 5, 165, 1990.

Krubitzer, L.A., Calford, M.B., and Schmid, L.M., Connections of somatosensory cortex in megachiropteran bats: the evolution of cortical fields in mammals, *J. Comp. Neurol.*, 327, 473, 1993.

Logothetis, N.K. et al., Functional imaging of the monkey brain, *Nature Neurosci.*, 2, 555, 1999.

Logothetis, N.K. et al., Neurophysiological investigation of the basis of the fMRI signal, *Nature*, 12, 150, 2001.

Maunsel, J.H. and van Essen, D.C., The connections of the middle temporal visual area (MT) and their relationship to a cortical hierarchy in the macaque monkey, *J. Neurosci.*, 3, 2563, 1983.

Mishkin, M., Analogous neural models for tactual and visual learning, *Neuropsychologia*, 17, 139, 1979.

Moore, C.I. et al., Segregation of somatosensory activation in the human rolandic cortex using fMRI, *J. Neurophysiol.*, 84, 558, 2000.

Nelson, R.J. et al., Representations of the body surface in postcentral parietal cortex of *Macaca fascicularis*, *J. Comp. Neurol.*, 192, 611, 1980.

Ogawa, S. et al., Brain magnetic resonance imaging with contrast dependent on blood oxygenation, *Proc. Natl. Acad. Sci. U.S.A.*, 87, 9868, 1990.

Penfield, W. and Rasmussen, T., *The Cerebral Cortex of Man: A Clinical Study of Localization of Function*, Hafner Publishing, New York, 1968.

Perlmutter, J.S. et al., PET measured evoked cerebral blood flow responses in an awake monkey, *J. Cereb. Blood Flow Metabol.*, 11, 229, 1991.

Pons, T.P. et al., The somatotopic organization of area 2 in macaque monkeys, *J. Comp. Neurol.*, 241, 445, 1985.

Posner, M.I. and Raichle, M.E., The neuroimaging of human brain function, *Proc. Natl. Acad. Sci. U.S.A.*, 95, 763, 1998.

Rees, G., Friston, K., and Koch, C., A direct quantitative relationship between the fucntional properties of human and macaque V5. *Nature Neurosci.*, 3, 716, 2000.

Robinson, C.J. and Burton, H., Organization of somatosensory receptive fields in cortical areas 7b, retroinsula, postauditory, and granular insula of *M. fascicularis*, *J. Comp. Neurol.*, 192, 69, 1980a.

Robinson, C.J. and Burton, H., Somatotopographic organization in the second somatosensory area of *M. fascicularis*, *J. Comp. Neurol.*, 192, 43, 1980b.

Roberts, T.P.L. et al., Quantification and reproducibility of tracking cortical extent of activation by use of functional MR imaging and magnetoencephalography, *Am. J. Neuroradiol.*, 21, 1377, 2000.

Slutsky, D.A., Manger, P.R., and Krubitzer, L., Multiple somatosensory areas in the anterior parietal cortex of the California ground squirrel (*Spermophilus beecheyii*), *J. Comp. Neurol.*, 416, 521, 2000.

Stefanacci, L. et al., fMRI of monkey visual cortex, *Neuron*, 20, 1051, 1998.

Teale, P. et al., Magnetic auditory source imaging in macaque monkey, *Brain Res. Bull.*, 33(5), 615, 1994.

Tootell, R.B. et al., Functional analysis of human MT and related visual cortical areas using magnetic resonance imaging, *J. Neurosci.*, 15, 3215, 1995.

Vanduffel, W. et al., Visual motion processing investigated using contrast agent-enhanced fMRI in awake behaving monkeys, *Neuron*, 32(4), 565, 2001.

Whitsel, B.L., Pertrucelli, L.M., and Werner, G., Symmetry and connectivity in the map of the body surface in somatosensory area II of primates, *J. Neurophysiol.*, 32, 170, 1969.

Wikstrom, H. et al., Effects of interstimulus interval on somatosensory evoked magnetic fields (SEFs): a hypothesis concerning SEF generation at the primary sensorimotor cortex, *Electroencephalogr. Clin. Neurophysiol.*, 100, 479, 1996.

Wu, J. and Okada, Y.C., Physiological bases of the synchronized population spikes and slow wave of the magnetic field generated by a guinea-pig longitudinal CA3 slice preparation *Electroencephalogr. Clin. Neurophysiol.*, 107, 361, 1998.

6 Pharmacologic Magnetic Resonance Imaging (phMRI)

Bruce G. Jenkins, Yin-Ching Iris Chen,
and Joseph B. Mandeville

CONTENTS

0-8493-0122-X/03/$0.00+$1.50
© 2003 by CRC Press LLC

6.1 INTRODUCTION

6.1.1 OVERVIEW

The technique of functional magnetic resonance imaging (fMRI) using relative cerebral blood volume (rCBV), blood oxygenation level-dependent (BOLD), and T_1-based cerebral blood flow (CBF) techniques led to a revolution in brain mapping.[1-3] These techniques are based on the coupling of neuronal activity, metabolism, and hemodynamics (discussed further in Chapters 4 and 5) leading to changes in signal intensity sensitive to these parameters. Similar studies were performed with positron emission tomography (PET) as discussed in Chapter 9.

The possibility that fMRI may help us understand the organization and flow of information in the brain generated great excitement. The past few years have witnessed an explosion in the number of facilities dedicated to performing fMRI. In addition to the interest in fMRI from the neuroscience community, clinical medicine may benefit from the development of fMRI techniques such as perfusion studies of stroke, presurgical planning for conservation of eloquent cortex during brain surgery, and investigation of motor systems in movement disorders. Most fMRI studies used task activation such as photic stimulation or finger movements or cognitive challenge to induce neuronal activity. However it is also possible to elicit neuronal activity with pharmacologic ligands, and this technique may allow us to generate maps of the metabolic consequences of receptor stimulation of relevance to a large number of cerebral disorders.

Studies of receptor binding can be performed *in vivo* using PET imaging or performed *postmortem* using autoradiography. These techniques use direct agonists or antagonists to map out the receptor binding parameters or density of these sites in the brain. Such studies are currently of diagnostic value for examination of dopamine receptor depletion in Parkinson's disease (PD) and have great potential for studying drug abuse and schizophrenia.

Autoradiographic and PET studies have also examined metabolic changes (blood flow and glucose utilization) after neurotransmitter stimulation using, for example, amphetamine.[4] fMRI is well suited to study these metabolic changes.[5] Early reports of the use of MRI to study the acute effects of amphetamine,[5-7] cocaine and cocaine analogs,[5,8,9] apomorphine or L-dopa,[10-12] nicotine,[13] heroin,[14] and serotonin ligands[15] have already appeared. Nonetheless, a number of issues render interpretation of the induced signal changes more difficult than in conventional task-related fMRI. Because drugs are used as the stimuli of interest and can exert effects very different from functional activation tasks, we coined the term pharmacologic MRI (*phMRI*) to describe these experiments.[5]

Unlike conventional task-related fMRI studies that allow time courses of the stimuli to be controlled at will, the time course of phMRI is determined by the pharmacodynamic profile of the drug administered to induce the signal changes. Since most drugs can be anticipated to have rather long time courses compared to task-related stimuli (several minutes or more compared to seconds for conventional fMRI), data collection and analysis schemes become important for accurate determination of metabolically induced signal changes after pharmacologic stimulus. Some of the approaches to this problem will be discussed in Section 6.2.

The first of two types of phMRI is the technique discussed in the papers cited above. This method is most often used in drug challenge studies in which MR signal changes are monitored after acute administration of the drug of interest. Clearly, the basic model has many permutations including antagonism of the effects of one drug with another or examining the acute effects of one drug on the chronic effects of another (useful perhaps for studying cocaine addiction). The second type of phMRI is the observation of the modulatory effects of a pharmaceutical on a conventional task-related fMRI study, for example, to determine the effects of D2 agonists upon cognitive tasks.[16] This type of study will be considered for the purposes of this chapter as a variation on conventional fMRI and is covered in more detail in Chapters 4 and 5. The effects of such drug administration must be kept in mind in the course of interpreting the hemodynamic changes because the drug itself may exert modulatory effects on the hemodynamics. We will now compare the possibilities of studying neuroreceptors using MRI techniques with the more traditional techniques such as PET and autoradiography.

6.1.2 COMPARISON OF PHMRI, PET, AND AUTORADIOGRAPHY

For those accustomed to studying neuroreceptors using PET or autoradiography, the possibility of measuring specific receptor parameters based on simple hemodynamic changes seems remote. At best, one might hope to verify the assumption that the hemodynamic changes observed after administration of a particular drug correlate with the activation of the receptor systems targeted by the drug; and seek a pharmacologically induced "metabolic" coupling entirely analogous to the metabolic coupling usually assumed in standard fMRI studies. Such correlations can be made empirically using techniques capable of measuring receptor binding, receptor distribution, and the attendant metabolic circuitry.

These in turn can be correlated with electrophysiologic data and companion metabolic studies. Such correlations might entail measuring BOLD signal changes and correlating them with changes in the cerebral metabolic rate of glucose utilization (CMRglc), evoked potentials, and perhaps even EEG or magnetoencephalography (MEG) data. In such a manner one can painstakingly verify which correlations determine BOLD signal, knowing that we all stand on firmer ground when trying to interpret BOLD signal changes. Such studies are now under way in many laboratories around the world.

Monitoring hemodynamic changes after administration of a drug will lead to three obvious general outcomes. First, one may obtain no response or correlation whatsoever with other measured parameters. The only conclusion to be drawn in that case is that a drug targeted toward a specific receptor has no hemodynamic effect. This does not mean that it has no behavioral or metabolic effect, for example, the vasodilatory and vasoconstrictive properties of the drugs may cancel one another. The second possible outcome is a hemodynamic effect that is measurable but does not correlate with any obvious pattern of receptors. Another is that the targeted receptors have such a widespread distribution that distinguishing nonspecific from specific effects is quite difficult. We have observed such effects with caffeine and theophylline. Activation (more precisely, negative rCBV change) was seen over almost the entire brain, mirroring the distribution of adenosine A1 receptors. A variation on this basic scenario is that the hemodynamic effects resulting from administration of the drug are complicated enough that specific correlation with a receptor system is not possible. In this regard, a phMRI study can be anticipated to mirror a PET measurement of glucose utilization or CBF. This situation is encountered in almost every fMRI study. The neurovascular coupling serves as a type of "black box" and the interpretation of the hemodynamic patterns is anatomic or contextual in nature. The third and most satisfactory possibility is a very good correlation between the hemodynamic changes induced by the drug and a given receptor distribution. This situation is most likely when the administered drug causes release of a vasoactive molecule reflective of the targeted receptor system or when the pattern of vascular targets is reflective of the receptor targets in the brain tissue.

The probability of any one of these scenarios occurring alone is less likely than not, but one may get closer or further to any of these three extremes. We will examine the three possibilities discussed above in much more detail later. But in this section we will compare PET, autoradiography, and phMRI assuming that phMRI studies are useful for examining neuroreceptors. Shown in Table 6.1 is a comparison of PET and MRI with the relative advantages and disadvantages of each considering the types of information that can be obtained from the techniques and issues related to the data collection. As shown in Table 6.1, PET can examine both the metabolic response to neuronal stimulation (usually performed using measures of glucose accumulation with ^{18}F-fluorodeoxyglucose or CBF using ^{15}O-labeled water) as well as the direct binding of the compound to its targets. PET has the added advantage of utilizing either tracer-level doses of the ligand or can examine the metabolic coupling evoked by behaviorally-relevant doses as MRI can. MRI is better, in general, at examining the hemodynamic changes possessing superior temporal resolution and spatial resolution if one considers the BOLD effect (the relative advantages of CBF measurements are more murky given the low sensitivity of arterial spin-labeling). MRI is also better at examining changes in rCBV. PET is obviously superior at examining changes in glucose utilization, although this can be examined using MR spectroscopy (both ^{13}C and proton spectroscopy of the glucose peak at 5.23 ppm) with its inferior spatial and temporal resolution compared to PET. The superior temporal sampling characteristics of MR in general, make examination of

TABLE 6.1

Comparisons of PET and phMRI: Complementary Techniques

Parameter	phMRI	PET
In-plane spatial resolution	0.25–3 mm	1.5–12 mm
Direct drug binding	No	Yes
Metabolic coupling	rCMRO$_2$, rCBV, CBF	rCMRglc, rCMRO$_2$, CBF
Drug time course (hemodynamic)	Yes	No
Drug time course (binding)	Maybe	Yes
Multiple studies	Yes	Sometimes
Tracer level doses	No	Yes
Behaviorally relevant doses	Yes	Yes

drug time courses more flexible than with PET, though both techniques are clearly useful.

Using PET imaging to examine receptor populations requires administration of drugs that bind specifically to a given receptor population. Data interpretation is not as straightforward as might be anticipated. A complicated multicompartmental model is derived with compartments for the free, specifically bound, nonspecifically bound, and plasma components with transfer coefficients for the compartments as shown in Figure 6.1. To render so many parameters experimentally tractable, a number of assumptions are made. For instance, in the case of dopamine receptors, it is usually assumed that the cerebellar time activity curves represent only the nonspecifically bound compound and that the specifically bound curves in other brain regions such as striatum can be fitted using parameters for the plasma, transfer coefficients, and nonspecifically bound compartments derived from the cerebellar curves. We will demonstrate the possibility for determining such parameters from phMRI data sets in favorable circumstances.

The obvious advantage to MRI of having no requirement for radioactivity (or a cyclotron or PET scanner, both of which are less available than MR machines) is that repeated studies of the same subject are more feasible. Nonetheless, it is better to characterize PET and MR as complementary techniques that have much to offer in studies of pharmaceutical interactions.

Autoradiographic techniques have the obvious "terminal" barrier to overcome. Autoradiography can measure the full complement of parameters measurable by PET and can also examine mRNA expression levels, receptor protein levels, and direct ligand binding to the receptors. The large array of parameters that can be examined with autoradiography make it an attractive complement to PET or phMRI. Interestingly, in discrete brain regions, a direct relationship between mRNA expression levels and ligand binding or protein expression levels is not always found.[17–19] This means that selection of a "gold standard" for comparison of a phMRI or PET activation pattern can be problematic. Also, because phMRI is in its infancy, the empirical determination of patterns of activity that can be observed after administration of various drugs is a work in progress and will likely be very different for different classes of drugs targeted toward various neurotransmitter systems.

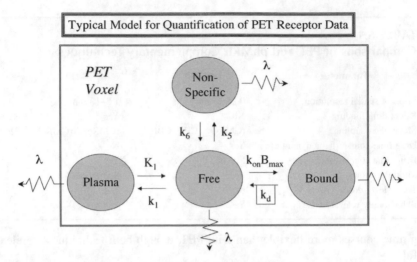

FIGURE 6.1 Schematic of data from a PET study. Rate constants are determined by fitting time activity curves corrected for both arterial input function and radioactive decay (λ). The cerebellum is often used to provide a measure of nonspecific binding parameters for studying dopaminergic drugs. The B_{max} is the total number of receptors. The k's represent transfer coefficients and rate constants for binding to the receptor.

We will consider specific correlations between receptor densities measured with PET or autoradiography and those determined by phMRI. As an introduction, let us examine a hypothetical phMRI procedure following injection of drug X targeted toward the dopaminergic system. Obviously, the first step is to determine the regional pattern of hemodynamic changes elicited by the drug. For the dopaminergic system, the drug might be an agonist or antagonist of a specific dopamine receptor subtype. It might also be a compound targeted toward the dopamine transporter. If the drug produced a hemodynamic consequence (not a foregone conclusion), the spatial pattern of hemodynamic changes it induced can be compared with a number of autoradiographic parameters. Is the pattern similar to that of receptor mRNA expression levels? Is it similar to the pattern of drug binding measured autoradiographically? Is it similar to the immunohistochemical distribution of receptor proteins? Is it similar to the pattern of CMRglc induced around the brain? These are good questions, and in an ideal animal study, they could be addressed but, as yet, no such study has been performed. It is not as easy to perform such studies on postmortem human tissue, but we can examine PET data for both CMRglc and direct drug binding. No one has performed such a study.

Histologic and autoradiographic studies produce exquisite spatial resolution, but quantitative measurements of mRNA expression and protein levels can be problematic. Quantitative studies such as CBF with iodoantipyrene and CMRglc attempt to take a metabolic snapshot by allowing enough time for accumulation of labeled compound (the required time for glucose can be 45 minutes) in a system where the metabolic parameters may change dynamically. This may account for the differences between phMRI and autoradiographic measurements of CMRglc.

6.1.3 Neurovascular Coupling

Changes in neuronal activity have long been known to lead to changes in metabolic activity. The mechanisms of the coupling of metabolic and hemodynamic changes and the locations where these changes occur are the subjects of intense research. Most of the existing data and models were developed to describe changes in cortical glutamatergic neuronal systems.

Many of the unifying principles of the glutamatergic system may not be universal across neurotransmitter systems. One example is that the reuptake of glutamate released during firing occurs through astrocytes. In the dopaminergic system, most reuptake occurs at the presynaptic neuron, so the coupling mechanisms of these systems may well be different.

The concept of increases in neuronal activity coupling to increased metabolic and hemodynamic changes goes back over 100 years to the pioneering work of Roy and Sherrington who postulated a coupling between brain activity and blood flow. More recently, much work has gone into developing models of what happens during firing of a glutamatergic neuron. Most of the work focused on what happens to glucose metabolism as a surrogate marker for neuronal activity. Early work investigated the subcellular distribution of glycolytic enzymes and led to the conclusion that much of the glycolytic apparatus is localized in nerve terminals rather than in cell bodies.[20–22] This work was followed by experiments of Sokoloff and others showing that the localization of increased glucose utilization during neuronal activity was in the terminal regions rather than in the perikarya.[23–25]

These early experiments led to the paradigm most elegantly articulated by Magistretti and Pellerin[26–28] and supported by others[29] in which a cycle of glutamate release from the presynaptic terminal is followed by reuptake of the synaptic glutamate by the astrocyte. The glutamate is then converted into glutamine and lactate is also produced for transport back to the neuron to use as a fuel. This model makes two important predictions: (1) since transport of glutamate (along with Na^+) into the glia is fueled by $Na^+K^+ATPase$ and the neurons consume lactate, most of the glucose utilization must happen in the glial cells and not the neurons and (2) this model predicts, consistent with the experimental data, that most increased glucose utilization happens at the synaptic level. Much of the increased glucose utilization cannot be defined as pre- or postsynaptic because it occurs in the glia. The simplified story to emerge from these results is that increased metabolic response happens at the level of the synapse rather than at the cell bodies. The question of how increased glucose consumption at the astrocyte is coupled to an increase in CBF is still unknown. Uptake of glutamate through astrocytes has been shown to be coupled *in vitro* to release of vasoactive molecules such as arachidonic acid and vasoactive intestinal peptide.[30,31] What happens *in vivo* is not known.

This principle will not necessarily generalize to other neurotransmitter systems such as the dopaminergic for the simple reason that most dopamine reuptake occurs on the presynaptic side of the dopamine neuron via dopamine transporter protein (DAT). This system is reviewed in Cooper et al.[32] The control of dopamine synthesis and uptake is, to a large degree, controlled by presynaptic D2 autoreceptors that are more sensitive than postsynaptic dopamine receptors to the effects of dopamine and apomorphine. These data seem to suggest that the metabolic changes are mediated via the presynaptic dopamine neurons. We investigated this hypothesis using unilateral lesioning of the nigrostriatal dopamine tracts and 6-hydroxydopamine.[5] The hemodynamic changes induced by amphetamine or CFT were ablated by the presynaptic lesioning, and this was consistent with PET data from the same animals.

These data were also consistent with prior 2-deoxyglucose autoradiographic measurements of glucose utilization rates after stimulation with either amphetamine or cocaine in the same lesion model.[33,34] Nonetheless, these experiments do not prove that the hemodynamic response is driven presynaptically because the experiments also destroyed the ability of the neurons to synthesize dopamine. Whether metabolic changes are induced at the presynaptic neurons or derive from astrocytes, the important question related to understanding neurovascular coupling in a quantitative manner is which molecules actually mediate the coupling between neurotransmitter reuptake, metabolic change, and a change in hemodynamics.

One confound to completely dissecting neurovascular coupling is that most neurotransmitters are also vasoactive. Many neurotransmitters have receptors on the vasculature. Several different brain neurotransmitters have axonal projections to the microcirculature in many brain regions. Many amino acid neurotransmitters, in particular glutamate, appear to couple to changes in blood flow via nitric oxide (NO).[35–37] As discussed earlier, this coupling is thought to arise at the astrocyte level. Serotonin took its name because it is a potent vasoconstrictor — a fact discovered before its role as a neurotransmitter was known.[38] Acetylcholine also has vasoactive properties.[39] A coupling of cholinergic M5 receptors on the vasculature apposed to NO neurons (which are vasodilatory) in the basal forebrain provides control of cerebral microcirculation.[40,41] Confounding the neurovascular coupling is the fact that cholinergic activation of the substantia innominata (SI) leads to increased CBF in the absence of increases in glucose utilization.[42] Strong histological evidence indicates that dopamine neurons are intimately associated with microvasculature in brain parenchyma.[43,44] It has recently been suggested on the basis of such data that much of the hemodynamic change observed in neuronal activation may be dopaminergic in origin.[45]

A study by Krimer et al.[45] showed direct immunocytochemical evidence for termination of central dopaminergic neurons on penetrating arterioles and the pericytes of capillaries. The pericytes are the contractile motors that regulate capillary flow. The highest density of dopaminergic innervation of these microvessels was in areas of cortex known to be high in dopaminergic innervation in the parenchyma, for example, the frontal cortex. Thus, control of microvascular flow via dopamine release is certainly important in regulating changes induced by dopaminergic drugs. Dopammine is vasoactive in many other areas of the body. Adenosine is another neurotransmitter whose vasoactive properties are well known — especially in the heart. Adenosine antagonists such as caffeine and theophylline can increase energy metabolism and decrease CBF at the same time.[46] The list of vasoactive molecules in the brain also includes many important neuropeptides.[47]

Table 6.2 lists neurotransmitter systems amenable to analysis using phMRI based on their known activation of CBF, common drugs, and disease states relevant to those molecules. A wide array of molecules appear amenable to analysis. This does

TABLE 6.2
Neurotransmitter Systems Amenable to phMRI Analysis

System	Clinical Targets	Common Drugs with phMRI Potential
Glutamatergic	Drug abuse, schizophrenia	Ketamine, phencyclidine (PCP)
Dopaminergic	Drug abuse, schirophrenia, Parkinson's disease	Cocaine, amphetamine, L-dopa, apomorphine, haldol
Cholinergic	Alzheimer's disease, cigarette addiction	Nicotine, scopolamine, tacrine
Opioid	Drug abuse, pain research	Fentanyl, morphine
GABAergic	Epilepsy, anxiety	Vigabatrin, flumazenil, diazepam
Serotinergic	Drug abuse, sleep disorders	2-Bromo-LSD, MDMA (ecstasy)
Adenosinergic	Neurodegeneration, coffee and tea consumption	Caffeine, theophylline

not, however, guarantee that all molecules targeted to a given neurotransmitter system may have vasoactive properties. Isolating the neurovascular coupling interactions in the face of such a daunting array of vasoactive molecules can be complicated. In the case of stimuli that may ultimately drive different brain regions, it is likely that numerous neurotransmitters may be involved in coupling metabolic changes to increases in CBF. phMRI may be a very good way to isolate some of these interactions and coupling relationships.

Our laboratory has collected a great deal of data on the dopaminergic system that may be of interest because it is quite different from the cortical glutamatergic and GABAergic systems usually examined in most fMRI studies. It has long been known that dopaminergic ligands can increase CBF. Measurement of CBF using autoradiography after amphetamine stimulus showed regionally specific increases in dopamine-rich brain areas.[4] Increases in cerebral glucose utilization rates after dopaminergic stimulus are also found in similar brain regions.[4,48–50] It is not surprising that MRI techniques sensitive to hemodynamics can measure changes due to stimulation with amphetamine or cocaine. One question that naturally arises is what agents and synaptic activities actually mediate the coupling between the receptor activation and blood flow? Obviously, the question is complicated. It has not been completely answered for any of the phenomena that modulate cerebral hemodynamics such as hypercapnia, hypoxia, or neuronal activation. Nonetheless, great strides have been made in this direction.

Consider the events that may occur after stimulation of the dopaminergic system using substances such as amphetamine or cocaine. Amphetamine has a two-fold mechanism. First, it reverses the dopamine transporter protein to provide reverse transport of the dopamine from the presynaptic neuron to the synaptic cleft.[51] Second, it apparently can render the vesicular environment alkaline to enhance vesicular release of dopamine and reverse transport.[52] Cocaine is a member of a family of drugs (including nomifensene and methylphenidate) that block the dopamine transporter (DAT), thus blocking reuptake of dopamine. The product of these two mechanisms is an increase in synaptic dopamine concentrations. As the dopamine concentration increases, the dopamine diffuses both across the synapse and away from the synapse.

Since we have evidence of dopamine receptors on the vasculature, it is reasonable to assume that some dopamine will directly affect the vessels. In addition, the postsynaptic dopamine neurons will be stimulated. These neurons control afferent output via the striatum and globus pallidus to the thalamus and hence to cortex. In addition to the effects of dopamine released directly upon the vasculature, dopamine has the potential to produce downstream effects in areas it metabolically activates. Since reuptake of dopamine, like uptake of glutamate, is coupled to energy demands mediated by $Na^+K^+ATPase$, changes in metabolism may also lead to further hemodynamic changes at the presynaptic dopamine neurons. Changes in hemodynamics elicited in the downstream areas are likely to be coupled via other vasoactive substances. These two perspectives are illustrated as follows:

Mechanism I: Drug $\rightarrow \Delta DA \rightarrow \Delta CBV$

Mechanism II: Drug $\rightarrow \Delta DA \rightarrow \Delta$Metabolism $\rightarrow \Delta$Substance X $\rightarrow \Delta CBV$

It is likely that a combination of these mechanisms is operative with a relative weighting determined by the brain region and local conditions. Separation of vascular from metabolic effects may be analyzed by using phMRI to obtain hemodynamic effects and PET or autoradiography of glucose utilization to determine metabolic changes. Such comparisons may be difficult to make based on the different time courses of the techniques.

Figure 6.2 is a simple diagram of the perspective we believe is reasonable with regard to regulation of blood flow or volume in the brain. It shows the baseline state in which vascular volume and flow are under the control of any number of vasoactive molecules (some vasoconstrictive and some vasodilatory). After administration of a drug such as amphetamine, the dopamine concentration increases to the point where dopamine is the "biggest hammer" and drives a vasodilatory response, thereby increasing CBV, CBF, and the BOLD effect.

Interestingly, this type of model allows for the fact that other substances might antagonize the CBV effects of amphetamine, without actually changing the dopaminergic neurotransmission. We hypothesized earlier that dopamine may drive hemodynamic changes based on the strong temporal correlation between the time course of the dopamine release measured by microdialysis and the changes in BOLD or rCBV. Figure 6.3 shows such a correlation. It shows the time course of dopamine release after administration of 2 mg/kg amphetamine to a halothane-anesthetized animal and the time course of rCBV changes in a different animal. The phMRI data was set to have the same temporal resolution of the microdialysis (10 min).

Detailed study of stimulation of neurotransmission, however, quickly leads to the conclusion that no neurotransmitter is alone. Many neurotransmitters in a given brain region are coupled. Increasing the level of stimulation to one leads to reciprocal changes in the coupled system to maintain homeostasis. As an example, we will examine the interactions of the dopaminergic and adenosinergic systems in the brain.

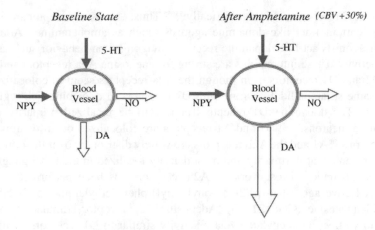

FIGURE 6.2 Illustration of a plausible situation for hemodynamic changes. In this model many vasoactive substances control baseline flow. A large increase in one of the molecules (in this case dopamine) may be responsible for driving hemodynamic change due to administration of a drug like amphetamine.

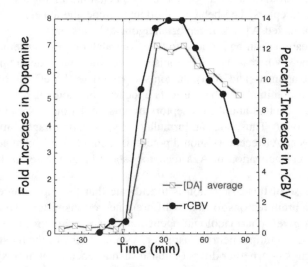

FIGURE 6.3 Comparison of microdialysis data from dorsal lateral striatum and percent change in rCBV in the same region in another rat after administration of 2 mg/kg amphetamine. Both data sets were collected under 1% halothane anesthesia. The time courses are nearly identical except for a reproducible earlier rise in rCBV.

A large body of literature exists on interactions of dopamine and glutamate, dopamine and serotonin, and dopamine and GABA.

Although the dopamine–adenosine story is not concluded, the considerable literature and experimental findings paint a fairly consistent picture of the importance of interactions of adenosine and dopamine in regulation of dopaminergic tone. It is clear from pharmacological and behavioral studies that dopamine receptors and adenosine A2 receptors act antagonistically.[53–55] Thus, adenosine receptor antagonists (such as caffeine) act like dopamine agonists (such as amphetamine). Adenosine receptor agonists act like dopamine receptor antagonists on behavior such as locomotor activity. These interactions are strong for adenosine A2a receptors and dopamine D2 and D1 receptors even though the A2a receptors seem to colocalize only on the same striatopallidal neurons with D2 receptors in dopamine-rich regions of the brain. The dopamine D1 receptors appear to be localized primarily on the striatonigral neurons.[56–58] D1 and A1 receptors are colocalized on strioentopenduncular neurons.[59] A1 and the A2b receptors are widely distributed over the brain while the A2a receptors are primarily and most densely localized in the basal ganglia and olfactory tubercule.[55] Most work on A2a receptors has been performed with the potent, selective agonist 2-[p-(2-carbonyl-ethyl)-phenylethylamino]-5′-N-ethylcarboxamidoadenosine (CGS 21680). Adenosine A2a receptor stimulation exerts a stimulatory effect on adenylate cyclase activity similar to D1 receptors, while adenosine A1 receptors cause inhibitory effects on adenylate cyclase activity similar to dopamine D2 receptors. The vasodilatory effects of adenosine are well known, and adenosine antagonists such as caffeine are vasoconstrictive.

Thus, it is not unlikely to expect that hemodynamic changes observed after dopaminergic stimulation with cocaine or amphetamine might also be modulated by adenosine receptors. The behavioral effects of cocaine appear to be potentiated by caffeine, a mixed A1, A2 receptor antagonist.[60] Rats unilaterally lesioned with 6-hydroxydopamine can be induced to turn contralaterally by systemic administration of caffeine,[61] whereas the A2a agonists reduce the contralateral turning induced by D2 or D1 agonists and A2a antagonists potentiate the effects of D1 and D2 agonists in these animals.[62] These effects appear to be modulated via the opposing effects of D2 receptors and A2a receptors upon stimulation-evoked GABA release of striatal neurons.[63] Thus, one can formulate a hypothesis: antagonism of adenosine A2a or adenosine A1 receptors should potentiate hemodynamic changes induced by cocaine, whereas activation of A2a receptors should antagonize the hemodynamic effects of cocaine.

The purpose of this discussion is to indicate that these phenomena are likely to be found in brain regions for many different neurotransmitters. Thus, the administration of a given pharmacologic agent may have to be considered in light of interactions with multiple neurotransmitter systems. Many of the most behaviorally efficacious drugs — whether drugs of abuse such as cocaine or antipsychotics such as clozapine — target multiple neurotransmitter systems. Cocaine clearly blocks the serotonin and dopamine transporters. Clozapine may be one of the "dirtiest" drugs ever studied because of its activities at multiple serotonin receptors, dopamine D4 receptors, and adrenergic receptors. One must interpret potential phMRI data with an eye to conservative interpretation of the data, especially in human studies in which separation of all the competing hemodynamic interactions is not likely possible. Those conducting animal studies have no excuse for such a lack of thoroughness.

6.2 METHODOLOGIES

6.2.1 MAGNETIC RESONANCE TECHNIQUES FOR COLLECTING HEMODYNAMIC DATA

This section will discuss various techniques in the order of increasing contrast-to-noise ratios (CNRs). The CNR is a logical way to describe the relative merits or demerits of functional and pharmacological MRI due to the relatively low sensitivities of these techniques in general. Thus, sensitivity becomes a logical criterion by which to arrange the techniques. Brief descriptions of the major MR methods follow. They are arranged in the order of increasing CNRs used to follow changes in brain activity as a result of task or pharmacologic stimulation. These techniques are all based on hemodynamic metrics. Section 6.2.2 will describe a few nonhemodynamic techniques.

6.2.1.1 The Original Technique: First Pass Bolus Mapping of Changes in rCBV

The first functional magnetic resonance images were collected by Belliveau and colleagues at Massachusetts General Hospital in 1989 and 1990 and published in 1991.[1] They chose to use a technique pioneered at Massachusetts General[64] involving intravenous administration of a bolus of paramagnetically labeled salt, Gd(DTPA).[2-] This technique allows measurement of relative cerebral blood volume (rCBV) based on the retention of the contrast agent in the intravascular space. Because the contrast agent is chosen for its high magnetic susceptibility, large gradients are induced between the blood and brain tissue. These gradients spread out far beyond the actual spatial volume distribution of the blood vessels. They in turn decrease the T_2^* relaxation rates of the water spins that diffuse through the gradients, thereby affecting a relatively large proportion of the total water signal (in excess of the cerebral blood volume or CBV). This renders the technique more sensitive than it might otherwise be, but at a cost of only being able to measure the relative rather than absolute CBV.

At common concentrations of agents with common imaging parameters, the total signal loss observed as the bolus passes through the brain can be as high as 100%. The signal rapidly returns to baseline. Standard tracer kinetic analyses can be applied to the signal to derive parameters related to cerebral hemodynamics. The area under the curve is roughly proportional to CBV; the peak drop is roughly proportional to CBF. The main limitations of this technique are two-fold. First is the requirement to inject at least two doses of contrast agent (before and after stimulus). Even though Gd(DTPA)[2-] is nontoxic, it still carries minimal risk. Second, in order to collect multiple time points, multiple injections are required. This quickly becomes prohibitive and dramatically limits the statistical power of the technique. Since the technique is no longer used for functional imaging experiments, we will not consider it further. Interested readers can get further details from the original reports[1,65] The technique is still widely used for measuring hemodynamic parameters for stroke and tumor patients in clinical settings.

6.2.1.2 CBF-Based Techniques

The early brain functional imaging experiments using PET/SPECT methods were based on increases in CBF[66] or glucose utilization.[67–69] CMRglc is likely to be a more direct marker of synaptic activity than techniques based on hemodynamics. Nonetheless, a number of studies indicated relatively tight couplings between increases in CMRglc and CBF during neuronal activation.[70–73] Thus, CBF appears a logical choice for MR studies of brain function given the limitations of measuring glucose utilization with MR.

A number of techniques have evolved to measure changes in absolute and relative CBF. These techniques became a veritable "alphabet soup" of acronyms, but they all rely on changes of apparent longitudinal relaxation time (T_1) by blood spins flowing into voxels, based on the fact that they have attained different saturation levels compared to the intravoxel spins. In principle, all these methods are similar to other tracer kinetic methodologies that appeared over the years. In this case, instead of diffusion of a labeled substance such as iodoantipyrene used in autoradiographic measurements of CBF, water is used as a freely (or almost freely) diffusible tracer. The origins of the method go back many years to studies of flow using MR spectroscopy.[74] The physics principles are similar to those used in MRI for time-of-flight angiography.[75]

The first practical demonstration of this method in the brain was by Detre and Koretsky et al.[76] The first demonstration of the effect for functional brain imaging was by Kwong et al.[2] who noted it in the same paper that demonstrated BOLD imaging. This technique was also used in one of the first phMRI studies of increased CBF caused by administration of 20 mg/kg amphetamine (a nearly lethal dose) in rats.[6] Numerous variations have appeared and this section will not cover all of them because they have lower CNRs than techniques such as BOLD and IRON and are not likely to prove as useful. Nonetheless, the ability to measure absolute flow with these methods makes them worth mentioning.

We will discuss the general principles behind arterial spin labeling but a more detailed description can be found in Chapter 2. Flowing spins will alter the effective T_1 within a voxel. It can be assumed that the flow of spins in and out of a voxel will alter the magnetization in the following manner (we follow the approach of Detre et al.).[76]

$$\frac{dM_z(t)}{dt} = \frac{M_0 - M_z(t)}{T_1} + \frac{f}{\lambda} M_a(t) - \frac{f}{\lambda} M_z(t)$$

where f is the perfusion (in ml/g/min), λ is the tissue:blood partition coefficient (ml/g; usual brain value of 0.88), M_a is the arterial magnetization, M_0 is the equilibrium longitudinal magnetization, and $M_z(t)$ is the longitudinal magnetization at time t. The incoming spins to a voxel can be altered using saturation, where $M_a(t) = 0$, or inversion, where $M_a(t) = -M_0$. One assumption of this approach is that water is a freely diffusible tracer such that the incoming spins are effectively incorporated into the voxel and the outgoing spins come from the voxel. This assumption has been tested to be reasonable under all but very high flow conditions. This allows equilibration such that $M_v(t) = M_a(t)$. By applying a long period of labeling, a steady state is attained:

$$\frac{dM_z(t)}{dt} = \frac{M_0 - M_z(t)}{T_1} + \frac{f}{\lambda} M_a(t) - \frac{f}{\lambda} M_z(t) = 0$$

Solving and rearranging with the appropriate boundary conditions leads to:

$$f = \frac{\lambda(M_{ss} - M_0)}{T_1(M_a - M_{ss})}$$

where M_{ss} is the apparent steady-state magnetization in the presence of continuous arterial spin labeling. The time to reach steady state is on the order of 5 secs at most field strengths. The amount of perturbation of inflowing spins is defined as:

$$\alpha = \frac{M_0 - M_a}{2M_0}$$

where perfect inversion would mean $\alpha = 1$. Typically, efficiencies can be achieved using a single surface coil on the neck for inversion of $\alpha = 0.7 - 1$. The longer the transit time from the labeling site to the voxel of interest, the smaller α gets. Thus, spin labeling the neck of a giraffe would likely result in very small labeling in a brain voxel of interest. The true α is $\alpha_{voxel} = {}_{label} \exp(-\Delta t/T1_{blood})$. In practice, this is not a problem except in regions of very low flow. Combining the two previous equations leads to:

$$f = \frac{\lambda(M_{ss,control} - M_{ss,label})}{T_1(M_{ss,label} + (2\alpha - 1)M_{ss,control})}$$

where M_{ss}, label, or control is the steady-state magnetization in the control and continuously labeled states. This equation allows for calculation of the absolute CBF, assuming we can measure α and we assume or measure λ.

This technique relies on differences between labeled and unlabeled images to achieve CBF contrast. The typical signal differences are small, leading to rather low CNR. However, one might wish to use the technique in a number of circumstances. First, as shown elegantly in a number of papers, interleaving BOLD and CBF imaging may allow measurement (albeit indirectly) of relative changes in cerebral oxygen consumption ($rCMRO_2$). Secondly, one might wish to determine the absolute flow change in order to separate components of neurovascular coupling. This might occur in a case of a large increase in flow in the absence of a concomitant increase in glucose utilization. Such a situation can occur, for instance, in stimulation of the cholinergic neurons in the basal forebrain.[42] One might anticipate a change in glucose utilization in the absence of a flow change.[46] Measurement of absolute CBF can be of great value in working with these two phenomena. In most situations however, one anticipates a good coupling of glucose utilization and oxygen utilization.

6.2.1.3 BOLD Techniques

BOLD contrast was named by Ogawa in 1990 after he used the technique at high magnetic field (11T) to detect contrast in veins in rat brains due the intrinsic magnetic susceptibility of deoxyhemoglobin.[77] Hemoglobin is paramagnetic in the deoxy state and diamagnetic in the oxy state. Others subsequently used the method to detect changes in brain parenchyma during perturbations such as hypoxia.[77,78] After the original fMRI paper by Belliveau and colleagues,[1] a number of groups applied the BOLD technique to examine changes in brain activity as a result of photic or motor stimulation. In 1992, papers by Bandettini et al.,[79] Kwong et al.,[2] and Ogawa et al.[3] created a stir when it became apparent that brain activity could be mapped by simple, noninvasive, gradient echo MRI. Thus, any facility with MRI equipment could perform functional brain imaging (although the technique requires high speed imaging, such as echo planar imaging, to attain reasonable statistical power).

This technique is discussed elsewhere in this book (Chapters 4 and 5). We will discuss potential use of BOLD imaging to determine relative tissue oxygen consumption ($rCMRO_2$). While BOLD imaging has the advantage of ease of use, it has the disadvantage that the main parameter measured (percent signal change that can be converted to $\Delta R2^*$) has no direct physiologic relevance. Thus, interpretation of BOLD contrast is problematic. BOLD contrast most accurately reflects the tissue concentration of deoxyhemoglobin. In cases where increases in CBF outstrip increases in $CMRO_2$ the result will be increased signal on images sensitive to T_2^*.

A number of papers discuss modeling approaches using the relative balance between CBF and BOLD contrast to determine $rCMRO_2$ changes induced by brain stimulation.[80–82] The principles of the approaches are quite simple. Following the approaches of Davis et al., Mandeville et al., and Ogawa et al.,[80,81,83] we can write the R2* changes induced by a stimulus as:

$$\Delta R2^*{}_{BOLD}(t) \propto VF(t)\left(\frac{CMRO_2(t)}{CBF(t)}\right)^{\beta} - VF(0)\left(\frac{CMRO_2(0)}{CBF(0)}\right)^{\beta}$$

where R2* (t) represents the BOLD R2* changes, VF is the blood volume fraction, and CBF and $CMRO_2$ are the blood flow and oxygen consumption at times 0 and t. One first determines in the same subject and brain region the increase in CBF in a stimulus where no increase in $CMRO_2$ is expected. Such a stimulus is found in hypercapnia (increased CO_2 concentration). This determines the coupling of $\Delta R2^*$ to a given increase in CBF under conditions of constant $CMRO_2$.

These experiments employed interleaved CBF and BOLD imaging to determine simultaneous responses of the given brain tissue. The next step was determining response to a neuronal stimulus where increases in $CMRO_2$ are expected. In this situation, the BOLD percent signal increases (and $\Delta R2^*$) will be less than those observed under conditions of the same CBF increase due to the increased tissue $CMRO_2$:

$$rCMRO_2(t) = \left(\frac{CBF(t)}{CBF(0)}\right)^{1-\alpha/\beta} \left(1 - \frac{B(t)-1}{M}\right)^{1/\beta}$$

where $rCMRO_2$ is the relative $CMRO_2$, $B(t)$ is the fractional BOLD signal change, α is 0.38 determined from the Grubb relationship between CBV and CBF ($CBV \approx CBF^\alpha$), and M is the parameter that represents the maximal BOLD signal change from the baseline state determined from the changes induced via hypercapnia (i.e., when the change in $CMRO_2 = 0$).

$$M = \frac{B(t)-1}{1 - \left(\frac{CBF(t)}{CBF(0)}\right)^{-(\beta-\alpha)}}$$

The reason for discussing these issues is that a pharmacological stimulus may very well alter relative changes in CBF or $CMRO_2$ differently in the BOLD imaging experiment. We discussed just such a finding in the case of cholinergic stimuli above. Thus, use of such techniques may allow for discrimination of the origins of the BOLD signal changes and also allow for separation of pure vascular stimuli from stronger metabolic changes.

Such studies produced remarkable consistencies in estimates of $CMRO_2$ changes induced by forepaw stimulation in rats[81] or photic stimulation in humans.[80,82] All these studies and more recent ones indicate that $CMRO_2$ increases about a factor of two less than CBF. In most of these experiments, the increase in $CMRO_2$ was about 20%. This is in contrast to the earlier PET studies where increases of about 5% were noted.[84] More recent studies show changes of about the same magnitude (25%). These numbers are in conflict with magnetic resonance spectroscopy studies of ^{13}C in rats where changes on the order of 300% were noted.[85,86] The $CMRO_2$ measurements using PET and ^{13}C are considerably less sensitive than BOLD imaging. The original PET observations determined correctly that the increase in CBF was considerably greater than that in $CMRO_2$. The discrepancy with the ^{13}C data is harder to reconcile although recent ^{13}C data in humans revealed an upper limit for the increase in $CMRO_2$ of about 30% for photic stimulation.[87] This value is consistent with the other MRI studies.

6.2.1.4 CBV Mapping

This technique is a relatively recent entry to brain imaging, although its principles were first demonstrated in the 1980s.[64] The idea is to inject an intravascular contrast agent with high magnetic susceptibility to sensitize the images to relative CBV. Functional imaging is then performed using drugs or tasks to cause increases in

CBF and CBV. The much higher magnetic susceptibility of the contrast agents compared to deoxyhemoglobin leads to a much bigger effect than is seen with BOLD contrast.

The contrast agents used for this technique are primarily based on iron oxide nanoparticles. Thus, we dubbed the technique increased relaxation with iron oxide nanoparticles (IRON) to distinguish it from BOLD.[88] The technique was used simultaneously in a number of laboratories in 1998.[89–91] Further explorations have proven that the method provides a huge increase in CNR compared to BOLD imaging at most field strengths.[88,92] Because the CNR produced by the various techniques is so important, we discuss it in in a separate section.

Two other major differences distinguish this technique from BOLD. First, the very high magnetic susceptibility renders the T_2^* of the intravascular signal so short that the intravascular signal essentially disappears. This is in sharp contrast to BOLD imaging where the venous intravascular signal is an important confound of the signals observed. Second, the magnetic susceptibility of the contrast agent is constant, whereas the magnetic susceptibility of deoxyhemoglobin constantly changes due to variations in oxygen extraction in the tissue. This has the effect of rendering BOLD contrast a mixed parameter with no unique physiologic signature. The contrast agent allows one to continually monitor changes in rCBV. These are the major features of IRON CBV mapping.

A typical experimental IRON protocol would be performed by collecting a series of baseline images before injection of the contrast agent. Depending on the expected time course of the pharmacologic stimulus, one can tailor the imaging time accordingly, trading off temporal resolution for spatial resolution if the expected duration is long enough. This point cannot be emphasized strongly enough, and is one compelling reason to use IRON mapping for pharmacologic stimulus instead of BOLD imaging. Because the intrinsic CNR of the BOLD effect is rather small, achieving the requisite statistical power usually necessitates using a rapid technique such as echo planar imaging. A large number of images per unit time then provides the requisite increase in CNR over a slower, higher spatial resolution technique. With IRON imaging, a large increase in CNR means that one can use a slower, higher spatial resolution technique.

Figure 6.4 shows a typical time course of an IRON protocol after injection of a hypothetical drug that induces a CBV increase compared to a typical BOLD experiment. After obtaining a series of baseline images, a new baseline is acquired; the signal changes observed are proportional to relative CBV as originally outlined in Villringer.[64] One converts the signal decrease observed after injection of iron oxide contrast agent to $\Delta R2^*$ values as $\Delta R2^* = -\ln (S/S_0)/TE$ and $rCBV = K\Delta R2^*$ where K is a constant that scales the R2* values with the regional CBV. In cases where K might be known, it would be possible to calculate the absolute CBV. In practice, this is very difficult, although validation studies performed over the years have verified that the measures of relative CBV are consistent with what is expected. No true "gold standard" has evolved for the determination of absolute CBV. In a typical experiment one might use the following:

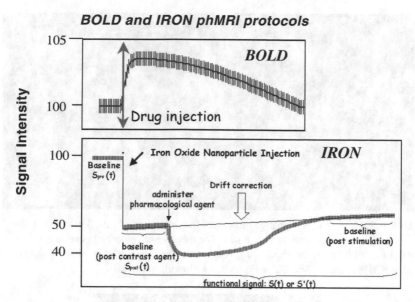

FIGURE 6.4 Typical protocols for BOLD (top) and IRON (bottom) phMRI experiments. IRON requires injection of a contrast agent with high magnetic susceptibility and a long plasma half-life. This in turn renders the images sensitive to relative cerebral blood volume (rCBV).

$$\frac{\Delta rCBV(t)}{rCBV_0} = \left(\frac{\Delta R2^*(t)}{\Delta R2_0^*} \right) - 1$$

Our contention is that use of intravascular contrast agents with high magnetic susceptibility that allow mapping of rCBV will greatly improve phMRI compared to BOLD imaging. Figure 6.5 maps amphetamine-induced activation in a control rat. Figure 6.6 shows two typical statistical maps of amphetamine activation in the striatal region using IRON phMRI (bottom) and BOLD phMRI (top). These data were acquired at a magnetic field strength of 4.7 T. The BOLD effect is much stronger at that strength than at typical clinical magnetic fields like 1.5 T. Nevertheless, it is clear that use of the contrast agents produced a much "cleaner" functional map due to greater statistical power. IRON phMRI increased CNR in the striatum relative to the BOLD method by a factor of about three for CFT and amphetamine. In order to produce a functional map of similar appearance to the map obtained in a single animal using the IRON method, BOLD data from about six rats would have to be averaged.

A number of different iron oxide agents with slightly different magnetic properties have been used for this purpose and reviewed.[88] Most of these agents are nontoxic; one is currently in clinical trials as a method for coronary angiography[93] or liver imaging[94] at doses as high as 1.7 mg iron/kg. The typical doses in animal studies ranged from 4 to 10 mg/kg. Further advantages and disadvantages of this method are discussed below.

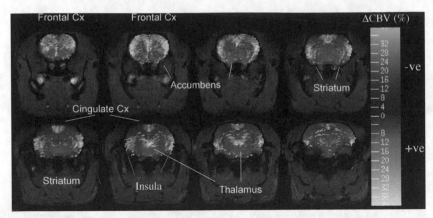

FIGURE 6.5 Map of rCBV changes in a rat after injection of 3mg/kg amphetamine. The primary brain structures activated are noted. The map is not smoothed (spatial resolution was $0.2 \times 0.2 \times 1$ mm) and is thresholded for rCBV changes ranging from –40 to 40%. Note few negative rCBV changes. See Color Figure 6.5 following page 210.

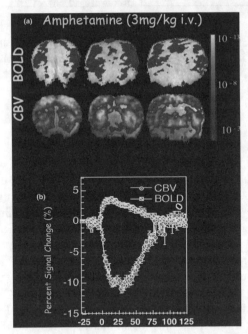

FIGURE 6.6 (a) Comparison of BOLD and IRON images at the same statistical threshold derived from a Student's t-test after administration of 3 mg/kg amphetamine in a rat. Note the nearly 10 orders of magnitude decrease in the p-value for the IRON technique compared to the BOLD technique (both data sets were collected with the same number of images). (b) Plot of the percent changes induced by the same stimulus for BOLD (top) and IRON images. Note the increased rCBV after amphetamine induces a negative percent signal change during IRON imaging. The huge increase in the area under the curve for the IRON is largely responsible for the increase in statistical power of this technique. See Color Figure 6.6 following page 210.

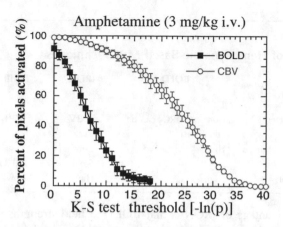

FIGURE 6.7 Percent of the striatum activated at a given statistical threshold for a BOLD and IRON study of 3 mg/kg amphetamine stimulus in seven rats. It illustrates the great increase in statistical power of the IRON technique.

Another way to judge the relative statistical powers of these imaging methods is to compare volumes of striatum that exceed a statistical threshold for "activation." Figure 6.7 compares the percent of striatum activated as a function of the statistical threshold (log of the p value) for BOLD and IRON phMRI. When IRON phMRI selects almost 100% of the striatum, the BOLD method selects only about 33%. At a threshold such that less than 10% of the striatum is selected by the BOLD method, about 33% of the striatum is activated using the IRON method.

It thus appears clear that following injection of amphetamine, IRON phMRI provides an increase of CNR in the striatum. These results lead us to make the following contentions about comparisons of BOLD and IRON phMRI: (1) CNR should be increased everywhere in the brain for pharamacological stimuli, (2) the magnitude of the increase in CNR will vary regionally, with subcortical structures generally benefitting more than cortical structures from a larger increase in CNR, (3) the percent change in CBV should correlate regionally with the percent change in the concentration of deoxyhemoglobin (dHb), and (4) CNR in draining veins should be amplified by the BOLD method and attenuated by the IRON method.

6.2.2 ADVANTAGES AND DISADVANTAGES OF MR TECHNIQUES: THE BRAIN–VEIN CONTROVERSY REVISITED

The BOLD technique is the most common method for fMRI and phMRI studies for a number of reasons. It is the easiest to implement, provides higher contrast-to-noise ratio than CBF-based fMRI techniques, and requires no injection of contrast agents as do CBV methodologies. Nonetheless, conventional BOLD techniques have a number of disadvantages. No direct physiologic parameter can be measured. Aside from the obvious increase in CNR obtained with contrast agents, contrast methods provide certain benefits. Unlike conventional BOLD imaging, contrast methods produce direct measurement of a physiologically relevant parameter: CBV.

TABLE 6.3
Comparisons of Hemodynamic-Based MRI Techniques

	BOLD	IRON	FAIR	ASL
MR Parameter	T_2^*	T_2^*	T_1	T_1
Physiologic parameter	None (rCMRO$_2$ can be modeled)	rCBV	rCBF	CBF
Spatial vascular weighting	High	Low	Low	Low
Relative CNR	1	5	≈ 0.25	≈ 0.5
Temporal resolution	High	High	Low	Low

A further advantage of IRON is that BOLD at field strengths such as 4.7 and 1.5 T shows a high degree of spatial weighting toward large veins. Mandeville et al.[92] showed that BOLD is embedded with a vascular weighting factor and the activation map is shifted toward larger vessels than brain tissues. Because of the ring of arachnoid vessels surrounding the rat brain, the BOLD activation map tends to shift outward toward the edge (compare the BOLD and IRON images in Figure 6.6). The IRON technique, however, can be optimized to have the maximal sensitivity in tissue rather than in vessels and thus show the location of neuronal activation more accurately. For the larger vessels, the very short intravascular T_2^* led to very little signal on the gradient echo images we used, and hence less vascular weighting. For BOLD imaging, such a feature may appear at very high magnetic field strengths such as 9.4 T or likely even higher. Relative comparisons of the BOLD and IRON techniques are outlined in Table 6.3. The relative CNR comparisons in the table are approximate only for field strengths from 1.5 to 4.7 T. The CNR advantage of IRON over BOLD at these field strengths is about eight at 2 T and about three at 4.7 T.[88,92]

One last potential advantage of the IRON technique relates to the problem of "physiologic noise."[95-98] Our preliminary observations suggest that potential fluctuations due to cardiac motion and other vascular activities[88] may be decreased after injection of an intravascular contrast agent. Such a contention is confirmed by measurements of root mean square (rms) peak-to-peak fluctuations compared to baseline signal intensities before and after injection of contrast agent.

Preliminary measurements (BOLD vs. IRON) of the standard deviation of the baseline divided by the mean in seven animals in region of interests (ROIs) led to the following: 3.9 ± 1.5 vs. striatum $2.5 \pm 0.5\%$ (striatum); 3.8 ± 1.1 vs. 2.3 ± 0.6 (frontal cortex); and 7.9 ± 2.8 vs. striatum 4.8 ± 2.8 (sagittal sinus). This effect has two potential explanations. The incredibly short T_2^* of the vessels after injection leads to a complete loss of intravascular signals and any fluctuations due to intravascular signals will be lost. Second, the large gradients set up around the small vessels tend to lead to intervoxel spatial smoothing; with bold BOLD imaging, physiologic vascular "noise" tends to reflect the relative intervoxel vascular density. A complete understanding of this effect requires further study. Nonetheless, it indicates another potential advantage of the IRON technique and may yield further insight into the origins of physiologic noise.

Clearly, the biggest disadvantage to the IRON technique is the large amount of iron that must be used. Since the optimal signal changes and CNRs will attain when the signal loss is approximately $1/e$,[90] a typical injection is 3 to 10 mg/kg of total iron per dose, depending on the agent used. While iron is relatively nontoxic, such an increase in body iron load may represent an unwarranted cost for the relative benefit of the MR exam. We noted no toxicity with the relatively high doses we used. The superparamagnetic blood pool agent we used produced R2* changes with 4.5 mg/kg similar to what MION produced with 10 mg/kg.[88] In our prior studies in a rodent model of Parkinson's disease, we noted no toxicity due to the injection of the SPBPA agent even after multiple studies in the same animals over the course of 1 year.[12] Further studies are required to determine potential for use in humans.

6.2.3 DATA ANALYSIS TECHNIQUES

Data processing applied to fMRI studies attracts greater numbers of investigators every year. A number of processing schemes based on PET experiments and protocols targeting the unique features of MRI data have been developed. The analysis of phMRI data can be approached using the tools developed for conventional fMRI studies.

The SPM (statistical parametric mapping) web site (http://www.fil. ion.ucl.ac.uk/spm/) describes such tools in detail. We will cover only two topics here. First, we will develop a framework for understanding CNR, then see how BOLD data analysis can lead to shifts in statistical or parametric maps (e.g., CBV) that may be generated. Second, we will describe how to model phMRI data based on pharmacologic principles.

6.2.3.1 Theoretical Framework for CNR

It is convenient to think of CNR at spatial location $\mathbf{r}$ and time t as the product of the signal-to-noise ratio (SNR), a vascular weighting function (W), and a term that depends on functional changes (Φ) and is independent of baseline physiology:

$$CNR(\mathbf{r},t) = SNR(\mathbf{r})\ W(\mathbf{r})\ \Phi\ (\mathbf{r},t) \qquad (6.1)$$

A theoretical framework for quantitatively comparing BOLD and CBV CNR can be developed by making simplifying assumptions. For CBV phMRI, these assumptions include (1) changes in the transverse relaxation rate of the MRI signal after injection of a contrast agent are linearly proportional to the blood volume fraction (V) at spatial location $\mathbf{r}$ and time t, $\Delta R_2^*(\mathbf{r},t) = K\ V(\mathbf{r},t)$, where K depends upon contrast agent dose, (2) noise does not depend on contrast agent dose, and (3) a sufficient amount of contrast agent is used so that BOLD contributions to relaxation rate changes during functional challenges can be neglected.

For BOLD phMRI, we assume (1) the transverse relaxation rate is a linear function of the voxel concentration of deoxygenated hemoglobin, $\Delta R_2 = K\ \Delta[dHb]$, (2) the small arterial blood volume fraction (~10 to 15%) can be neglected, and (3) a tight linear regional relationship exists between resting state values of CBF and $CMRO_2$, as consistently measured by PET studies. Under these assumptions, the

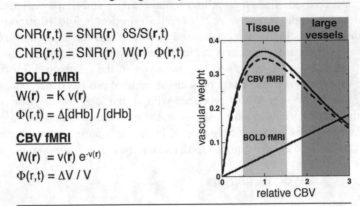

Vascular weighting theory (2T)

$CNR(\mathbf{r},t) = SNR(\mathbf{r})\ \delta S/S(\mathbf{r},t)$

$CNR(\mathbf{r},t) = SNR(\mathbf{r})\ W(\mathbf{r})\ \Phi(\mathbf{r},t)$

BOLD fMRI

$W(\mathbf{r}) = K\ v(\mathbf{r})$

$\Phi(\mathbf{r},t) = \Delta[dHb]\ /\ [dHb]$

CBV fMRI

$W(\mathbf{r}) = v(\mathbf{r})\ e^{-v(\mathbf{r})}$

$\Phi(\mathbf{r},t) = \Delta V\ /\ V$

FIGURE 6.8 Relative vascular weighting functions (proportional to CNR) for BOLD and IRON imaging at 2 T. The relevant equations describing the graph are at left. BOLD imaging has its greatest sensitivity in large veins. IRON imaging has its greatest sensitivity in tissues and has little in large veins. The dotted line in the IRON curve indicates the decrease in weighting from signal *increases* due to the BOLD effect. The effects at 4.7 T can be scaled essentially by increasing the slope of the BOLD curve by 4.7/2 or 2.35, leaving the IRON curve unchanged.

expressions for the CNR of BOLD fMRI and CBV fMRI can be derived, and the respective functions of Equation 6.1 are as follows:

$$W_{BOLD}(\mathbf{r},t) \approx T_E\ R_2^{*BOLD}(\mathbf{r}_0,0)\ v(\mathbf{r}),\quad \Phi_{BOLD}(\mathbf{r},t) \approx -\Delta[dHb](\mathbf{r},t)/[dHb](\mathbf{r},0)$$

$$W_{CBV}(\mathbf{r},t) \approx e^{-v(\mathbf{r})}\ v(\mathbf{r}),\quad \Phi_{CBV}(\mathbf{r},t) \approx -\Delta V(\mathbf{r},t)/V(\mathbf{r},0) \qquad (6.2)$$

where $R_2^{*BOLD}(\mathbf{r}_0,0)$ is the BOLD part of the resting state transverse relaxation rate at some location $\mathbf{r}_0$, T_E is the gradient echo time of the BOLD imaging sequence, V is the blood volume fraction, and v is the resting state blood volume with respect to the point $\mathbf{r}_0$ ($v(\mathbf{r}) = V(\mathbf{r},0)/V(\mathbf{r}_0,0)$). In a comparison of the CNR of the two methods, a point $\mathbf{r}_0$ must be selected such that injection of contrast agent drops the signal intensity to about e^{-1} of the preinjection value; this location depends on both the contrast agent and the local blood volume fraction.

The forms of the weighting functions for these MRI methods differ due to injection of contrast agent, which reduces SNR proportional to a decreasing exponential of relative blood volume. Figure 6.8 shows weighting functions vs. the negative log of the ratio of signal intensities before (S_{BOLD}) and after (S_{CBV}) injection of contrast agent; this quantity is proportional to the product of resting CBV and contrast agent dose. The dependence of CNR on resting state blood volume is expected to be much stronger for BOLD phMRI than for IRON phMRI, where CNR is insensitive to small changes in resting state CBV about the point v = 1 and decreases when the magnitude of resting state CBV deviates in either direction from this value. In contrast, BOLD CNR changes with a roughly linear dependence on

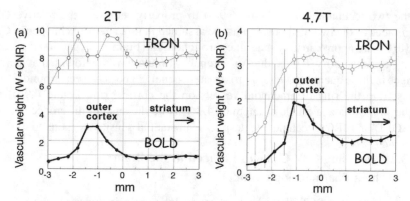

FIGURE 6.9 Estimates of the relative contrast-to-noise ratios of BOLD phMRI (closed circles) and IRON phMRI (open circles) at magnetic field strengths of 2 T (a) and 4.7 T (b) proceeding from the cortical rim toward the striatum. For equal percent changes in CBV, estimates are shown for the relative BOLD. CNR has been normalized to 1 in striatum at each field strength. CNR is expected to increase in striatum by factors of about 8 and 3 at 2 and 4.7 T, respectively. The peaks seen around −1 mm arise from the cortical rims of arachnoid vessels in the rat brain. The peaks are negative for the IRON technique due to the short T_2^* of the blood after injection of contrast agents.

resting state blood volume, exacerbating the "brain vs. vein" ambiguity due to CNR amplification in large veins.

Equation 6.2 suggests a way to compare CNR for the BOLD and IRON methods that will help illuminate functional couplings during an acute pharmacological challenge. By computing the CNR for BOLD and CBV phMRI separately (e.g., using a t statistic) and then dividing the two CNR maps, the result should be of the form:

$$CNR_{BOLD}/CNR_{CBV} = K \; e^{v(r)} \{\% \; \Delta[dHB]/\% \; \Delta CBV\} \qquad (6.3)$$

If we assume that the percent change in dHb and the percent change in CBV scale together across different brain regions, the ratio in Equation 6.3 should produce the appearance of a blood volume map, since $e^{v(r)} \sim e^1 \; v(r)$ for small change in CBV about the point r_0. By comparing this ratio with a blood volume map created as $v = -\ln(S_{CBV}/S_{BOLD})$ following injection of the contrast agent, the hypothesis can be tested that the percent change in CBV and percent change in dHb scale regionally together.

Figure 6.9a provides a theoretical estimate for the increase in CNR in cortex and striatum at magnetic field strengths of 2 and 4.7 T. The figures show dorsal-ventral projections through forepaw somatosensory cortex. Closed circles are measured blood volume fractions, computed as $v = -\ln(S_{BOLD}/S_{CBV})$, where S_{BOLD} and S_{CBV} are the MRI signal intensities before and after injection of an iron oxide contrast agent at an iron dose of 12 mg/kg and a fixed echo time. The open circles are gamma functions of the relative blood volume fraction (v) as defined in Equation 6.2. The relative magnitude between the curves for BOLD and CBV phMRI was set according to a value of $R_2^{*(BOLD)}$ experimentally determined in rat somatosensory cortex.[90] The vascular weights shown in Figure 6.9(a) represent approximate CNR values obtained for the two techniques. For Figure 6.9(a) to properly represent the relative CNR magnitudes of the two methods, it must be assumed that the percent changes in CBV and [dHb] are approximately the same throughout the brain. For functional changes in rat somatosensory cortex due to forepaw stimulation, we found that percent changes in these quantities were approximately equal.[90] The peak seen around −1 mm comes from the ring of arachnoid vessels on the cortical rim. Figure 6.9(b) is a similar plot of data at a field strength of 4.7 T. Note the smaller difference between the BOLD and IRON techniques, despite a substantial sensitivity gain.

6.2.3.2 Modeling CBV Changes Induced in the Brain by a Pharmacologic Model

Data analysis of a PET pharmacology study inherently includes all the different pharmacodynamic parameters of interest. The intent is to determine the concentration of drug in the brain or the kinetic parameters associated with its binding. No such analysis is usually attempted, perhaps wisely, for hemodynamic measures. The reason for this was discussed earlier in this chapter: the number of molecules responsible for the hemodynamic change is so large that any model is likely to contain enough "garbage" to make extraction of quantitative parameters difficult. Nonetheless, under favorable circumstances, some useful models may be derived. If the drug in question has a PET tracer analog, one could combine parameters derived from the PET model to extract the lifetime of the drug in the brain, then postulate that the hemodynamic effects of the drug will be directly proportional to its concentration in the brain. We can describe the model as:

$$\frac{dCBV}{dt} = K \frac{d[Drug]}{dt}$$

where the rate of change of CBV is proportional to the rate of change of the drug in the voxel of interest. If such a relationship can be validated, one might, under controlled circumstances (blood gases, breathing rate, etc.), extract the drug concentration in the brain or the relative drug concentration in the brain after empirical estimates of K and determining where such a relationship might break down.

In the case of a drug like amphetamine that increases synaptic and extrasynaptic dopamine concentrations we can further predict that, at least in the striatum, the release of dopamine may directly lead to vasodilation (see Figure 6.3). In this case, the equation above can be rewritten as:

$$\frac{dCBV}{dt} = K * C_{free}^{Da}(t) = R(t) - U(t)$$

where C_{free}^{Da} is the free dopamine concentration as a function of time that is the balance between release R(t) and reuptake U(t). The latter is usually modeled as Michaelis-Menton kinetics for the dopamine transporter. Figure 6.10 shows such a possibility incorporating the phMRI and PET data with microdialysis data, incorporating all the kinetic terms that might be needed for the simplest description. Since

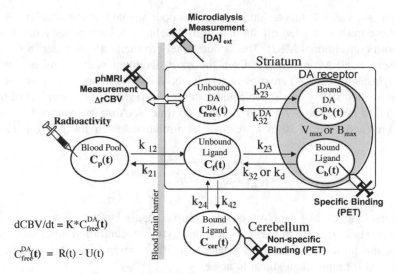

FIGURE 6.10 Combined hypothetical compartmental analysis of PET, phMRI, and microdialysis data using the dopamine system as an example. The syringes represent points where data is collected by each technique. The other kinetic parameters, such as transfers across the blood–brain barrier, k_{12}, and k_{21}, are modeled from the data. The DA receptors may be DAT or postsynaptic D2 receptors. In this model, the extracellular dopamine and the ^{11}C-labeled ligand compete to bind to the DA receptor. Therefore, the extracellular space includes compartments for the free unbound dopamine and for the free unbound ^{11}C ligand. The binding and dissociation rates (ks) are as shown. We assumed here that the vasoactive effects of dopamine on the vasculature allowed us to determine a free dopamine concentration similar to that of microdialysis. Such a study has yet to be performed.

such a study has not yet been published, further discussion here would be premature. Such modeling often produces solutions to differential equations that represent the difference of two exponentials (characteristic of a phMRI time course). Fitting noisy BOLD data to such a model often leads to nonunique solutions at best and nonsense at worst.

6.2.4 NONHEMODYNAMIC MR TECHNIQES OF POTENTIAL USE FOR phMRI

Two other MR techniques have been used to investigate brain activation. We will briefly discuss both techniques because they have proved very useful for examining pharmacologic stimuli and have more potential to reveal alternative physiologic parameters than the simple hemodynamic metrics discussed above. The first technique is magnetic resonance spectroscopy (MRS). The other is T_1-weighted imaging of accumulation of manganese due to neuronal stimulation.

6.2.4.1 Magnetic Resonance Spectroscopy

This technique is widely used for research into brain disorders and clearly has potential for studying pharmacologic challenges. However, even at high field strengths such as 4 T, this technique produces poor spatial and temporal resolutions (and these must be traded off starting from baselines that are already much lower than with conventional MRI). This is due largely to the fact that water in the brain is present at 80 M in protons. Even the most abundant neurochemicals such as N-acetylaspartate (NAA) are present at only about 25 mM in protons. If we compare the relative sensitivity of a T_2-weighted water image (assuming a water T_2^* of 65 ms and a TE of 100 ms at 4.7 T) and a short echo time NAA image (with a T_2 for NAA of 250 ms and a TE of 20 ms), we arrive at a relative sensitivity of NAA/H_2O of:

$$\frac{0.025 \text{ M} * \exp^{-(0.02/0.25)}}{80 \text{ M} * \exp^{-(0.1/.065)}} = 0.0013$$

where the longer T2 of the NAA methyl group compared to that of water adds back (via exp(-TE/T2)) some of the signal lost due to the concentration difference. Nonetheless, this represents a factor of greater than 700 or an increase in averaging time of 500,000 for equivalent signal to noise.

A number of studies examined photic stimulation using magnetic resonance spectroscopy. They focused on detection of increased lactate during photic stimulation[99] and changes in glucose utilization.[87,100,101] Changes in glucose utilization can be measured in two ways. The first is observing glucose resonances directly (optimally at 5.23 ppm[102]) and measuring their decline during photic stimulation.[101] This technique has the advantage of being a direct measure of glucose utilization, thus avoiding many of the modeling problems inherent in PET. On the other hand, the low sensitivity leads to low spatial and temporal resolution.

The other method is to utilize ^{13}C-labeled glucose and observe its metabolic transformation through the TCA cycle to glutamate and other metabolites.[87,100,103,104] This technique has the advantage of providing incredible metabolic specificity, but it also suffers from poor spatial and temporal resolution. Increases in both spatial and temporal resolution utilizing echo planar spectroscopy,[105–107] especially at higher magnetic fields such as 7 or 9.4 T and with phased array surface coils, may lead to more practical pharmacologic spectroscopy studies. At these high field strengths, with reasonable averaging times, we might hope to achieve spatial resolution on the order of a clinical PET scanner (about 3 to 4 mm in plane).

A number of studies examined metabolic response to pharmacologic stimulation. The effects of the glutamate antagonist MK-801 were examined using proton and phosphorus spectroscopy.[108] The authors showed increased lactate after MK-801 administration, indicative of nonoxidative glycolysis. Increased brain GABA concentrations were noted in occipital cortex after administration of vigabitrin (an inhibitor of GABA-transaminase) to epileptic patients.[109] We examined the effects of amphetamine stimulation on brain TCA cycle flux in frontal cortex using ^{13}C MRS.[110] We found an increase in labeling of C2-glutamate of about 34% indicative of increased CMRO$_2$ of the same magnitude (interestingly the rate of C4-labelin, often taken as a surrogate marker for TCA cycle flux, was much faster). These data are averages over about 90 minutes. It is unlikely that the metabolic profile is constant over this period. Higher field strengths and better carbon-edited proton observation techniques may improve temporal and spatial resolution.

6.2.4.2 Manganese-Enhanced MRI (MEMRI)

The other nonhemodynamic technique, pioneered in the laboratory of Dr. Alan Koretsky, is the injection of paramagnetic manganese (after opening the blood–brain barrier with mannitol) to detect brain activity.[111] This technique relies on the ability of manganese to substitute for calcium. Cells that have increased uptake of calcium during brain stimulation will selectively accumulate manganese. This, in turn, leads to a decrease in T_1 that is readily detectable using conventional T_1-weighted imaging. In principle, this technique has high sensitivity and exquisite spatial resolution. One study compared the focus of activation of BOLD fMRI to MEMRI at 9.4 T and showed the foci of the two techniques were within 200 μm of one another.[112] This lends credence to the utility of BOLD imaging.

The MEMRI technique suffers from a number of problems that render it less compelling than it might otherwise appear. First, the blood–brain barrier must be opened since Mn^{++} will not enter the brain otherwise.[113] Opening the barrier with mannitol often leads to great interanimal variability. Another problem is that not all neurons accumulate Ca^{++} during stimulation. Reuptake of dopamine, for instance, on presynaptic neurons is not Ca^{++} dependent. Second, accumulation of Mn^{++} in the globus pallidus and selectively in dopamine neurons[113] may confound results. Nonetheless, this technique shows great promise for animal models. It has the potential of very high spatial resolution, comparable to that attained in MR microscopy. This results from the fact that the stimulus can be performed outside the magnet where the manganese will accumulate at the active sites, and then the animal can be placed in the magnet for imaging. Since the images are not time-dependent over a short time, one can spend most of the imaging time averaging to obtain ultrahigh spatial resolution.

6.2.5 Confounds of Respiratory Gases and Anesthesia

Most phMRI studies are and will continue to be hemodynamic. Changes in respiratory gases during such a study can represent a major confound in interpretation of the signal changes whether the parameter measured is CBF, rCBV, or BOLD. This is true also for fMRI studies. Changes in breathing rate can easily change CO_2 levels in the blood. For instance, hyperventilation will drop pCO_2 from about 38 to 20 in less than a minute. Figure 6.11 plots changes in end tidal CO_2 ($EtCO_2$) and BOLD percent signal change in a human subject hyperventilated for 3 minutes.

Note how rapidly the $EtCO_2$ changes. The changes are mirrored by a decrease in BOLD signal due to the decreased CBF. The $EtCO_2$ takes much longer to return to baseline (about 5 minutes). Such changes have been shown to alter the response of visual cortex to photic stimulation and paradoxically decrease the BOLD signal.[114] In situations where awake humans are administered drugs such as cocaine and amphetamine, it is imperative to simultaneously measure $EtCO_2$ to determine the effects of changes. Intravenous cocaine administration reportedly decreases

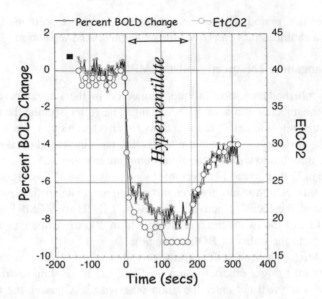

FIGURE 6.11 Comparison of changes in BOLD signal (echo planar images; TR/TE 2500/45 ms; 1.5 T) from multiple gray matter regions in the cortex vs. end tidal CO_2 ($EtCO_2$) measured simultaneously in a normal human control before, during, and after 3 minutes of hyperventilation. Note the tight correlation between the BOLD signal and $EtCO_2$, the short time to drop the CO_2, and the much longer time to return to baseline. Measurement of such changes is critical during drug stimulation, e.g., a short burst of hyperventilation can exert a much longer term effect on signal changes.

$EtCO_2$,[115] likely due to hyperventilation. Changes in blood pressure can also affect hemodynamics, but studies of autoregulation suggest that maintenance of CBF in the face of decreased arterial pressure occurs over a fairly wide range of pressures. Recent measurements of simultaneous CBV and CBF using MRI suggest that CBF and CBV are constant between 65 and 140 mm Hg pressure.[116]

Another study simultaneously monitored changes in BOLD contrast and blood pressure during a blood withdrawal protocol under varying anesthesia conditions.[117] This study suggested a regionally heterogeneous correlation between the two parameters. It is thus imperative to measure these parameters during imaging. Many drugs of interest can cause changes in mean arterial blood pressure.

The confounds of anesthesia are even more profound than those of changes in systemic physiologic variables. The latter effects can be readily measured and potentially corrected for, whereas those of anesthesia can often selectively affect different neurotransmitter systems. Furthermore, the goal of any good anesthetic is retention of systemic involuntary responses such as respiration, while blunting cortical responsivity. This requirement is often in conflict with the goals of a functional or pharmacologic study. Many studies investigated the effects of differing anesthetics on the coupling of cerebral metabolism and anesthetic dose.[118] They will not be reviewed here except to note the very large differences in the CBF increases observed for the same stimulus with different anesthetics.[119]

These studies have not generally examined the neurovascular coupling problem with respect to the differing neurotransmitter systems selectively affected by various anesthetics. For a number of anesthetics such as halothane or isoflurane, the exact mechanisms are not known. It is therefore difficult to predict *a priori* which receptor systems will be most affected. What is clear from studies of the mechanisms of action of halothane is that there is good evidence for influence on multiple systems including glutamate uptake, glucose utilization, phospholipid methylation, glycine receptor antagonism, decreased calcium channel binding sites, etc.

Urethane is capable of inducing anesthesia without affecting neurotransmission in various subcortical areas and the peripheral nervous system. Urethane, like the volatile anesthetics, is thought to target multiple neurotransmitter systems through potentiation and inhibition of neurotransmitter-gated ion channels.[120] For a number of anesthetics, however, the target neurotransmitter systems are known. Ketamine, a common anesthetic for animal surgery, is a noncompetitive glutamate N-methyl-D-aspartate antagonist[121,122] that can also potentiate dopamine release after administration of drugs like amphetamine.[123] Like MK-801, it can induce regionally selective changes in brain metabolism. Morphine sulfate is another anesthetic used for functional studies, and it obviously targets the opioid receptors. α-Chloralose is another common anesthetic for fMRI studies; it preserves functional metabolic coupling in the cortex.[124]

Forepaw stimulation in α-chloralose-anesthetized rats showed increases of regional cerebral metabolic rate of glucose (CMRglc) measured with autoradiography,[124] and CBF and CBV measured by fMRI[90] in the forelimb (FL) area of somatosensory cortex. However, α-chloralose has been shown to depress the activities of the dopaminergic neurons.[125] Halothane, in contrast to α-chloralose, attenuates the functional metabolic coupling in the cortex[124] but preserves dopamine activity in the striatum.[125] We showed that α-chloralose can turn off the effects of cocaine and amphetamine in the brain.[126]

Clearly, each neurotransmitter system must be carefully investigated — preferably with multiple anesthetics — before one can be confident of the results. The effects of anesthesia are not always negative confounds, however. The phMRI response to the antipsychotic agent clozapine can be selectively modulated by different anesthetics. Use of α-chloralose allows one to turn off the dopamine-related components, whereas use of halothane retains them.[126]

6.2.6 Basic Drug Challenge Designs

6.2.6.1 Acute Model

The most basic form of a phMRI experiment is to monitor acute signal changes (via BOLD or IRON) using a baseline condition followed by administration of the drug of interest. The relative nature of the signal changes measured by both BOLD or IRON CBV methods means that comparisons to absolute changes in metabolism are difficult or impossible. The ability to measure an absolute metabolic parameter makes one capable of monitoring the chronic effects of a drug challenge, for example,

PET studies of the effects of haloperidol (a rather dirty dopamine D2 antagonist) revealed decreases in glucose metabolism after chronic administration of the drug.

Optimally, a technique that can measure absolute changes in the parameter of interest (CBV, CBF, CMRglc, etc.) is required. The only MR technique envisioned as useful for this purpose is arterial spin labeling, a method capable of measuring absolute CBF. However, its low sensitivity has precluded its full exploration in that context. In situations where changes might be regional, it is possible that measurements of relative CBV might be of some value. Thus, most studies will likely continue as acute drug challenges.

Another point should be made with regard to the acute drug challenge model. A scientist is often interested in the pattern of receptor alterations induced by a drug, not in the metabolic perturbations that may have resulted from its administration. Our studies of the dopamine system led to the conclusion that the dynamics and populations of the dopamine receptors exert major influences on the metabolic changes induced by acute administration of a dopaminergic drug such as amphetamine. Thus, one can interpret the acute administration of a drug as a means of indirectly probing the population and circuitry involved with a particular receptor population. Clearly this type of interpretation must be proven for each new ligand and receptor system. Once such a conclusion can be made, the acute drug challenge becomes a means to probe such circuitry.

Figure 6.4 is a typical example of data from an IRON experiment. The baseline signal is measured in a number of images, then an iron oxide contrast agent is administered. This leads to a loss of signal (an increase in R2*) proportional to the CBV. Amphetamine is injected while imaging proceeds continuously. The signal changes are monitored for as long as one anticipates the drug of choice will have an effect. In cases where that period is unknown, it may be useful to image as long as the animal remains physiologically stable. Increasing the number of images will obviously increase the statistical power of the experiment, assuming of course that parameters are stable. Signal drift that occurs over a long period must be accounted for.

The pharmacodynamic profiles of drugs can often be very different even when they are targeted to the same receptor system. For instance, cocaine and amphetamine exert similar effects on synaptic dopamine concentration, but cocaine has a much shorter time course. In addition, cocaine effects are extremely sensitive to the method of administration. A similar effect on synaptic dopamine changes and hemodynamic changes that occurs for cocaine at an intravenous dose of, say, 1 mg/kg requires about 10 mg/kg orally or intraperitoneally. For amphetamine, the relative difference of intraperitoneal vs. intravenous challenge is about 30% less for intraperitoneal administration compared to a factor of 10 for cocaine. The importance of understanding as much as possible about the pharmacodynamic effects of the drug of choice before performing an experiment cannot be stressed enough. Perhaps phMRI will become a useful adjunct for performing such pharmacodynamic screening. It may be useful to note that the dissociation between direct vascular effects of the drug of choice and stimulation of the receptors must be examined. The acute hemodynamic effects of a drug may be different from those that occur when, for instance, the drug reaches its peak concentration in brain tissue.

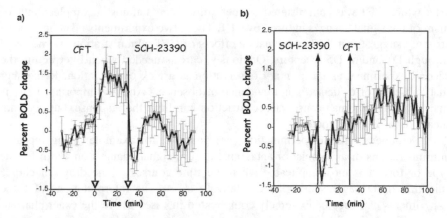

FIGURE 6.12 Effect of D1 antagonism on signal changes evoked by a dopamine transporter blocker. Averaged BOLD phMRI time courses from rat striatum after administration of (a) CFT (0.5 mg/kg) followed by SCH-23390 (0.6 mg/kg (n = 7) or (b) pretreatment with SCH-23390 (0.6 mg/kg) followed by CFT (0.75 mg/kg (n = 7). In both cases the D1 antagonist turns off or blocks signal changes induced by CFT. The arrows indicate administration of SCH-23390 or CFT.

A permutation on the basic acute drug challenge is repeated administration of a drug with a relatively short time course. In this case, one can study, for instance, the effects of acute tolerance. Such experiments are feasible with drugs such as cocaine and nicotine whose hemodynamic effects last about 20 minutes. It is not necessarily feasible with drugs such as amphetamine that have very long time courses.

6.2.6.2 Agonism and Antagonism of Acute Drug Challenges

Many other permutations on the basic framework of the simple acute drug challenge study exist. One of the most basic and important, especially in initial phases of investigating a new drug, is the study of the antagonism and agonism of drug effects. Let us examine one such experiment using another dopaminergic ligand. We utilized CFT (a potent and selective blocker of the dopamine transporter protein). CFT causes a very similar activation profile to that elicited by amphetamine.

Figure 6.12 shows two curves with the protocol specified. These data were collected using the BOLD technique. We administered 0.5 mg/kg of CFT followed 30 minutes later (left), after hemodynamic changes began to plateau, by administration of 0.6 mg/kg of a dopamine mixed D1/D5 antagonist (SCH23390). The signal changes were followed for the same time period over which the experiment might have continued for CFT alone (CFT alone takes about 70 minutes to return to baseline). The D1 antagonist immediately blocked the BOLD signal changes.

It is sometimes possible, however, that the signal turns off for reasons unrelated to administration of the antagonist, so the antagonist can be administered before the drug of choice. Figure 6.12(b) shows inversion of the prior protocol and administration of the D1 antagonist before the CFT. This signal was followed for 20 minutes, after which CFT was administered. As before, we noted almost a complete antagonism of the signal changes induced by CFT. These two experiments taken in concert strongly suggest that the hemodynamic effects of CFT administration are mediated through D1 and/or D5 receptors. Obviously, care is needed when interpreting the second experiment as the primary observation is a lack of activation. Remember that "absence of evidence is not evidence of absence." Another important issue is that any drug that may cause vasoconstriction can limit the response, but does not mean that it is an atagonist.

A number of further permutations are possible, for example, using repeated administrations of an agonist or antagonist to turn signal changes on and off. This type of format is most applicable when the time courses of the drugs of choice (nicotine or D1 agonists, e.g., are relatively short. The interpretations of these experiments can become extremely complicated in cases where the exact pharmacodynamics and brain distributions of the chemicals are not known. In such cases, alternative techniques must be employed to make such determinations to aid in interpretation of the results. However, such studies should be performed anyway. Use of any technique in isolation often leads to the classic paradox of the blind men examining an elephant. Approaching a problem with the mindset that "every problem is a nail to a man with a hammer" is a hazard in the MRI community.

6.2.6.3 Acute Model for Examining Effects of Chronic Drug Administration

It may appear that the acute drug challenge model has severe limitations for examining the effects of chronic drug changes. Such changes are of crucial importance for understanding receptor dynamics in clinical situations.

Two important examples stand out. The first is the effect of chronic administration of antipsychotic medications in schizophrenic populations. Drugs such as haloperidol, olanzapine, and clozapine often require some time before they attain full efficacy. A second salient example comes from study of chronic abusers of such drugs as cocaine or ecstasy. Abusers often experience a tolerance to the effects of these drugs and this implies changes in populations of receptors that modulate the pharmacology of the drug of abuse. Thus, it appears that the acute drug challenge may not provide an adequate model for examining receptor dynamics. However, many ways exist to construe the acute drug challenge model. The most valuable method is to view such challenges as means to probe snapshots of receptor populations and their associated circuitry.

One possibility is using a different ligand as a challenge agent if it has a more powerful effect on the receptor system in question than the therapeutic agent. As an example, chronic cocaine abuse has been reported to lead to alterations in the populations of dopamine transporters and dopamine D2 receptors.[127,128] One could use a drug challenge with amphetamine or apomorphine to probe dopaminergic circuitry with more efficacy than cocaine (the short time course of the hemodynamic effects of cocaine makes it less than optimal in this case). One hypothesis might be that the decrease in dopamine transporter might lead to a much smaller effect of amphetamine than would be observed in a control population. This is because the effects of amphetamine are predicated on reverse transport of the vesicular pool of dopamine via the dopamine transporter. Such an experiment might be tried to assay the effects of cocaine use and chronic haloperidol use for schizophrenia or methylphenidate (Ritalin) treatment for attention deficit hyperactivity disorder.

6.3   CURRENT AND FUTURE APPLICATIONS OF PHMRI

As discussed earlier, the coupling of pharmacologic stimulation, neural activity, and a hemodynamic change is very complicated. Therefore, when performing an initial phMRI experiment with a given drug or neurotransmitter system, one should take great pains to determine that the hemodynamic changes observed are due to the neurotransmitter or receptor system in question. This should not be assumed as a foregone conclusion without proof. Otherwise, to paraphrase Lord Kelvin, the ability to interpret signal changes observed is of a meager and insubstantial nature. This is especially true in systems where the neurotransmitter may also be vasoactive. As noted earlier, most neurotransmitters are vasoactive.

We will now outline steps that demonstrate that hemodynamic changes observed are due to stimulation of the neurotransmitter system in question. Stimulation may activate the specific neuronal subtype targeted by the pharmacologic ligand and may also include downstream circuitry that will likely involve other neurotransmitter systems. With this in mind, we outline some of the criteria that should be fulfilled. Many of these experiments can only be performed in animals, possibly in support of subsequent human studies. The following criteria help demonstrate that hemodynamic changes induced by a given ligand are specific to the neurotransmitter in question:

1. phMRI signal changes should not correlate with changes in systemic physiologic parameters (e.g., pCO_2, blood pressure).
2. phMRI signal changes should be correlated with distribution of receptors of the neurotransmitter in question and/or downstream circuitry measured with autoradiography or PET.
3. Selective lesioning of the receptor system in question should modulate phMRI signal changes in predictable ways.
4. Administration of agonists and antagonists of the receptor system should modulate the signal in a manner consistent with the proposed mechanisms of action of the agonists and antagonists.
5. phMRI signal changes should correlate with behavioral and/or neurotransmitter dynamics (the latter measured, e.g., with microdialysis).

The first criterion may appear obvious, but in a number of circumstances the relationship between regional changes in systemic parameters and specific activation of a given neurotransmitter may be correlated. For instance, administration of adenosine receptor agonists can produce decreases in blood pressure. If the drops are large enough, they may alter local tissue hemodynamic parameters, as discussed in Section 6.2.5. Such a drop may also be correlated with direct action of the ligand on adenosine receptors. Since adenosine A1 receptors are found throughout the brain, separating these two phenomena may be impossible. Generally, if uniform changes occur over the entire brain and they correlate with changes in systemic physiologic variables, it will be difficult to determine which effects are specific to the neurotransmitter system in question in the absence of other information. To give this confound a positive spin, we could also say that these types of data may be of some use in determining hemodynamic effects of systemic changes in something like CO_2.

The second criterion can be considered *sine qua non* if phMRI is to be considered a useful neuroreceptor mapping tool. As we stated earlier, the various metrics that might be chosen to correlate with phMRI data are somewhat open to interpretation. However, the general distributions of most of the major neurotransmitters in the brain are known with some degree of specificity. The issue of the downstream circuitry is important and has been encountered in all fMRI studies of task activation. The metabolic effects of stimulation of a given set of neurons lead to local changes and changes in the attendant circuitry. This question must be reframed in light of the specific distribution of vascular receptors. Less is known about the distribution of vascular receptors than is known about the distribution of parenchymal receptors. Also the spatial correlation between vascular and parenchymal receptors is not well known. Again, disentangling the neurovascular coupling problem is a complex matter. If the pattern of activation induced by a given drug is *not* consistent with any known receptor distributions of the drug administered, the interpretation of the phMRI data is much less interesting than it would otherwise be. The likely place to look in such a situation is for specific vascular phenomena, for example.

The third criterion is important. It helps demonstrate that the phMRI activation observed is specific to the neurotransmitter system studied. If a lesion is made to ablate a neurotransmitter, for example, the response induced by a drug targeted to that neuroreceptor system should also be reduced. This will be described in more detail below.

The fourth criterion is important for the same reason. By examining the responses of a given receptor system to both agonists and antagonists, it is possible to gain a better understanding of the effects of hemodynamic coupling. One could postulate that administration of a dopamine receptor D1 agonist might increase CBV (this is the case). Simple logic might suggest that administration of a dopamine D1 antagonist would decrease CBV (this is also the case). Thus, one can immediately suggest that signal increases noted after administration of nonspecific ligands such as amphetamine are driven largely by D1 agonism. Such a criterion should always be included in planning animal studies.

Finally, the last criterion is important for a number of reasons. In PET imaging one is often interested in the regional binding of a tracer level of a given ligand. This gets at the receptor distribution. In phMRI, in order to get a measurable response, one must typically inject a high enough dose that there are measurable systemic effects. Such doses are usually behaviorally active — hence the phMRI data should correlate, temporally and spatially, with the behavioral data. In this context these studies can be considered to be similar to what is observed with task activated fMRI studies where the behavioral response in general correlates spatial and temporally with the fMRI response (although in practice one is usually performing the inverse solution of manipulating a behavior and solving for the brain signal changes).

In order to make these criteria more concrete, we will review the steps taken in animal studies of the dopamine system to show how hemodynamic changes observed after stimulation with dopaminergic drugs were truly due to stimulation of dopamine receptors. Luckily, in the case of the dopamine system, a large body of literature enabled us to cross-validate the phMRI studies.

6.3.1 APPLICATIONS TO DOPAMINERGIC SYSTEM

We used two injected drugs to stimulate activity in an acute challenge design. The first was amphetamine, a drug that causes reverse transport of dopamine through the dopamine transporter and increases dopamine release from presynaptic vesicles.[51] The second drug was β-CFT (2β-carbomethoxy-3β-(4-fluorophenyl)tropane), a selective blocker of the dopamine transporter that decreases reuptake of presynaptic dopamine. The first animal experiment might require injection of a target drug and observation of hemodynamic changes. It is possible to simultaneously measure both mean arterial blood pressure (MABP) and pCO2 in the same animal, thereby assuring that hemodynamic changes are not due to changes in systemic physiologic parameters. This is a good start, but it is hardly sufficient. We showed that injections of amphetamine and β-CFT produced transient systemic increases in MABP. The increases were of much shorter duration than BOLD or rCBV changes induced by these drugs[5] — a dynamic that was already known for amphetamine.[129]

The next step might be to compare how the spatial patterns of BOLD or rCBV changes compare to known distributions of dopaminergic neurons. Dopamine D1 and D2 receptors have the highest densities of expression in the striatum, nucleus accumbens, substantia nigra, ventral tegmental area, and prefrontal cortex.[32] They also produce extremely high densities in the large olfactory areas of rats. Thus, the observed signal changes generally correlate with the known spatial patterns of dopamine receptors although the correlation is not perfect. A very large induced phMRI signal change occurs in the thalamus, an area not ordinarily considered to have high dopamine receptor density (except for D5 receptors). The thalamus is, however, the output circuit to the cortex from the striatum. Thus it is not surprising that activation might be seen there.

In the dopamine system, a number of well described and specific lesion models already existed for selective ablation of the nigral-striatal dopamine tracts using 6-hydroxydopamine toxin.[130] These lesion models can be utilized unilaterally (see Figure 6.13). The unlesioned side is essentially normal, and can be used as a control. This then allows one to determine whether signal changes are indeed due to dopamine, as other related aminergic neurotransmitters such as norepinephrine and noradrenaline and acetylcholine are spared in this model. Comparing the BOLD and rCBV changes induced by amphetamine or CFT indicates that the signal changes are largely restricted to the intact side. The intact side looks similar to a conventional amphetamine scan (Figure 6.14).[5,8,12]

A simple behavioral test correlates well with the degree of lesioning. After a dose of amphetamine, a unilaterally lesioned animal will turn repeatedly to its contralateral side. The time course of the turning correlates well with the time course of the phMRI signal changes in the striatum. Not surprisingly, it also parallels the

Unilateral 6-OHDA Parkinson's Model

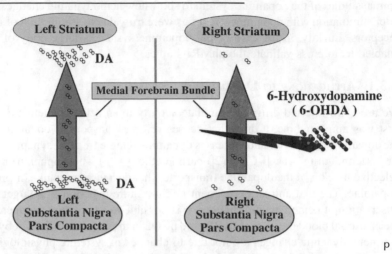

FIGURE 6.13 Schematic of unilateral destruction of nigral-striatal dopamine tracts using 6-hydroxydopamine toxin. This well characterized model provides a way to study the effects of dopaminergic depletion while the other side of the brain remains relatively normal. In this model, the noradrenergic and cholinergic neurons are spared.

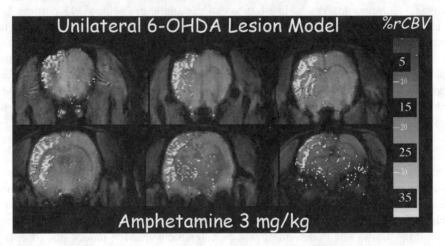

FIGURE 6.14 IRON imaging of the percent rCBV changes induced by 3 mg/kg amphetamine in a rat with a unilateral 6-OHDA lesion. Note the nearly complete loss of hemodynamic changes on the lesioned side, including the downstream thalamic circuitry, frontal cortex, and striatum. See Color Figure 6.14 following page 210.

release of dopamine induced by amphetamine. This time course is the same on the intact side in a lesioned animal and in a control animal. Figure 6.13 also showed the correlation of dopamine release and the phMRI time course (BOLD and rCBV) in a control animal. The time course of dopamine release clearly parallels that of the hemodynamic changes for amphetamine and CFT. These results suggest that dopamine may drive the hemodynamic response.

One more experiment provides additional evidence that the phMRI signal changes are due to stimulation of dopamine neurons. Transplantation of fetal dopamine cells into the unilaterally lesioned striatum restored the behavioral profile (stopping the animals from turning after injection with amphetamine). It also restored the binding of CFT as measured by PET scans and the phMRI response at the same location as the graft. This was readily verified by postmortem histology.[8] The technique may prove useful for study of fetal and stem cell grafting in Parkinson's disease.[8,131] It is discussed in more detail in Section 6.3.3.

In summary, hemodynamic changes induced by dopaminergic ligands are specific to dopamine in the striatum. phMRI signal changes do not correlate with pCO_2 or blood pressure changes. Signal changes are lost by destruction of dopaminergic fiber innervation even when cholinergic, glutamatergic, adenosynergic, GABAergic, and adrenergic innervation is intact. phMRI response is restored by transplantation of dopaminergic neurons. It correlates spatially and temporally with dopamine efflux measured via microdialysis and is strongest in areas with high dopamine innervation, as measured by PET or autoradiography. Signal magnitude correlates with ability to release dopamine.

6.3.2 Applications of phMRI to Studies of Drug Abuse

Drugs of abuse such as nicotine, cocaine, and heroin are major problems in the industrialized world. While each of those substances targets a different neurotransmitter system (cholinergic, dopaminergic, and opioid systems, respectively), the general consensus is that most of the rewarding effects of the drugs act through the meso-cortical-limbic dopaminergic system that includes the sublenticular extended amygdala, hypothalamus, nucleus accumbens, striatum, and frontal cortex. This reward pathway is common in alcohol and other types of substance abuse and in potentially addictive behaviors involving sex,[132] video games,[133] and even music.[134]

A number of approaches can be taken when investigating drugs of abuse using fMRI or phMRI. One is studying the effects of drugs of abuse on cognitive or visual tasks by targeting brain regions of interest. The effects can be chronic or can be studied during administration of the drug.[135-137] It is essential when investigating effects during drug administration to understand the vascular effects of the drug in the absence of cognitive challenge.

Another potentially revealing study would focus on the effects of tasks targeting the reward circuitry in control and addicted populations.[138,139] Such studies may be useful in explaining imbalances in such circuitry that may precipitate or predispose individuals toward abuse. It is essential to pay attention to potentially adaptive changes that may take place in, for example, the dopaminergic system as consequences of the abuse of drugs. This condition may be probed via the acute challenge methodology discussed above. We believe the acute challenge method is most sensitive to the basal state of the target receptors in the brain, and hence can be likened somewhat to a PET study of receptor populations.

We will now summarize some of the acute challenge phMRI literature concerning animal and human studies. More papers on this subject appear every year. We will try to focus on what may be learned from such studies rather than cataloguing the findings.

6.3.2.1 Dopaminergic Drugs

Dopaminergic drugs have been studied extensively using phMRI methods. Cocaine, its analogs, and amphetamine have been studied in humans and animals. The animal data on such drugs are reasonably consistent, in that an increased CBV or BOLD signal is generally noted in the basal ganglia.[5,7,9,140] More or less cortical activation is seen with different drugs in dopaminergically related brain areas such as frontal and insular cortex similar to prior studies with PET and autoradiography. Data on humans is more difficult to interpret for a number of reasons. Studies in humans are restricted to analyzing the BOLD effect (or the even less sensitive imaging of CBF by MRI). Data from primary sensory stimuli such as photic stimulation are often greater than those obtained with cognitive stimuli, and the cocaine-induced effects (given the relatively small doses around 0.5 mg/kg used in human studies compared to the 1 mg/kg doses used in rodent studies) are relatively small. Work from Hans Breiter's laboratory has shown that expectancy is a severe confound of BOLD signal in, for instance, the nucleus accumbens as it may determine the amplitude of the baseline BOLD signal.[138]

A number of other confounds remain in the human data. Acute administration of cocaine can lead to vasoconstriction and subsequent decreases in CBV or BOLD in many different brain regions.[115,141] It also increased BOLD in limbic areas such as the nucleus accumbens.[142] A study by Kaufman et al.[141] revealed significant differences in rCBV after administration of 0.4 mg/kg cocaine in both men and women and significant differences among women as a function of menstrual cycle. However, as discussed earler (Section 6.2.5), many decreases in BOLD and rCBV may be related to hyperventilation. After infusion of cocaine under double-blind conditions, cocaine-dependent subjects demonstrated significant increases in heart rate and mean arterial blood pressure and decreases in $ETCO_2$.[142] Correlation maps of signal changes induced by infusion of cocaine with behavioral measures (euphoria or craving) showed dramatic differences. Craving tended to be associated with activation in the nucleus accumbens and amygdala and the "rush" or euphoria tended to correlate with activity in the anterior cingulate, basal forebrain, and ventral tegmental areas. Administration of cocaine in a double-blind fashion (where neither the subject nor investigator knew whether the subject received cocaine or placebo) is required to eliminate the possibility that cues about the substance injected will change expectancy, and thereby modulate the signal. Figure 6.15 illustrates a pattern of activity induced by a single intravenous dose of 0.6 mg/kg of cocaine administered in a double-blind fashion or a dose of saline. The images indicate that the expectancy of receiving the cocaine (whether or not the subject receives cocaine or saline) causes increased BOLD signal in the ventral nucleus accumbens. In the case of the cocaine infusion, unlike the saline, activation is seen in the dorsal-medial accumbens and the subcallosal complex.[142]

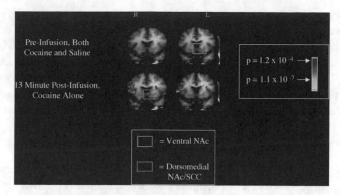

FIGURE 6.15 BOLD phMRI (1.5 T) of double-blind infusion of a single intravenous dose of cocaine (0.6 mg/kg) or saline. The expectancy of receiving cocaine (regardless of whether the subject receives cocaine or saline) causes increased BOLD signal in the ventral nucleus accumbens. In the case of cocaine infusion, activation is seen in the dorsal-medial accumbens, and the subcallosal complex.[142] (Courtesy of Dr. Hans Breiter, Massachusetts General Hospital.) See Color Figure 6.15 following page 210.

Other studies of brain regions involved in cocaine craving focused on fMRI response to visual cues of cocaine use to stimulate craving.[143,144] Areas such as the anterior cingulate, dorsolateral prefrontal cortex, and caudate were significantly activated in cocaine-abusing subjects in response to visual cues. These studies indicate that response to a relatively small injection of cocaine is a complicated effect of several cognitive and emotional responses in addition to its direct pharmacologic and vasoactive effects.

Most of these studies successfully demonstrate the utility of phMRI for evaluation of acute drug challenges to dopaminergic reward circuitry. However, no one has yet combined a study to evaluate changes in the dopamine system as a function of the addictive process with withdrawal and therapy. Such a combination could, for example, evaluate the effects of addiction and withdrawal on the D2 system since decreases in D2 binding have been associated with increased cocaine craving and self-administration.[145,146] Another study might analyze the changes associated in cocaine-induced activation by pretreatment with D2 agonists or antagonists. Another possibility is examining changes to the dopamine transporter protein — the primary target of cocaine and amphetamine.

Further correlation of temporal changes in the acute challenge model such as repeated acute challenges longitudinally with temporal changes in molecules such as CREB and Δ-FosB[147] would be invaluable in determining whether time courses are correlated. Such a study would have the potential to associate changes in brain circuitry with molecular events known to correlate with behavioral profiles. For example, increased CREB activity in the 25 days after cessation of cocaine has been shown to correlate with an acute anhedonic effect. Buildup of Δ-FosB over later times correlated with potentiation of the abuse potential.[146] Such a study in animals would be of great value when combined with behavioral and phMRI studies. Luckily, repeated injections of cocaine to humans in a laboratory setting do not seem to influence future abuse.[148]

We discussed above the correlations between extracellular dopamine and the phMRI signal changes. Interestingly, in rhesus monkeys there were no correlations of extracellular dopamine with drug-seeking activity in response to visual cues. There were, however, huge increases in extracellular dopamine induced by the cocaine.[149] This is an important factor to keep in mind when trying to assess the origins of increased BOLD or CBF in the brain reward circuitry. Another very important confound is discussed below with respect to nicotine administration.

6.3.2.2 Nicotine

Nicotine has been the subject of many studies. Like the dopaminergics, nicotine can exert specific vascular effects, most notably vasodilation. However, much of the observed vasodilatory effect appears to be mediated via NO.[41] Intravenous administration of nicotine to human subjects led to increased BOLD signal in nucleus accumbens, amygdala, cingulate, and frontal lobes, all areas associated with reward circuitry.[13] In addition, the primary sites of activation appear to correspond well with the distribution of nicotine cholinergic binding sites seen using PET ^{11}C-nicotine binding.[150] The highest concentration of sites is found in the frontal, cingulate, and insular lobes of the cortex and in the thalamus and basal ganglia. These results are somewhat different from PET measurements of changes in regional CBF. Nicotine reduced rCBF in the left anterior temporal cortex and right amygdala. Increases were noted in the right anterior thalamus.[151,152] Nicotine was administered intravenously in the MRI study and nasally in the PET studies. How these two administration routes affect the observed signal changes is not known.

Separation of the components of activation due to reward circuitry vs. components produced by direct stimulation of the cholinergic receptors has not been attempted, nor have systematic investigations of the effects of other cholinergic antagonists and agonists on nicotine-induced hemodynamic changes. Breiter et al.[138] cited an additional confound related to activation of reward circuitry vs. the direct effects of the drug on its target receptors in their studies of monetary rewards. They noted positive and negative BOLD signal changes in the nucleus accumbens in response to the same stimulus, depending on the subject's expectation of the stimulus. Thus, in studies where the drug is not administered in double-blind fashion, it is conceivable that the expectation of the subject may dramatically influence the activation seen in accumbens. This is likely to be a confound in cases where a drug of interest such as nicotine does not produce a large change in dopamine release in the dopaminergic elements of the reward circuitry.

6.3.2.3 Heroin

A few studies have appeared examining the effects of heroin. One study examined the effects of an acute heroin dose upon visual activation using fMRI. Not surprisingly, there was decreased activation after heroin in all the subjects.[136] Another study followed visual drug cues in heroin users with an actual drug dose to evaluate different brain patterns associated with cues for use. The "urge to use" correlated strongly with increased regional blood flow (rCBF) in the inferior frontal and orbitofrontal cortex regions implicated in conditioning and reward.[153] Autoradiographic studies of changes in blood flow in rats after acute doses of heroin showed increased CBF in many different brain regions that could be blocked by naloxone.[154,155] One phMRI study of heroin has appeared in rats.[14] In this study there was a large difference between spontaneously breathing and artificially-ventilated rats with the former showing widespread decreases in BOLD. In the latter case there were systematic increases in BOLD signal regions consistent with the distribution of opiate mu-receptors in rat brain. These increases were blockable using naloxone.

The confounds of changes in respiratory gases are pointed out by a number of the studies discussed above. It is clear that simultaneous measurement of blood gases is critical. However, this brings up the interesting point that changes in global hemodynamic states induced by changes in blood gases may be overridden in select brain regions by direct action of other vasoactive neurotransmitters. Such a complicated set of dynamics means that simple corrections of drift in phMRI signals may not always be useful or even feasible.

The use of phMRI for investigations related to drug abuse is only in its infancy. Nonetheless, MRI lends itself well to multiple longitudinal studies that will be of great value for studying the effects of withdrawal and therapy. In addition, the high temporal and spatial resolution of MRI may well allow for better discrimination of subtle pharmacodynamic effects than is possible with other techniques.

6.3.3 APPLICATIONS TO STUDIES OF NEURODEGENERATION

Neurodegenerative disorders such as Alzheimer's disease (AD) and Parkinson's disease (PD) are devastating progressive illnesses. Much is known about their pathology and much less is known about their etiology. Most of these illnesses have few therapeutic options, and the therapies used to date eventually stop working after some period of time. Many of these diseases target specific neurotransmitter systems or selectively damage specific brain regions. Cholinergic neurons seem to be selectively vulnerable in AD. Dopamine neurons are the primary targets in PD. This selectivity with respect to neuronal populations makes the use of phMRI a potentially valuable adjunct for addressing questions of etiology, natural history, and progression.

PET studies have investigated many of the same metabolic and neurotransmitter questions one would like to address with phMRI in various neurodegenerative conditions. These studies often show decreased glucose utilization in the parts of the brain undergoing selective degeneration. In addition, degeneration of dopamine neurons in PD and cholinergic neurons in AD can be shown using ligands selective for those neurotransmitter systems. We will not review this literature here. We will discuss phMRI studies of the dopaminergic system in PD models.

Unlike the situation for many neurodegenerative conditions, good PD animal models have existed for many years. With the advent of transgenic mouse models, more neurodegenerative diseases will be the subjects of animal studies. The PD models were based on neurotoxins that are selective for dopamine neurons. The first model was based upon 6-hydroxydopamine, a compound selectively taken up by dopamine neurons where it generates toxic hydroxyl radicals. It has been used for many years in rats via direct injection of 6-OHDA into the substantia nigra or medial forebrain bundle to destroy the nigro-striatal or nigro-frontal dopaminergic projections.

One helpful feature of such a model is the ability to produce unilateral lesions and keep one side of the animal relatively intact as a control. Such lesions generate characteristic behavioral profiles because injections of amphetamine cause the animals to rotate when dopamine is released on the intact sides. This behavior has been well characterized over the years and the amount of dopamine cell loss is quantitatively related to the number of rotations over a threshold value.[156]

Another permutation is to inject 6-OHDA into the striatum and follow the retrograde transport into, and subsequent degeneration of, the substantia nigra. Another toxin model is capable of producing the selective destruction of dopamine neurons that is the hallmark of PD. It was discovered when adulterated synthetic heroin caused a number of 20-year old individuals to develop symptoms almost entirely reminiscent of idiopathic PD. The contaminant was a compound known as MPTP. It is converted via monoamine oxidase-B (MAO-B) into N-methyl-4-phenylpyridinium (MPP$^+$).[157] MPP is an extremely selective inhibitor of complex I in the electron transport chain that inhibits ATP production. Its selectivity for the dopaminergic system is thought to arise from selective uptake of MPTP via the dopamine transporter. The model has been most often studied in primates and can generate the PD model with systemic injections. Rats have little MAO-B. They convert very little MPTP into MPP$^+$ and thus suffer little dopamine cell loss. We will discuss rat and monkey PD models and cover aspects of pathology and therapy rather than perform a literature review.

6.3.2.4 Unilateral Rat Models of PD

We have extensively studied 6-OHDA in a rat PD model using phMRI.[5,8,12] Figure 6.13 is a schematic of such a model. Our studies were geared toward multiple objectives. We wanted to show that the hemodynamic effects of amphetamine or β-CFT (a selective dopamine transporter blocker similar to cocaine or methylphenidate) were due to dopamine release, not to some other neurotransmitter.

Careful lesioning led to selective dopamine cell loss, whereas cholinergic and noradrenergic neurons were preserved. We found a loss of hemodynamic response on the lesioned side, while the phMRI response was preserved on the intact side.[5,8] Figure 6.14 illustrates these effects.

We also showed that the behavioral profile of the rotational behavior after administration of amphetamine correlated quite nicely with the phMRI time course. This lends credence to the utility of the technique for assessment of the behavioral consequences of the disease model. It also indicates that phMRI will be a useful marker for following potential therapies. We showed this possibility where recovery of the dopaminergic response occurred after transplantation with fetal dopamine cells in the striatum. The recovery correlated with the temporal pattern of the rotational behavior, the spatial distribution of ^{11}C-CFT binding (a ligand selective for DAT), and histology results.[8] These experiments were conducted with BOLD phMRI. Later experiments showed that IRON phMRI experiments (as expected)

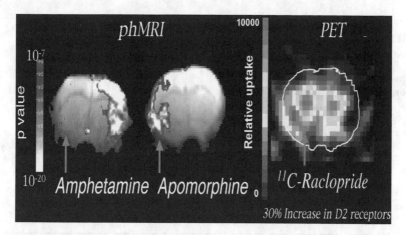

FIGURE 6.16 phMRI detection of postsynaptic dopamine receptor supersensitivity. Left: IRON image of amphetamine activation in a rat with a unilateral 6-OHDA lesion. As shown in Figure 6.14, the amphetamine produces rCBV increases on the intact side only. Administration of apomorphine, a dopamine agonist, to the same animal leads to increased rCBV on the lesion side only. PET imaging of D2 receptors using ^{11}C-raclopride in the same animal leads to an increase of about 30% on the lesioned side. The phMRI images have been averaged to produce average slice thicknesses comparable to the PET images (4.5 mm). See Color Figure 6.16 following page 210.

were even more sensitive and were able to show recovery of poststriatal cortical circuitry after the stem cell graft was able to successfully innervate the host.[131]

A third issue was the effect of receptor supersensitivity. It is well known that postsynaptic upregulation of dopamine receptors follows unilateral lesioning with 6-OHDA. This is referred to as supersensitivity because it leads to unusual behavioral sensitivity to the effects of dopamine. This phenomenon has been shown for other neurotransmitter systems as well. Injection of amphetamine in unilaterally lesioned animals produced the expected loss of phMRI response on the lesioned side. Injection of apomorphine, a nonselective dopamine agonist, produced increased rCBV on the lesioned side and very little on the intact side.[12] Another parameter of interest is supersensitivity caused by upregulation of postsynaptic dopamine receptors. It is possible to inject apomorphine, a nonspecific dopamine agonist, to elicit a large response on the lesioned side while the intact side shows no response to the apomorphine. The endogenous dopamine competes with (and wins over) apomorphine for binding to receptors on the intact side. This is not possible on the lesioned side, so a large increase in CBV occurs after apomorphine injection. Apomorphine was a very sensitive marker for supersensitivity.[12] Other studies have shown decreases in R2* after administration of L-dopa in an MPTP-lesioned primate model.[10] This effect is similar to that noted with apomorphine, although the changes were smaller due to the relatively low increases in synaptic dopamine levels caused by L-dopa.

This finding correlated well with postsynaptic PET measurements of upregulation in D2 receptors in the same animals (see Figure 6.16). These studies add credence to the belief that phMRI may be useful for investigating dopamine receptor dynamics in PD models and in studying PD. The studies amply demonstrate that

TABLE 6.4
Dopaminergic Decline in PD Assessed via PET or phMRI

Physical Effect or Symptom	Receptor Parameter	PET Marker	phMRI Marker
Loss of presynaptic DA terminals	Loss of DAT	^{11}C-CFT binding decreased	Amphetamine or cocaine phMRI response decreased
Loss of DA synthesis	Loss of DA cell bodies	Decreased ^{18}F-dopa uptake	Decreased response to amphetamine?
Supersensitivity or dyskinesias	Upregulation of postsynaptic D2 receptors	Increased binding potential of ^{11}C-raclopride	Large phMRI response to apomorphine or L-dopa

phMRI is a useful tool for investigating dopamine cell loss, dopamine cell recovery using fetal and stem cell transplantation, and measurement of receptor supersensitivity. The primate studies discussed below confirm the value of phMRI.

One question left unresolved is the comparison with PET. Hemodynamic measurements made with phMRI are indirect. PET directly measures dopamine receptor binding and dopamine metabolism using ^{18}F-labeled dopa. We will compare PET and phMRI for measuring dopamine cell loss, dopamine cell recovery, and receptor supersensitivity. Table 6.4 compares the parameters measured by using PET or phMRI to study dopamine cell loss in PD. PET measurements of dopamine cell loss seem to be best reflected in ligands specific for DAT.[158] These ligands provide markers for presynaptic dopamine terminals that are depleted in PD. By comparison, amphetamine stimulus reflects the amount of dopamine that can be released. Loss of the dopamine transporter will lead to a loss of an effect after amphetamine stimulus or stimulation with a DAT blocker such as β-CFT. The lack of effect from an amphetamine stimulus arises because dopamine concentrations are depleted (less is available for release) and because the reverse transport of dopamine into the synaptic cleft induced by amphetamine requires invagination of the DAT. Compounds such as β-CFT are also ineffective at evoking increases in dopamine levels due to the lack of target DAT. We found a good correlation between PET measures of decreased CFT binding in unilaterally lesioned rats with both amphetamine- and CFT-induced phMRI changes.[5,140]

These results clearly indicate the utility of phMRI for assessing various components of dopaminergic function. Separating some of these effects into their components may be difficult, but carefully designed experiments using animal models may well do this. For instance, deciding whether a loss of DAT or simply a loss of presynaptic dopamine stores occurred can be accomplished by considering the differences between CFT and amphetamine. If neither compound can produce a signal increase in the lesioned brain, DAT targets are probably depleted. Existing experiments do not indicate whether the synthesis and presynaptic dopamine stores are intact (although the models indicate they are not). The use of L-dopa as a challenge may prove to be quantitatively related to the amount of presynaptic dopamine that can be released. It may be possible to administer L-dopa in conjunction with a DAT blocker such as cocaine or CFT to potentiate the effects of the L-dopa.

Pharmacological MRI also makes a good tool for following therapeutic interventions in lesion models. We showed a good recovery of dopamine cell loss following transplantation of fetal dopamine cells and stem cells.[8,131] The sizes of the grafts were shown by phMRI to be consistent with grafts seen in PET scans and in subsequent histology studies. phMRI has the potential to become a useful clinical tool if and when such therapies prove to be efficacious for PD.

ACKNOWLEDGMENTS

We would like to acknowledge the contributions of our many colleagues, especially M. Flint Beal, Hans Breiter, Anna-Liisa Brownell, Anthony J-W. Chen, Keith Chiappa, Ji-Kyung Choi, Ole Isacson, Ekkehard Kuestermann, John B. Moore, T. Van Nguyen, and Bruce R. Rosen.

REFERENCES

1. Belliveau, J.W. et al., Functional mapping of the human visual cortex by magnetic resonance imaging, *Science,* 254, 716, 1991.
2. Kwong, K.K. et al., Dynamic magnetic resonance imaging of human brain activity during primary sensory stimulation, *Proc. Natl. Acad. Sci. U.S.A.,* 89, 5675, 1992.
3. Ogawa, S. et al., Intrinsic signal changes accompanying sensory stimulation: functional brain mapping with magnetic resonance imaging, *Proc. Natl. Acad. Sci. U.S.A.,* 89, 5951, 1992.
4. Carlsson, C., Hagerdal, M., and Siesjo, B.K., Influence of amphetamine sulfate on cerebral blood flow and metabolism, *Acta Physiol. Scand.,* 94, 128, 1975.
5. Chen, Y.I. et al., Detection of dopaminergic neurotransmitter activity using pharmacologic MRI: correlation with PET, microdialysis, and behavioral data, *Mag. Res. Med.,* 38, 389, 1997.
6. Silva, A.D. et al., Multislice MRI of rat brain during amphetamine stimulation using arterial spin labelling, *Mag. Res. Med.,* 33, 1995.
7. Zhang, Z. et al., Pharmacological MRI mapping of age-associated changes in basal ganglia circuitry of awake rhesus monkeys, *Neuroimage,* 14, 1159, 2001.
8. Chen, Y.I. et al., Detection of dopaminergic cell loss and neural transplantation using pharmacological MRI, PET and behavioral assessment, *Neuroreport,* 10, 2881, 1999.
9. Marota, J.J. et al., Cocaine activation discriminates dopaminergic projections by temporal response: an fMRI study in rats, *Neuroimage,* 11, 13, 2000.
10. Chen, Q. et al., Mapping drug-induced changes in cerebral R2* by multiple gradient recalled echo functional MRI, *Mag. Res. Imaging,* 14, 469, 1996.
11. Zhang, Z. et al., Functional MRI of apomorphine activation of the basal ganglia in awake rhesus monkeys, *Brain Res.,* 852, 290, 2000.
12. Nguyen, T.V. et al., Detection of the effects of dopamine receptor supersensitivity using pharmacological MRI and correlations with PET, *Synapse,* 36, 57, 2000.
13. Stein, E.A. et al., Nicotine-induced limbic cortical activation in the human brain: a functional MRI study, *Am. J. Psychiatr.,* 155, 1009, 1998.

14. Xu, H. et al., Heroin-induced neuronal activation in rat brain assessed by functional MRI, *Neuroreport*, 11, 1085, 2000.

15. Scanley, B.E., Kennan, R.P., and Gore, J.C., Changes in rat cerebral blood volume due to modulation of the 5-HT(1A) receptor measured with susceptibility enhanced contrast MRI, *Brain Res.*, 913, 149, 2001.

16. Kimberg, D.Y. et al., Cortical effects of bromocriptine, a D-2 dopamine receptor agonist, in human subjects, revealed by fMRI, *Hum. Brain Mapping*, 12, 246, 2001.

17. Schalling, M. et al., Comparison of gene expression of the dopamine D-2 receptor and DARPP-32 in rat brain, pituitary and adrenal gland, *Eur. J. Pharmacol.*, 188, 277, 1990.

18. Pompeiano, M., Palacios, J.M., and Mengod, G., Distribution and cellular localization of mRNA coding for 5-HT1A receptor in the rat brain: correlation with receptor binding, *J. Neurosci.*, 12, 440, 1992.

19. Palacios, J.M. et al., Recent trends in receptor analysis techniques and instrumentation, *J. Chem. Neuroanat.*, 4, 343, 1991.

20. Knull, H.R., Association of glycolytic enzymes with particulate fractions from nerve endings, *Biochim. Biophys. Acta*, 522, 1, 1978.

21. Knull, H.R. and Fillmore, S.J., Glycolytic enzyme levels in synaptosomes, *Comp. Biochem. Physiol. B*, 81, 349, 1985.

22. Knull, H. and Minton, A.P., Structure within eukaryotic cytoplasm and its relationship to glycolytic metabolism, *Cell Biochem. Funct.*, 14, 237, 1996.

23. Kadekaro, M., Crane, A.M., and Sokoloff, L., Differential effects of electrical stimulation of sciatic nerve on metabolic activity in spinal cord and dorsal root ganglion in the rat, *Proc. Natl. Acad. Sci. U.S.A..*, 82, 6010, 1985.

24. Sokoloff, L., Measurement of local cerebral glucose utilization and its relation to local functional activity in the brain, *Adv. Exp. Med. Biol.*, 291, 21, 1991.

25. Sokoloff, L., Sites and mechanisms of function-related changes in energy metabolism in the nervous system, *Dev. Neurosci.*, 15, 194, 1993.

26. Pellerin, L. and Magistretti, P.J., Glutamate uptake into astrocytes stimulates aerobic glycolysis: a mechanism coupling neuronal activity to glucose utilization, *Proc. Natl. Acad. Sci. U.S.A.*, 91, 10625, 1994.

27. Pellerin, L. and Magistretti, P.J., Excitatory amino acids stimulate aerobic glycolysis in astrocytes via an activation of the Na^+/K^+ ATPase, *Dev. Neurosci.*, 18, 336, 1996.

28. Magistretti, P.J., Cellular bases of functional brain imaging: insights from neuron-glia metabolic coupling, *Brain Res.*, 886, 108, 2000.

29. Sokoloff, L. et al., Contribution of astroglia to functionally activated energy metabolism, *Dev. Neurosci.*, 18, 344, 1996.

30. Stella, N. et al., Glutamate-evoked release of arachidonic acid from mouse brain astrocytes, *J. Neurosci.*, 14, 568, 1994.

31. Sorg, O. and Magistretti, P.J., Characterization of the glycogenolysis elicited by vasoactive intestinal peptide, noradrenaline and adenosine in primary cultures of mouse cerebral cortical astrocytes, *Brain Res.*, 563, 227, 1991.

32. Cooper, J.R., Bloom, F.E., and Roth, R.H., *The Biochemical Basis of Neuropharmacology*, Oxford University Press, New York, 1996.

33. Lindvall, O., Ingvar, M., and Stenevi, U., Effects of methamphetamine on blood flow in the caudate-putamen after lesions of the nigrostriatal dopaminergic bundle in the rat, *Brain Res.*, 211, 211, 1981.

34. Lyons, D. and Porrino, L.J., Dopamine depletion in the rostral nucleus accumbens alters the cerebral metabolic response to cocaine in the rat, *Brain Res.*, 753, 69, 1997.

35. Iadecola, C., Regulation of the cerebral microcirculation during neural activity: is nitric oxide the missing link? *Trends Neurosci.*, 16, 206, 1993.
36. Fillenz, M. et al., The role of astrocytes and noradrenaline in neuronal glucose metabolism, *Acta Physiol. Scand.*, 167, 275, 1999.
37. Faraci, F.M. and Brian, J.E., Jr., Nitric oxide and the cerebral circulation, *Stroke*, 25, 692, 1994.
38. Cohen, Z. et al., Serotonin in the regulation of brain microcirculation, *Progr. Neurobiol.*, 50, 335, 1996.
39. Sato, A. and Sato, Y., Cholinergic neural regulation of regional cerebral blood flow, *Alzheimer Dis. Assoc. Disorders*, 9, 28, 1995.
40. Vaucher, E., Linville, D., and Hamel, E., Cholinergic basal forebrain projections to nitric oxide synthase-containing neurons in the rat cerebral cortex, *Neuroscience*, 79, 827, 1997.
41. El Husseiny, A. and Hamel, E., Muscarinic — but not nicotinic — acetylcholine receptors mediate a nitric oxide-dependent dilation in brain cortical arterioles: a possible role for the M5 receptor subtype, *J. Cereb. Blood Flow Metabol.*, 20, 298, 2000.
42. Barbelivien, A. et al., Neurochemical stimulation of the rat substantia innominata increases cerebral blood flow (but not glucose use) through the parallel activation of cholinergic and non-cholinergic pathways, *Brain Res.*, 840, 115, 1999.
43. Head, R.J. et al., Isolated brain microvessels: preparation, morphology, histamine and catecholamine contents, *Blood Vessels*, 17, 173, 1980.
44. Jones, B.E., Relationship between catecholamine neurons and cerebral blood vessels studied by their simultaneous fluorescent revelation in the rat brainstem, *Brain Res. Bull.*, 9, 33, 1982.
45. Krimer, L.S. et al., Dopaminergic regulation of cerebral cortical microcirculation, *Nature Neurosci.*, 1, 286, 1998.
46. Nehlig, A., Daval, J.L., and Debry, G., Caffeine and the central nervous system: mechanisms of action, biochemical, metabolic and psychostimulant effects, *Brain Res. Rev.*, 17, 139, 1992.
47. Gulbenkian, S., Uddman, R., and Edvinsson, L., Neuronal messengers in the human cerebral circulation, *Peptides*, 22, 995, 2001.
48. Orzi, F. et al., Comparative effects of acute and chronic administration of amphetamine on local cerebral glucose utilization in the conscious rat, *J. Cereb. Blood Flow Metabol.*, 3, 154, 1983.
49. Trugman, J.M. and James, C.L., D1 dopamine agonist and antagonist effects on regional cerebral glucose utilization in rats with intact dopaminergic innervation, *Brain Res.*, 607, 270, 1993.
50. Wechsler L.R., S.H., Sokoloff L., Effects of d- and l-amphetamine on local cerebral glucose utilization in the conscious rat, *J. Neurochem.*, 32, 15, 1979.
51. Jones, S.R. et al., Mechanisms of amphetamine action revealed in mice lacking the dopamine transporter, *J. Neurosci.*, 18, 1979, 1998.
52. Sulzer, D., Maidment, N.T., and Rayport, S., Amphetamine and other weak bases act to promote reverse transport of dopamine in ventral midbrain neurons, *J. Neurochem.*, 60, 527, 1993.
53. Ferre, S. et al., Antagonistic interaction between adenosine A2A receptors and dopamine D2 receptors in the ventral striopallidal system: implications for the treatment of schizophrenia, *Neuroscience*, 63, 765, 1994.
54. Latini, S. et al., A2 adenosine receptors: their presence and neuromodulatory role in the central nervous system, *Gen. Pharmacol.*, 27, 925, 1996.

55. Sebastiao, A.M. and Ribeiro, J.A., Adenosine A2 receptor-mediated excitatory actions on the nervous system, *Progr. Neurobiol.*, 48, 167, 1996.

56. Le Moine, C. et al., Dopamine-adenosine interactions in the striatum and the globus pallidus: inhibition of striatopallidal neurons through either D2 or A2A receptors enhances D1 receptor-mediated effects on c-fos expression, *J. Neurosci.*, 17, 8038, 1997.

57. Pollack, A.E. et al., Differential localization of A2a adenosine receptor mRNA with D1 and D2 dopamine receptor mRNA in striatal output pathways following a selective lesion of striatonigral neurons, *Brain Res.*, 631, 161, 1993.

58. Schiffmann, S.N. and Vanderhaeghen, J.J., Adenosine A2 receptors regulate the gene expression of striatopallidal and striatonigral neurons, *J. Neurosci.*, 13, 1080, 1993.

59. Ferre, S. et al., Dopamine D1 receptor-mediated facilitation of GABAergic neurotransmission in the rat strioentopeduncular pathway and its modulation by adenosine A1 receptor-mediated mechanisms, *Eur. J. Neurosci.*, 8, 1545, 1996.

60. Misra, A.L., Vadlamani, N.L., and Pontani, R.B., Effect of caffeine on cocaine locomotor stimulant activity in rats, *Pharmacol. Biochem. Behav.*, 24, 761, 1986.

61. Herrera-Marschitz, M., Casas, M., and Ungerstedt, U., Caffeine produces contralateral rotation in rats with unilateral dopamine denervation: comparisons with apomorphine-induced responses, *Psychopharmacology*, 94, 38, 1988.

62. Pollack, A.E. and Fink, J.S., Synergistic interaction between an adenosine antagonist and a D1 dopamine agonist on rotational behavior and striatal c-Fos induction in 6-hydroxydopamine-lesioned rats, *Brain Res.*, 743, 124, 1996.

63. Ferre, S. et al., The striopallidal neuron: a main locus for adenosine-dopamine interactions in the brain, *J. Neurosci.*, 13, 5402, 1993.

64. Villringer, A. et al., Dynamic imaging with lanthanide chelates in normal brain: contrast due to magnetic susceptibility effects, *Magn. Res. Med.*, 6, 164, 1988.

65. Frank, J.A. et al., Measurement of relative cerebral blood volume changes with visual stimulation by "double-dose" gadopentetate-dimeglumine-enhanced dynamic magnetic resonance imaging, *Invest. Radiol.*, 29, Suppl. 2, S157, 1994.

66. Henriksen, L., Paulson, O.B., and Lassen, N.A., Visual cortex activation recorded by dynamic emission computed tomography of inhaled xenon 133, *Eur. J. Nucl. Med.*, 6, 487, 1981.

67. Greenberg, J.H. et al., Metabolic mapping of functional activity in human subjects with the [18F]fluorodeoxyglucose technique, *Science*, 212, 678, 1981.

68. Phelps, M.E., Positron computed tomography studies of cerebral glucose metabolism in man: theory and application in nuclear medicine, *Semin. Nucl. Med.*, 11, 32, 1981.

69. Mazziotta, J.C. et al., Tomographic mapping of human cerebral metabolism: auditory stimulation, *Neurology*, 32, 921, 1982.

70. Baron, J.C. et al., Noninvasive measurement of blood flow, oxygen consumption, and glucose utilization in the same brain regions in man by positron emission tomography: concise communication, *J. Nucl. Med.*, 23, 391, 1982.

71. Lassen, N.A. and Ingvar, D.H., Brain regions involved in voluntary movements as revealed by radioisotopic mapping of CBF or CMR-glucose changes, *Rev. Neurol.* (Paris), 146, 620, 1990.

72. Fox, P.T. et al., Nonoxidative glucose consumption during focal physiologic neural activity, *Science*, 241, 462, 1988.

73. Grafton, S.T., PET: activation of cerebral blood flow and glucose metabolism, *Adv. Neurol.*, 83, 87, 2000.

74. Singer, J.R., Blood flow rates by nuclear magnetic resonance measurements, *Science*, 130, 1652, 1959.

75. Dixon, W.T. et al., Projection angiograms of blood labeled by adiabatic fast passage, *Magn. Res. Med.,* 3, 454, 1986.
76. Detre, J.A., Leigh, J.S., Williams, D.S., and Koretsky, A.P., Perfusion Imaging, *Mag. Res. Med.,* 23, 37, 1992.
77. Ogawa, S. et al., Brain magnetic resonance imaging with contrast dependent on blood oxygenation, *Proc. Natl. Acad. Sci. U.S.A.,* 87, 9868, 1990.
78. Turner, R. et al., Echo-planar time course MRI of cat brain oxygenation changes, *Mag. Res. Med.,* 22, 159, 1991.
79. Bandettini, P.A. et al., Time course EPI of human brain function during task activation, *Mag. Res. Med.,* 25, 390, 1992.
80. Davis, T.L. et al., Calibrated functional MRI: mapping the dynamics of oxidative metabolism, *Proc. Natl. Acad. Sci. U.S.A.,* 95, 1834, 1998.
81. Mandeville, J.B. et al., MRI measurement of the temporal evolution of relative $CMRO_{(2)}$ during rat forepaw stimulation, *Mag. Res. Med.,* 42, 944, 1999.
82. Hoge, R.D. et al., Investigation of BOLD signal dependence on cerebral blood flow and oxygen consumption: the deoxyhemoglobin dilution model *Mag. Res. Med.,* 42, 849, 1999.
83. Ogawa, S., Lee, R.M., and Barrere, B., The sensitivity of magnetic resonance image signals of a rat brain to changes in the cerebral venous blood oxygenation, *Mag. Res. Med.,* 29, 205, 1993.
84. Fox, P.T. and Raichle, M.E., Focal physiological uncoupling of cerebral blood flow and oxidative metabolism during somatosensory stimulation in human subjects, *Proc. Natl. Acad. Sci. U.S.A.,* 83, 1140, 1986.
85. Hyder, F. et al., Oxidative glucose metabolism in rat brain during single forepaw stimulation: a spatially localized 1H[13C] nuclear magnetic resonance study, *J. Cereb. Blood Flow Metabol.,* 17, 1040, 1997.
86. Hyder, F. et al., Increased tricarboxylic acid cycle flux in rat brain during forepaw stimulation detected with 1H[13C]NMR, *Proc. Natl. Acad. Sci. U.S.A.,* 93, 7612, 1996.
87. Chen, W. et al., Study of tricarboxylic acid cycle flux changes in human visual cortex during hemifield visual stimulation using (1)H-[(13)C] MRS and fMRI, *Mag. Res. Med.,* 45, 349, 2001.
88. Chen, Y.C. et al., Improved mapping of pharmacologically induced neuronal activation using the IRON technique with superparamagnetic blood pool agents, *J. Mag. Res. Imaging,* 14, 517, 2001.
89. van Bruggen, N. et al., High-resolution functional magnetic resonance imaging of the rat brain: mapping changes in cerebral blood volume using iron oxide contrast media, *J. Cereb. Blood Flow Metabol.,* 18, 1178, 1998.
90. Mandeville, J.B. et al., Dynamic functional imaging of relative cerebral blood volume during rat forepaw stimulation, *Mag. Res. Med.,* 39, 615, 1998.
91. Kennan, R.P. et al., Physiological basis for BOLD MR signal changes due to neuronal stimulation: separation of blood volume and magnetic susceptibility effects, *Mag. Res. Med.,* 40, 840, 1998.
92. Mandeville, J.B. et al., Regional sensitivity and coupling of BOLD and CBV changes during stimulation of rat brain, *Mag. Res. Med.,* 45, 443, 2001.
93. Taylor, A.M. et al., Use of the intravascular contrast agent NC100150 injection in spin-echo and gradient-echo imaging of the heart, *J. Cardiovasc. Mag. res.,* 1, 23, 1999.
94. Saini, S. et al., Multicentre dose-ranging study on the efficacy of USPIO ferumoxtran-10 for liver MR imaging, *Clin. Radiol.,* 55, 690, 2000.

95. Boxerman, J.L. et al., The intravascular contribution to fMRI signal change: Monte Carlo modeling and diffusion-weighted studies *in vivo, Mag. Res. Med.,* 34, 4, 1995.

96. Biswal, B., DeYoe, A.E., and Hyde, J.S., Reduction of physiological fluctuations in fMRI using digital filters, *Mag. Res. Med.,* 35, 107, 1996.

97. Buonocore, M.H. and Maddock, R.J., Noise suppression digital filter for functional magnetic resonance imaging based on image reference data, *Mag. Res. Med.,* 38, 456, 1997.

98. Purdon, P.L. and Weisskoff, R.M., Effect of temporal autocorrelation due to physiological noise and stimulus paradigm on voxel-level false-positive rates in fMRI, *Hum. Brain Mapping,* 6, 239, 1998.

99. Prichard, J. et al., Lactate rise detected by 1H NMR in human visual cortex during physiologic stimulation, *Proc. Natl. Acad. Sci. U.S.A.,* 88, 5829, 1991.

100. Chhina, N. et al., Measurement of human tricarboxylic acid cycle rates during visual activation by ^{13}C magnetic resonance spectroscopy, *J. Neurosci. Res.,* 66, 737, 2001.

101. Merboldt, K.D. et al., Decrease of glucose in the human visual cortex during photic stimulation, *Mag. Res. Med.,* 25, 187, 1992.

102. Gruetter, R. et al., Observation of resolved glucose signals in 1H NMR spectra of the human brain at 4 Tesla, *Mag. Res. Med.,* 36, 1, 1996.

103. Mason, G.F. et al., Simultaneous determination of the rates of the TCA cycle, glucose utilization, α-ketoglutarate/glutamate exchange, and glutamine synthesis in human brain by NMR, *J. Cereb. Blood Flow Metabol.,* 15, 12, 1995.

104. Gruetter, R., Seaquist, E.R., and Ugurbil, K., A mathematical model of compartmentalized neurotransmitter metabolism in the human brain, *Am. J. Physiol. Endocrinol. Metabol.,* 281, E100, 2001.

105. Posse, S. et al., *In vivo* measurement of regional brain metabolic response to hyperventilation using magnetic resonance: proton echo planar spectroscopic imaging (PEPSI), *Mag. Res. Med.,* 37, 858, 1997.

106. Hyder, F., Renken, R., and Rothman, D.L., *In vivo* carbon-edited detection with proton echo-planar spectroscopic imaging (ICED PEPSI): [3,4-(13)CH(2)]glutamate/glutamine tomography in rat brain, *Mag. Res. Med.,* 42, 997, 1999.

107. Guimaraes, A.R. et al., Echoplanar chemical shift imaging, *Mag. Res. Med.,* 41, 877, 1999.

108. Loubinoux, I. et al., Cerebral metabolic changes induced by MK-801: a 1D (phosphorus and proton) and two-dimensional (proton) *in vivo* NMR spectroscopy study, *Brain Res.,* 643, 115, 1994.

109. Petroff, O.A., and Rothman, D.L., Measuring human brain GABA *in vivo*: effects of GABA-transaminase inhibition with vigabatrin, *Mol. Neurobiol.,* 16, 97, 1998.

110. Kustermann, E.H.G. et al., Assessment of amphetamine induced stimulus using *in vivo* ^{13}C MRS in rat brain, in *Proc. Intl. Soc. Mag. Res. Med.,* 1998, p. 1362.

111. Lin, Y.J. and Koretsky, A.P., Manganese ion enhances T1-weighted MRI during brain activation: an approach to direct imaging of brain function, *Mag. Res. Med.,* 38, 378, 1997.

112. Duong, T.Q. et al., Functional MRI of calcium-dependent synaptic activity: cross correlation with CBF and BOLD measurements, *Mag. Res. Med.,* 43, 383, 2000.

113. Verity, M.A., Manganese neurotoxicity: a mechanistic hypothesis, *Neurotoxicology,* 20, 489, 1999.

114. Weckesser, M. et al., Functional imaging of the visual cortex with bold-contrast MRI: hyperventilation decreases signal response, *Mag. Res. Med.,* 41, 213, 1999.

115. Gollub, R.L. et al., Cocaine decreases cortical cerebral blood flow but does not obscure regional activation in functional magnetic resonance imaging in human subjects, *J. Cereb. Blood Flow Metabol.*, 18, 724, 1998.

116. Zaharchuk, G. et al., Cerebrovascular dynamics of autoregulation and hypoperfusion. An MRI study of CBF and changes in total and microvascular cerebral blood volume during hemorrhagic hypotension, *Stroke,* 30, 2197, 1999.

117. Kalisch, R. et al., Blood pressure changes induced by arterial blood withdrawal influence bold signal in anesthesized rats at 7 Tesla: implications for pharmacologic MRI, *Neuroimage,* 14, 891, 2001.

118. Stullken, E.H., Jr. et al., The nonlinear responses of cerebral metabolism to low concentrations of halothane, enflurane, isoflurane, and thiopental, *Anesthesiology,* 46, 28, 1977.

119. Lindauer, U., Villringer, A., and Dirnagl, U., Characterization of CBF response to somatosensory stimulation: model and influence of anesthetics, *Am. J. Physiol.*, 264, H1223, 1993.

120. Hara, K. and Harris, R.A., The anesthetic mechanism of urethane: the effects on neurotransmitter-gated ion channels, *Anesth. Analg.,* 94, 313, 2002.

121. Anis, N.A. et al., The dissociative anaesthetics, ketamine and phencyclidine, selectively reduce excitation of central mammalian neurones by N-methyl-aspartate, *Br. J. Pharmacol.,* 79, 565, 1983.

122. Thomson, A.M., West, D.C., and Lodge, D., An N-methylaspartate receptor-mediated synapse in rat cerebral cortex: a site of action of ketamine? *Nature,* 313, 479, 1985.

123. Hancock, P.J. and Stamford, J.A., Stereospecific effects of ketamine on dopamine efflux and uptake in the rat nucleus accumbens, *Br. J. Anaesth.,* 82, 603, 1999.

124. Ueki, M., Mies, G., and Hossmann, K.A., Effect of α-chloralose, halothane, pentobarbital and nitrous oxide anesthesia on metabolic coupling in somatosensory cortex of rat, *Acta Anaesthesiol. Scand.,* 36, 318, 1992.

125. Nieoullon, A. and Dusticier, N., Effects of α-chloralose on the activity of the nigrostriatal dopaminergic system in the cat, *Eur. J. Pharmacol.,* 65, 403, 1980.

126. Chen, Y.I. et al., Anesthetic filters for eliciting specific neurotransmitter effects in pharmacologic MRI, in *Proc. Intl. Soc. Mag. Res. Med.,* 2000, p. 967.

127. Kleven, M.S. et al., Effects of repeated injections of cocaine on D1 and D2 dopamine receptors in rat brain, *Brain Res.,* 532, 265, 1990.

128. Letchworth, S.R. et al., Effects of chronic cocaine administration on dopamine transporter mRNA and protein in the rat, *Brain Res.,* 750, 214, 1997.

129. Berntman, L. et al., Circulatory and metabolic effects in the brain induced by amphetamine sulphate, *Acta Physiol. Scand.,* 102, 310, 1978.

130. Perese, D.A. et al., A 6-hydroxydopamine-induced selective Parkinsonian rat model, *Brain Res.,* 494, 285, 1989.

131. Bjorklund, L.M. et al., Embryonic stem cells develop into functional dopaminergic neurons after transplantation in a Parkinson rat model, *Proc. Natl. Acad. Sci. U.S.A.,* 99, 2344, 2002.

132. Beauregard, M., Levesque, J., and Bourgouin, P., Neural correlates of conscious self-regulation of emotion, *J. Neurosci.,* 21, RC165, 2001.

133. Koepp, M.J. et al., Evidence for striatal dopamine release during a video game, *Nature,* 393, 266, 1998.

134. Blood, A.J. and Zatorre, R.J., Intensely pleasurable responses to music correlate with activity in brain regions implicated in reward and emotion, *Proc. Natl. Acad. Sci. U.S.A.,* 98, 11818, 2001.

135. Loubinoux, I. et al., Cerebral functional magnetic resonance imaging activation modulated by a single dose of the monoamine neurotransmission enhancers fluoxetine and fenozolone during hand sensorimotor tasks, *J. Cereb. Blood Flow Metabol.*, 19, 1365, 1999.

136. Sell, L.A. et al., Functional magnetic resonance imaging of the acute effect of intravenous heroin administration on visual activation in long-term heroin addicts: results from a feasibility study, *Drug Alcohol Depend.*, 49, 55, 1997.

137. Uftring, S.J. et al., An fMRI study of the effect of amphetamine on brain activity, *Neuropsychopharmacology*, 25, 925, 2001.

138. Breiter, H.C. et al., Functional imaging of neural responses to expectancy and experience of monetary gains and losses, *Neuron*, 30, 619, 2001.

139. Breiter, H.C. and Rosen, B.R., Functional magnetic resonance imaging of brain reward circuitry in the human, *Ann. NY Acad. Sci.*, 877, 523, 1999.

140. Chen, Y.I. et al., Improved mapping of pharmacologically induced neuronal activation using superparamagnetic iron blood pool agents, in *Proc. Intl. Soc. Mag. Res. Med.*, 1999, p. 348.

141. Kaufman, M.J. et al., Cocaine-induced cerebral vasoconstriction differs as a function of sex and menstrual cycle phase, *Biol. Psychiatr.*, 49, 774, 2001.

142. Breiter, H.C. et al., Acute effects of cocaine on human brain activity and emotion, *Neuron*, 19, 591, 1997.

143. Maas, L.C. et al., Functional magnetic resonance imaging of human brain activation during cue-induced cocaine craving, *Am. J. Psychiatr.*, 155, 124, 1998.

144. Garavan, H. et al., Cue-induced cocaine craving: neuroanatomical specificity for drug users and drug stimuli, *Am. J. Psychiatr.*, 157, 1789, 2000.

145. Volkow, N.D. and Fowler, J.S., Addiction, a disease of compulsion and drive: involvement of the orbitofrontal cortex, *Cereb. Cortex*, 10, 318, 2000.

146. Morgan, D. et al., Social dominance in monkeys: dopamine D2 receptors and cocaine self-administration, *Nature Neurosci.*, 5, 169, 2002.

147. Nestler, E.J., Molecular neurobiology of addiction, *Am. J. Addict.*, 10, 201, 2001.

148. Elman, I. et al., Clinical outcomes following cocaine infusion in nontreatment-seeking individuals with cocaine dependence, *Biol. Psychiatr.*, 49, 553, 2001.

149. Bradberry, C.W. et al., Impact of self-administered cocaine and cocaine cues on extracellular dopamine in mesolimbic and sensorimotor striatum in rhesus monkeys, *J. Neurosci.*, 20, 3874, 2000.

150. Nyback, H. et al., Attempts to visualize nicotinic receptors in the brain of monkey and man by positron emission tomography, *Progr. Brain Res.*, 79, 313, 1989.

151. Domino, E.F. et al., Nicotine effects on regional cerebral blood flow in awake, resting tobacco smokers, *Synapse*, 38, 313, 2000.

152. Zubieta, J. et al., Regional cerebral blood flow effects of nicotine in overnight abstinent smokers, *Biol. Psychiatr.*, 49, 906, 2001.

153. Sell, L.A. et al., Neural responses associated with cue evoked emotional states and heroin in opiate addicts, *Drug Alcohol Depend.*, 60, 207, 2000.

154. Trusk, T.C. and Stein, E.A., Effect of intravenous heroin and naloxone on regional cerebral blood flow in the conscious rat, *Brain Res.*, 406, 238, 1987.

155. Fuller, S.A. and Stein, E.A., Effects of heroin and naloxone on cerebral blood flow in the conscious rat, *Pharmacol. Biochem. Behav.*, 40, 339, 1991.

156. Robinson, T.E., Castaneda, E., and Whishaw, I.Q., Compensatory changes in striatal dopamine neurons following recovery from injury induced by 6-OHDA or methamphetamine: a review of evidence from microdialysis studies, *Can.J. Psychol.*, 44, 253, 1990.

157. Singer, T.P. and Ramsay, R.R., Mechanism of the neurotoxicity of MPTP: an update, *FEBS Lett.*, 274, 1, 1990.
158. Brownell, A.-L. et al., Cocaine congeners as PET imaging probes for dopamine terminals in normal and MPTP induced parkinsonism in nonhuman primate brain, *J. Nucl. Med.*, 37, 1186, 1996.

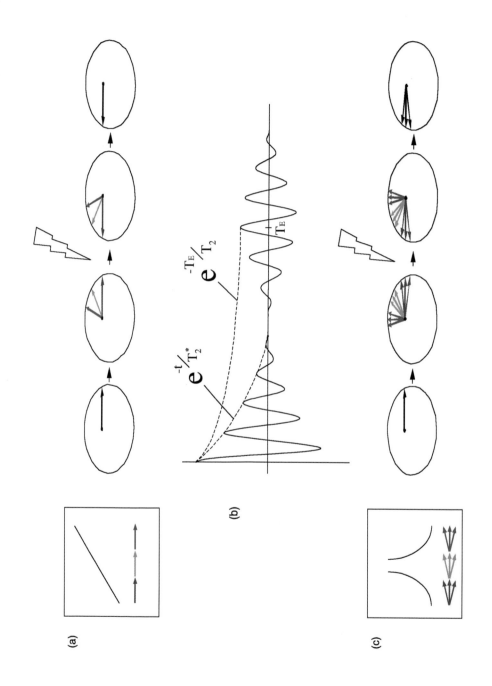

(a)

(b)

(c)

FIGURE 1.4 (a) In the presence of magnetic field heterogeneity (endogenous or via an applied external magnetic field gradient), excited nuclear spins acquire a resonant or precession frequency that depends on the external static magnetic field and on spatial position. Spatial coordinates with lower local magnetic fields will have lower frequencies (red arrows) and coordinates with higher local magnetic fields will have higher frequencies (blue arrows). An ensemble of such spins initially in phase (black arrow, far left cartoon) will subsequently dephase as individual spin vectors precess at these different frequencies (or rates). After application of a 180° RF pulse (jagged arrow), this dephased spin distribution has its magnetic orientation reversed in the transverse plane. However, spins continue to precess distributed in phase. Spins remain distributed in phase. Since these remain unchanged, the divergent spin distribution will ultimately rephase, momentarily forming an echo of the initial in-phase distribution (black arrow, far right cartoon). (b) In terms of NMR signal intensity, the initial dephasing of spins leads to a damped oscillation, with signal intensity (vector sum of spin vector distribution) diminishing rapidly. If the source of dephasing is endogenous magnetic field variation only, this decaying signal is called the FID (free induction decay) and its envelope can be described by an exponential decay time constant, T_2^*. A long T_2^* value implies low field heterogeneity and persistent signal. A short T_2^* implies rapid signal loss associated with greater field heterogeneity. Application of the 180° pulse leads to a rephasing of this decaying signal, then to the formation of an echo (at the echo time, TE, a time after the 180° pulse equal to the time between initial excitation and application of the 180° pulse. The amplitude of this spin echo is considerably restored (compared to the decaying FID), but is nonetheless smaller than that of the initial FID because of the incomplete rephasing of the spin distribution. This is because the rephasing relies on the precession of each spin at exactly the same rate after the 180° pulse as it did in the interval between initial excitation and the 180° application. To the extent that random spin–spin interactions lead to additional dephasing during either period, the echo is imperfectly refocused. Thus, the echo amplitude is dependent on the echo time and the time constant T_2, describing random spin–spin interactions. This description is rendered even more complex by the process of Brownian motion or random water diffusion. Although spins have resonant frequencies related to their local magnetic fields as shown in (c), as they diffuse through magnetic field heterogeneity, they also become distributed in phase (e.g., diverging red arrows, far at nominal low frequency locations). Since such diffusion is random, its effects also are imperfectly refocused (distributed black arrows, far right cartoon) by the mere 180° RF pulse and thus the spin echo amplitude is reduced further to an extent dependent on the rate of diffusion, the magnitude of field heterogeneities, and the echo time or TE.

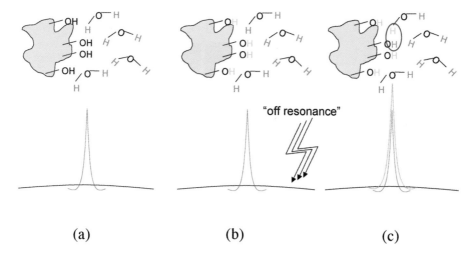

"off resonance"

(a)   (b)   (c)

FIGURE 1.9 Principle of magnetization transfer: (a) Protons in tissue are modeled as existing in two pools (free water and macromolecular). Magnetic resonance signal is derived almost entirely from the free water pool that has sharp resonance, compared to the broad resonance (short T_2) of the bound protons. (b) Off-resonance RF irradiation does not directly affect the narrow free water resonance peak (*off resonance* is sufficiently shifted in frequency to minimally impact nominal water resonance); in practice this radiation is typically applied at a frequency 1 to 2 kHz offset. This radiation impacts the broad resonance of the bound pool, leading to magnetic saturation of the protons. (c) Under appropriate chemical conditions (e.g., in myelin), protons from the bound pool and free water exchange carry saturated, noncontributory magnetization into the free pool and decrement the free water proton count available to generate the signal, leading to signal loss and diminished spectral peak. The process is called magnetization transfer and exists only when both (1) a macromolecular bound pool exists and (2) conditions are appropriate for proton exchange. The degree of magnetization transfer related signal loss can be quantified, e.g., as an index of myelin content.

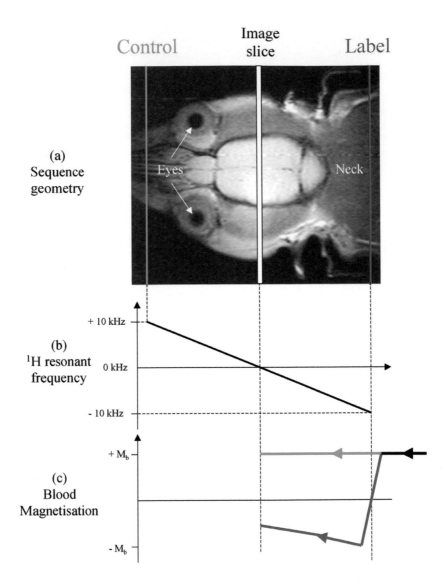

FIGURE 2.3 Continuous arterial spin labeling using flow-induced adiabatic fast passage. (a) Axial MR image through the rat brain shows the relative positions of the imaging (coronal) slice and the inversion (red) and control (green) planes. (b) The application of a magnetic field gradient causes the resonant frequency of water protons to constitute a linear function of position (over the range ~−10 kHz to +10 kHz). (c) By simultaneously applying a −10-kHz off-resonance RF pulse, blood water spins are inverted as they flow through the inversion plane (spin labeling). The control plane does not intersect any major arteries and does not cause spin labeling.

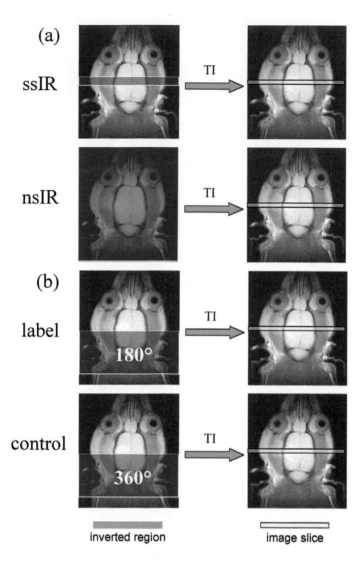

FIGURE 2.4 Pulsed arterial spin labeling using spatially restricted inversion pulses. (a) The flow-sensitive alternating inversion recovery [FAIR] approach acquires a pair of images, one following a slice-selective inversion pulse (upper) and the other following a global (nonselective) inversion pulse (lower). A difference between the images is caused by the difference in magnetization state of the inflowing blood water. (b) EPISTAR and signal targeting with alternating radio frequency also acquires a pair of images, although the difference in inflowing magnetization state is generated by inverting a volume of blood immediately proximal to the imaging slice (upper) or by applying a 360° pulse to this volume (leaving it effectively unaltered; lower). Images were acquired at a time *TI* after application of the inversion pulse.

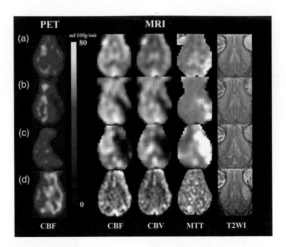

FIGURE 2.7 Comparison of CBF, CBV, and MTT maps produced from DSC-MRI and CBF images obtained by PET 6 hours after permanent MCAO or reperfusion. (a) Mild ischemia (CBF >30ml/100 g/minute in the ischemic cortex). (b) Moderate ischemia (CBF 12 to 30 ml/100 g/minute in the ischemic cortex). (c) Severe ischemia (CBF <12ml/100 g/minute in the ischemic cortex). (d) Postischemic hypoperfusion. Note the reliable correlation of DSC-MRI and PET. MTT clearly shows hemodynamic compromise. (From Sakoh, M. et al., *Stroke*, 31, 1958, 2000. With permission.)

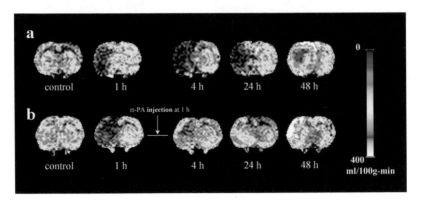

FIGURE 2.9 Cerebral blood flow (CBF) maps of coronal sections of an untreated (a) and a recombinant tissue activator (rt-PA)-treated (b) animal showing the evolution of changes in CBF, obtained before and during ischemia at 1, 4, 24, and 48 hours after embolization. After onset of embolization, a rapid decline in CBF was observed in the occluded MCA territory in both animals. CBF remained lower during the acute phase of ischemia (a). A return of CBF was observed in the cortex 48 hours after embolization (a). A rapid return of CBF was demonstrated after treatment with rt-PA 1 hour after injection of clot (b); rt-PA was administered 1 hour after embolization. (From Jiang, Q. et al., *J. Cereb. Blood Flow Metabol.*, 18, 758, 1998a. With permission.)

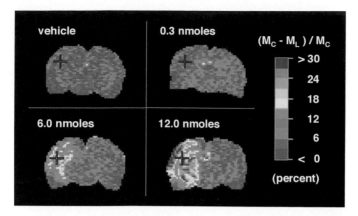

FIGURE 2.12 Pseudocolor images reflecting $100 \cdot (M_C - M_L) \cdot M_C - 1$ (where M_C is the magnetization intensity from the control image and ML is the magnetization from the labeled image) of a coronal slice at ~90 minutes after injection of saline vehicle or 2-chloroadenosine at 0.3, 6.0, or 12 nmoles. Injection of saline and 0.3 nmoles of 2-chloroadenosine produced no apparent effect on local perfusion. In contrast, injection of 6 nmoles of 2-chloroadenosine produced an obvious local increase in perfusion. Injection of 12 nmoles produced a marked increase in perfusion encompassing almost the entire hemisphere ipsilateral to injection. Plus signs indicate approximate locations of injection sites. (From Kochanek, P.M. et al., *Mag. Res. Med.*, 45, 924, 2001. With permission.)

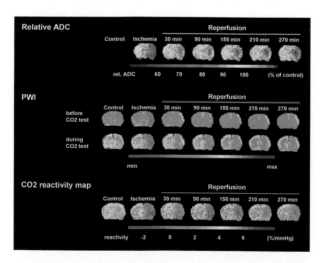

FIGURE 2.13 Time course of relative ADC (top row), PWI (middle row) before and during CO_2 reactivity, and quantitative CO_2 map (bottom row), during middle cerebral artery occlusion (ischemia), and at different time points of reperfusion. Note the inverse or low cerebrovascular reactivity during ischemia and the slow, incomplete improvement during reperfusion. (From Olah, L. et al., *Stroke*, 31, 2236, 2000. With permission.)

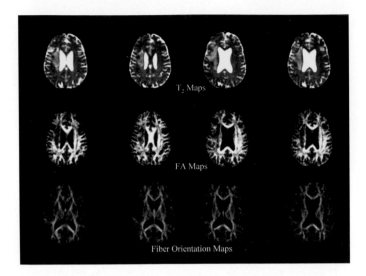

FIGURE 3.10 T$_2$, fractional anisotropy (FA), and color-coded direction maps of the brain acquired 2 weeks after a stroke. The maps of fiber orientation (bottom row) and FA (middle row) show reduced connectivity in regions that correspond to the lesion visible in the T$_2$ maps (top row). (Courtesy of Fernando Zelaya, Ph.D. and Derek Jones, Ph.D., Institute of Psychiatry, London.)

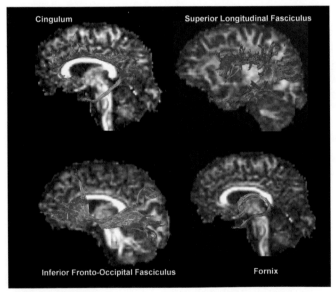

FIGURE 3.11 Example of fiber tractography applied to the human brain. Individual white matter tracts were extracted from DTI data with the use of a fiber tractography algorithm. (Courtesy of Derek Jones, Ph.D., Institute of Psychiatry, London.)

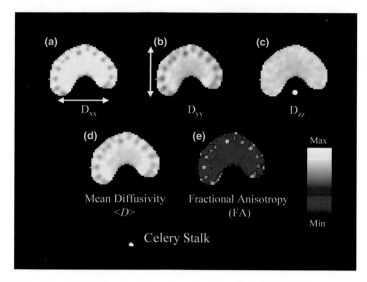

FIGURE 3.12 Diffusion tensor imaging of a celery stalk. Spatial maps of the rate of diffusion were measured perpendicular (a) and (b) and parallel (c) to the long axis of the stalk. The mean diffusivity (d) and fractional anisotropy (e) maps are rotationally invariant measures of isotropic and ansiotropic diffusion, respectively.

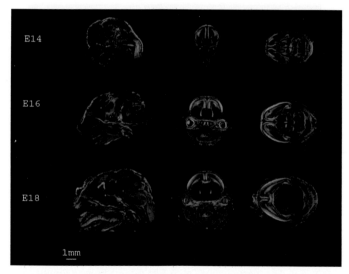

FIGURE 3.14 Diffusion tensor imaging of mouse brain development. *Ex vivo* imaging of a mouse brain at 14, 16, and 18 weeks of embryonic development. Brain samples were fixed by paraformaldehyde. RGB direction color coding: red = superior–inferior, green = right–left, and blue = anterior–posterior. Images were acquired at isotropic resolution of approximately 80 mm. (Courtesy of Susumu Mori, Ph.D., Johns Hopkins University, Baltimore.)

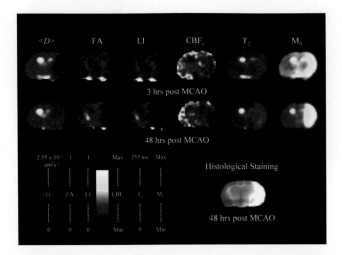

FIGURE 3.16 Spatial maps of mean diffusivity (*<D>*), fractional anisotropy (FA), lattice anisotropy (LI), cerebral blood flow index (CBF$_i$), T$_2$ and proton density (M$_0$) are shown for a cerebral ischemic lesion imaged at 3 and 48 hours after middle cerebral artery occlusion in a rat model of 60 minutes of transient ischemia. The corresponding postmortem TTC-stained slice is also shown.

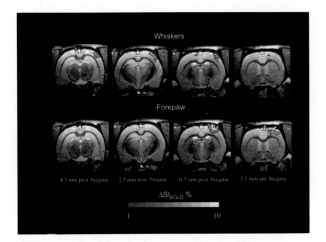

FIGURE 4.2 Coronal sections through the rat brain with the activated representation fields of the whisker barrel cortex (upper row) and the forepaw in the somatosensory cortex demarcated. fMRI activation data were obtained with EPI using a boxcar stimulation protocol and analyzing the data with STIMULATE software,[142] and superimposed on morphological high-resolution images. For whisker stimulation, a tape was stretched across all whiskers and moved by a pulse air stream. For forepaw stimulation, the electrical forepaw stimulation paradigm was applied.[28] The left whiskers or left forepaw were stimulated. The whisker representation area is more caudal and lateral than that of the forepaw.

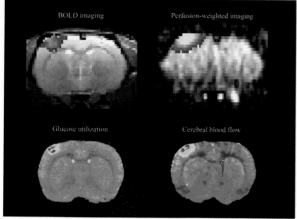

FIGURE 4.3 Coronal sections highlighting the activation of somatsosensory cortex by fMRI (upper) and autoradiographic (lower) techniques, respectively. fMRI data were obtained with BOLD and a perfusion-weighted sequence. Autoradiographic images reflect recording of the cerebral metabolic rate of glucose and cerebral blood flow. Note good spatial correspondence of activated areas of the four different techniques amplitudes (bottom) at increasing stimulation frequencies. SEP amplitudes were normalized to a 1.5-Hz value. Note the corresponding frequency behavior of BOLD fMRI and SEP amplitudes ($* = p < 0.05$; $** = < 0.01$; statistically different from data at 1.5 Hz). (From Brinker, G. et al., *Mag. Res. Med.*, 41, 469, 1999. With permission.)

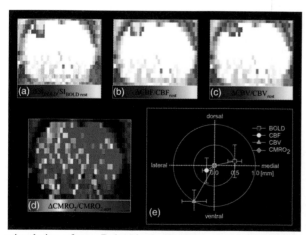

FIGURE 4.7 Coronal activation maps for BOLD (left), cerebral blood flow (center), and cerebral blood volume (right) for electrical forepaw stimulation of rats. Below is the $CMRO_2$ map, calculated pixelwise for pixels showing activation in individual parameter activation maps and following the algorithm appearing in Equation 4.1 in the text. Also shown are the average centers of mass for the three parameters, relative to the center of mass of the calculated $CMRO_2$ activation map. Note that the largest mismatch is observed for cerebral blood volume and BOLD changes. Cerebral blood flow changes are closest to the $\Delta CMRO_2$. (From Schwindt, W. et al., *Proceedings of Symposium on Brain Activation and CBF Control*, Tokyo, 2001. With permission.)

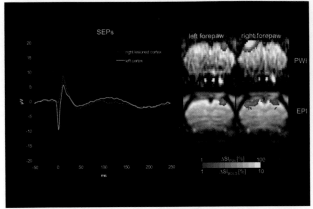

FIGURE 4.13 SEPs and simultaneously recorded EPI-based BOLD and PWI activation maps of adult rats that experienced cortical cold lesions of right hemispheres 1 day after birth. The activation area in the lesioned cortex is clearly reduced relative to cortex of the contralateral healthy hemisphere. In parallel, the corresponding SEP was strongly reduced and distorted.

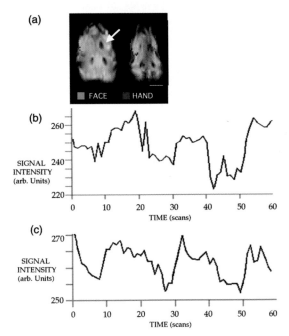

FIGURE 5.2 Cortical activation resulting from stimulation of the hands and face in the anesthetized macaque monkey. (a) Serial axial EPI slices (left = inferior, top = rostral) from stimulation of the hand (top row, red pixels) and the face (bottom row, green pixels). Arrow indicates the location of fluid-filled probe used for later superposition of anatomical and electrophysiological recording data (Disbrow, E.A. et al., 2000a). (b) Average change in signal intensity over time in voxels active in response to tactile stimulation of the hand (red pixels in (a)). (c) Time course of activity in response to identical tactile stimulation in an awake behaving human. Note the similarity in the percent signal change.

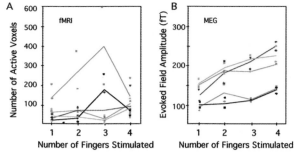

FIGURE 5.4 Extent of cortical activation in response to stimulation of an increasing number of digits. Subjects were scanned three times using fMRI and three times using MEG. (a) fMRI data show considerable within-subject variability (like colored dots) and between-subject variability (different colored lines), with no trend toward increasing area of activation with increasing number of stimulated digits. (b) MEG data indicate significantly less within-subject variability. While between-subject variability was still high, a significant correlation of magnetic field strength and number of digits stimulated was noted. For both (a) and (b), individual subject mean data are shown as solid lines.

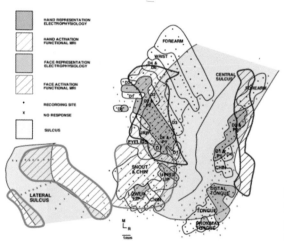

FIGURE 5.5 Correspondence between fMRI and electrophysiological maps obtained from macaque monkey cortex. Identical calibrated tactile stimuli were applied to digits or lips and tongue in both sets of experiments. Resulting maps are displayed on a flattened cortex. Dots represent recording sites in which neurons responded to tactile stimulation, Xs are sites where no response was elicited and black lines indicate borders of body part representations. In some instances, correspondence between the electrophysiological maps (solid red = hand, solid green = face) and the fMRI maps (striped red = hand, striped green = face) was good, e.g., the hand maps and one of the fMRI face maps (right). However, in 45% of the scans, the centroid of the fMRI map did not fall within the electrophysiologically defined map, as in the second face map (left).

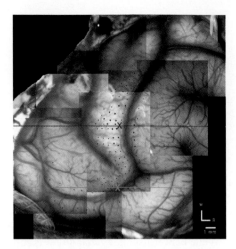

FIGURE 5.6 Variability of fMRI map location. A digital image of the macaque monkey cortex is used to display the anterior-posterior variability in the locations of map centroids. Dots indicate electrophysiological recording sites. Colors indicate penetrations in which cells responded to stimulation of the hand (red) or face (green). Colored Xs indicate mean locations of fMRI map centroids and colored lines indicate standard deviations of the means. Variability was largest in the anterior-posterior direction, perpendicular to major vessels.

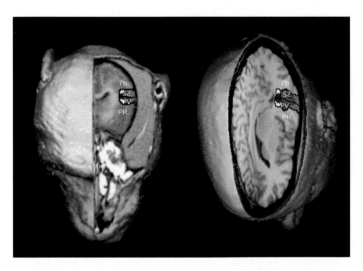

FIGURE 5.7 Schematic of the similarity of organization of higher order somatosensory cortex in the macaque monkey (left) and the human (right). Both species have mirror symmetric S2 and PV and more rostral areas (PR) and more caudal areas (7b) containing cells that respond to tactile stimulation. Macaque monkey data adapted from Krubitzer, L. et al., *J. Neurosci.*, 15, 3821, 1995. Human data adapted from Disbrow, E.A. et al., *J. Comp. Neurol.*, 418, 1, 2000b. With permission.

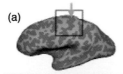

(a)

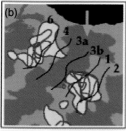

(b)

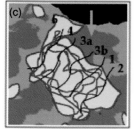

(c)

FIGURE 5.8 Activation patterns for tactile and kinesthetic/motor stimulation. (a) The location of activation in (b) and (c) shown on an inflated brain. (b) Average activation pattern from five subjects in response to tactile stimulation displayed on a flattened brain. Note the lack of activation in areas 3a and 2 and the sparse activation in motor area 4. (c) Average activation pattern for kinesthetic/motor stimulation resulting in the stimulation of deep receptors. Significant activation occurred in areas 4, 3a, and 2.

FIGURE 5.10 Somatotopic organization of S2 and PV. (a) Electrophysiological recording data from the upper bank of the lateral sulcus in the macaque monkey. S2 and PV are mirror symmetric, joined at the representations of the face hand and foot, with shoulder and hip representations flanking both sides. Adapted from Krubitzer, L. et al., *J. Neurosci.*, 15, 3821, 1995. With permission.

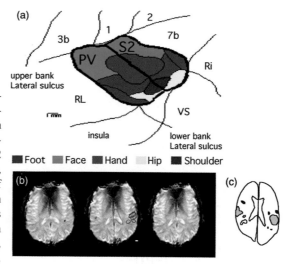

We used this data when examining human cortex, stimulating both distal (hands and feet) and proximal (hip and shoulder) body parts. The upper bank of the Sylvian fissure also contains two fields with similar organization. (b) Three axial slices showing activation from stimulation of the foot (left, red), hand (blue, center), and face (green, right). The positions of the foot and face activation are indicated on the center (hand representation) image, showing the medial-lateral organization of human cortex. The hip and shoulder representations of S2 and PV are located on both sides. (c) Schematic of activation of stimulation of the hand. Three areas of activation were observed, S2/PV in the center (gray), PR (anterior, black) and 7b (posterior, white). Adapted from Disbrow, E.A. et al., 2000b.

(a) Somatomotor Integration

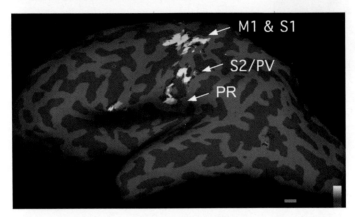

(b) Haptic Shape Discrimination

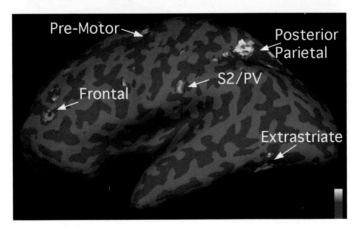

FIGURE 5.12 fMRI data from tasks based on cortico-cortical connections of S2 and PV in macaque monkeys. Because PV has connections with premotor cortex (Figure 5.11), we contrasted activation from somatosensory stimulation with activation from somatomotor stimulation (a). The large area of activation is seen in S2/PV and PR. S2 and PV are also active during haptic shape discrimination as contrasted to a tactile/motor control condition (b).

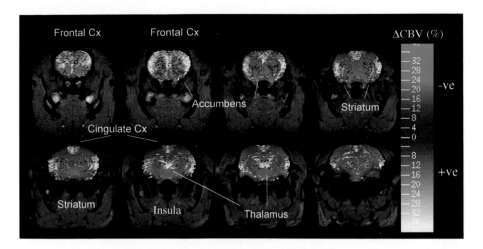

FIGURE 6.5 Map of rCBV changes in a rat after injection of 3mg/kg amphetamine. The primary brain structures activated are noted. The map is not smoothed (spatial resolution was 0.2 × 0.2 × 1 mm) and is thresholded for rCBV changes ranging from –40 to 40%. Note few negative rCBV changes.

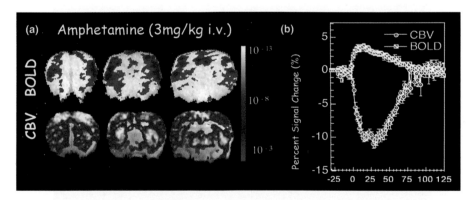

FIGURE 6.6 (a) Comparison of BOLD and IRON images at the same statistical threshold derived from a Student's t-test after administration of 3 mg/kg amphetamine in a rat. Note the nearly 10 orders of magnitude decrease in the p-value for the IRON technique compared to the BOLD technique (both data sets were collected with the same number of images). (b) Plot of the percent changes induced by the same stimulus for BOLD (top) and IRON images. Note the increased rCBV after amphetamine induces a negative percent signal change during IRON imaging. The huge increase in the area under the curve for the IRON is largely responsible for the increase in statistical power of this technique.

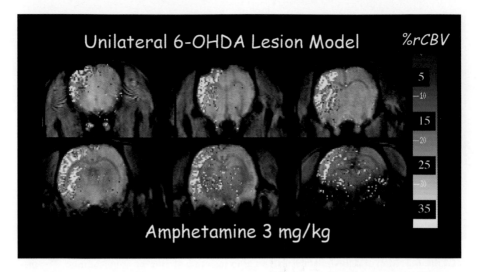

FIGURE 6.14 IRON imaging of the percent rCBV changes induced by 3 mg/kg amphetamine in a rat with a unilateral 6-OHDA lesion. Note the nearly complete loss of hemodynamic changes on the lesioned side, including the downstream thalamic circuitry, frontal cortex, and striatum.

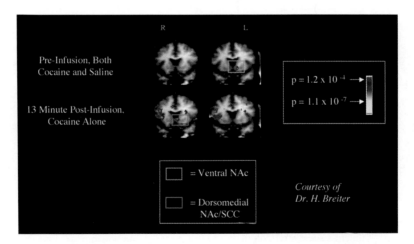

FIGURE 6.15 BOLD phMRI (1.5 T) of double-blind infusion of a single intravenous dose of cocaine (0.6 mg/kg) or saline. The expectancy of receiving cocaine (regardless of whether the subject receives cocaine or saline) causes increased BOLD signal in the ventral nucleus accumbens. In the case of cocaine infusion, activation is seen in the dorsal-medial accumbens, and the subcallosal complex.[142] (Courtesy of Dr. Hans Breiter, Massachusetts General Hospital.)

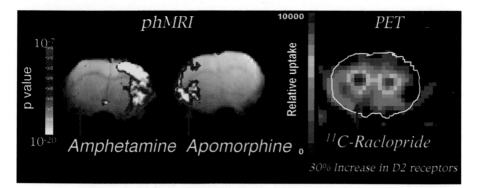

FIGURE 6.16 phMRI detection of postsynaptic dopamine receptor supersensitivity. Left: IRON image of amphetamine activation in a rat with a unilateral 6-OHDA lesion. As shown in Figure 6.14, the amphetamine produces rCBV increases on the intact side only. Administration of apomorphine, a dopamine agonist, to the same animal leads to increased rCBV on the lesion side only. PET imaging of D2 receptors using ^{11}C-raclopride in the same animal leads to an increase of about 30% on the lesioned side. The phMRI images have been averaged to produce average slice thicknesses comparable to the PET images (4.5 mm).

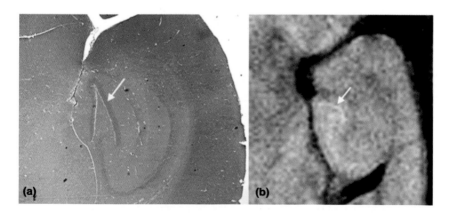

FIGURE 7.5 Hematoxylin and eosin stained C56Bl6/J mouse brain section at the level of the ventral hippocampus. (a) Corresponding diffusion-weighted in vivo MR microscopy image acquired at a spatial resolution of 0.0016 mm³. (b) The granule cell layer appears as a faint bright line in the diffusion-weighted image (arrow). MR microscopy data acquired from the Duke University Center for *In Vivo* Microscopy.

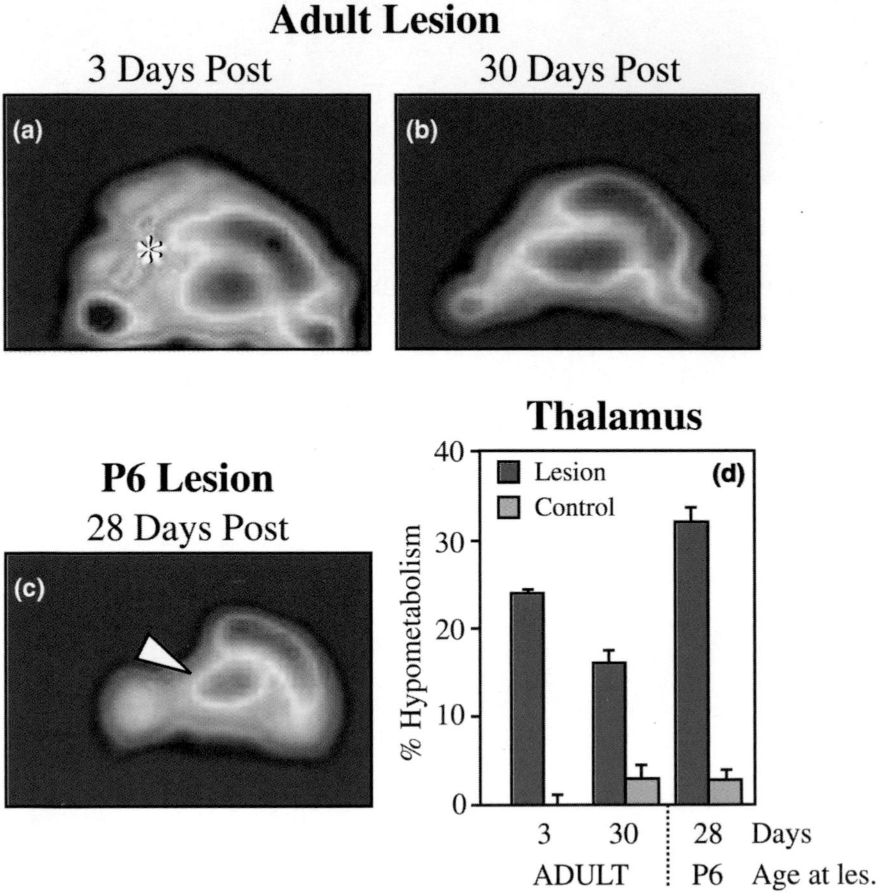

FIGURE 9.6 Effects of hemidecortication on thalamic metabolism studied by microPET. A and B are microPET images from an adult animal that underwent aspiration lesion of the left neocortex imaged 3 days (a) and 30 days (b) later. Note improvement in ipsilateral hypometabolism after 30 days. In an animal lesioned at 6 days of age and imaged 1 month later, imaging revealed severe hypometabolism in the ipsilateral thalamus (c). (d) shows quantitative data demonstrating the degree of thalamic hypometabolism in adults 3 and 30 days postlesion and P6 animals scanned 28 days postlesion.

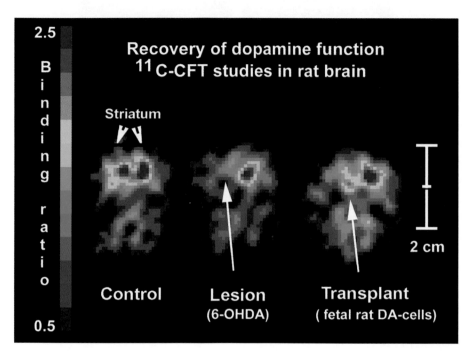

FIGURE 9.7 Imaging of dopamine terminals following 6-hydroxydopamine lesion and subsequent transplant using [^{11}C]-CFT. The left image shows uptake in the striatum of a control rat. The middle image shows loss of terminals following 6-hydroxy lesion. The right image demonstrates a return of function after transplantation of fetal dopaminergic neurons. Images were obtained on a PCR-1 tomograph. (Courtesy of Dr. A.L. Brownell, Harvard Medical School. With permission.)

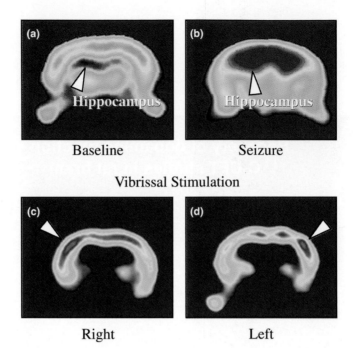

FIGURE 9.8 Detection of neuronal activation with FDG-microPET. (a) and (b) are images of an animal scanned prior to (a) and immediately following (b) kainic acid-induced seizure (uptake occurred during the seizure). Note the dramatic enhancement of signal in the hippocampus (arrow). (c) and (d) are images of animals scanned following an uptake period during which the right (c) or left (d) moustachial vibrissae were stimulated. Note slightly enhanced uptake of tracer in the vicinity of the barrel field cortex contralateral to the stimulation (arrows).

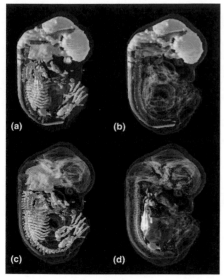

FIGURE 10.4 Three-dimensional "virtual mouse" embryo created from a volumetric *ex vivo* MR microscopic investigation. The computer model allows segmentation of all organs (a), the CNS (b), skeletal system (c), or a combination of systems (d). The ability to derive computer models of embryonic development and annotate these atlases will greatly benefit researchers investigating the influence of nature-versus-nurture developmental growth. (Adapted from Dhenain, M. et al., 2001. With permission.)

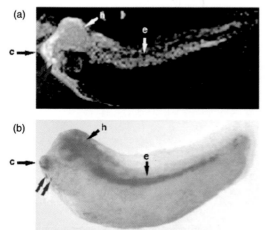

FIGURE 10.5 Detecting gene expression by MRI. The upper image (a) demonstrates a significant MR signal contrast change due to the presence of the smart contrast agent, EgadMe. This agent differentiates structures developed from cells modified to express the reporter gene lac Z from cells that did not carry the gene. The lower image (b) validates the presence of lac Z expression by traditional bright field histology. (Adapted from Louie, A.Y., et al., *Nature Biotechnol.*, 18, 321, 2000. With permission.)

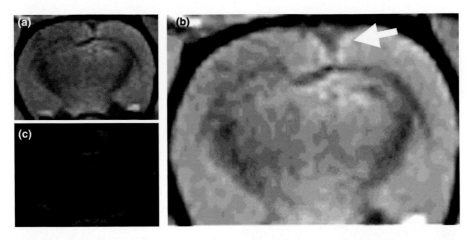

FIGURE 10.8 MRI visualization of a stem cell transplant in a rat with global ischemic brain damage. The visualization of transplanted stem cells was feasible by prelabeling cells *in vitro* with a bifunctional contrast agent, GRID. This allowed us to detect the transplant on both MRI (b) and fluorescent microscopy (a). An overlay of both images (right) provides corroborative evidence that both imaging modalities visualized the stem cell transplant. (Modo, M. et al, *Neuroimage*, 17(2), 803, 2002. With permission.)

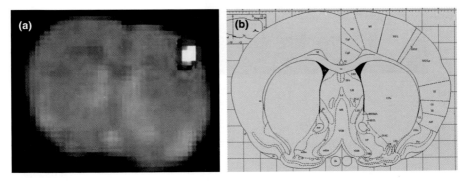

FIGURE 10.9 Detecting rodent brain function. Electrical stimulation of the rat forepaw was detected by BOLD-based fMRI in α-chloralose treated rats (a). The anatomical correlation of the functional activity corresponded to the area of the primary somatosensory cortex according to Paxinos' rat atlas (b). (Adapted from Lowe, A.S. et al., *Proc. 10th Annl. Mtg. Soc. Mag. Res. Med.*, 2002. With permission.)

7 Anatomical Studies in the Rodent Brain and Spinal Cord: Applications of Magnetic Resonance Microscopy

Helene Benveniste, Tom Mareci, and Steve Blackband

CONTENTS

0-8493-0122-X/03/$0.00+$1.50
© 2003 by CRC Press LLC

7.1 TECHNICAL OVERVIEW OF MAGNETIC RESONANCE MICROSCOPY

Several excellent texts now describe magnetic resonance imaging (MRI)[1-3] and magnetic resonance (MR) microscopy[4] in depth. In this overview, we will briefly discuss the aspects and characteristics of MR microscopy relevant to imaging studies of the rodent nervous system.

7.1.1 SIGNALS AND MAGNETS

MRI has become a mainstay of clinical medicine, offering excellent soft tissue contrast in a noninvasive procedure.[5,6] It involves mapping the distribution of signals from water in the tissues, specifically from the hydrogen nuclei. Although water produces the largest signals from the body due to its high abundance relative to other constituents, the MR signal is still quite small — on the order of microvolts or millivolts at best. Consequently, special care and effort are needed to maximize MR signals. This is especially important because the signals, or more correctly the signal-to-noise ratios (SNRs) obtained determine the image spatial resolution and acquisition time achievable for a given contrast as discussed below.

Multiple factors control the available SNR in MR experiments,[1] but the major determinants are (1) magnetic field strength (the SNR increases between linearly and quadratically with field strength), (2) the size of the signal detector or radiofrequency (RF) coil (the SNR increases linearly with decreasing coil diameter), and (3) the total data acquisition or so-called averaging time. With regard to rodent brain and spinal cord studies relevant to this chapter, horizontal bore magnets with bore sizes ≥15 cm (i.e., able to accommodate a rat body inside a gradient coil with a 5- to 10-cm internal diameter) are suitable for MR experiments.

Magnetic field strengths between 4 and 9.4 T are now common for rodent studies although some sites evaluate 11.7 T (33-cm and 40-cm bore) systems. The possibility of constructing magnets with even higher fields exists, although the costs are prohibitive (>$2 million). For smaller animals (mice) or *ex vivo* samples, higher fields are accessible through vertical bore magnets now commercially available up to 17.6 T (9 cm bore, reduced to approximately 6 cm with the gradients inserted) and 21.1 T (6 cm bore, reduced to 3 to 4 cm with gradients in place). Again, it is likely that even higher fields will be available in the near future.

As a rule, stronger magnetic fields provide increased SNR in MR imaging experiments (and are also beneficial for MR spectroscopy not to be discussed here). However, the technique requires other compromises in addition to the costs and physical siting issues. For example, susceptibility effects or image distortions caused by magnetic field inhomogeneities induced by the sample increase with an increase in magnetic field strength paradoxically can be either detrimental or beneficial in anatomical imaging studies and must be carefully considered. Further, at higher fields, the RF power requirements increase and RF coil construction at the higher frequencies become more difficult. Fortunately these obstacles are usually not a severe limitation on the small (rodent sized) scale at present field strengths and frequencies. Additionally, T_1 lengthens and T_2 shortens, both of which can alter image contrast. Despite these compromising factors, the benefits at higher magnetic field strengths outweigh the difficulties and the drive to continue increasing field strengths continues unabated.

7.1.2 IMAGING TIME, RADIOFREQUENCY COILS, SPATIAL RESOLUTION, AND GRADIENTS

Increasing the imaging time is an easy way to improve the image SNR, but it soon becomes a temporal and financial burden because the SNR increases as the square root of total acquisition time. Alternatively, the use of smaller RF coils leads to improved SNR (linear increases with decreases in coil diameter) at the expense of limiting examinations to smaller sample volumes. Although the magnetic field strength, RF coil size, and imaging time can all be manipulated (with compromises) to improve SNR, the major determinant of MR microscopic capabilities in terms of trading the improved SNR is spatial resolution. For an isotropic spatial resolution improvement (i.e., the same improvement in all three spatial dimensions), the SNR decreases as the cube of that improvement.

An isotropic resolution decrease from 100 μm to 50 μm reduces the voxel volume and hence the SNR in the imaging voxel by a factor of eight. At a given fixed magnetic field strength and RF coil design, this large signal loss is only recovered by manipulating acquisition times. Practical limits on spatial resolution can be determined very quickly and are outlined in the next section for rodent studies.

Also of practical interest in MR microscopy are the capabilities of the gradient coils used to spatially encode the MR signal. As the SNR improves and is traded for spatial resolution, stronger gradient coils are required to maximize the benefit of the increased SNR. Although this can be problematic on a large scale (i.e., on humans where the available gradient strengths are 1 to 4 G/cm), the gradient strength achievable increases as the gradient coil size decreases. Thus gradient strengths of 10 to 20 G/cm or better can accommodate rats and even higher gradient strengths (>100 G/cm) on smaller (<2 to 3 cm) samples. These are sufficient for most experiments.

7.1.3 MR MICROSCOPY ON RODENTS

High fields and small RF coils make the relatively small rodent brain accessible for high spatial resolution MRI. At the field strengths presently employed (4 to 11.7 T) and with RF volume coils fitting the animals' heads (2 to 5 cm in diameter), in-plane resolutions below 100 μm are readily obtainable in a few minutes (see Figure 7.1). At a level of spatial resolution below 100 μm in at least one spatial dimension, the imaging is often designated MR microscopy. Using surface coils on *in vivo* animals or smaller coils and/or much longer acquisition times on *ex vivo* samples (excised brains and spinal cords), resolutions of 50 μm and below can be achieved. In the extreme, small pieces of tissue can be examined in very small coils (<5 mm diameter) with relatively long acquisition times (hours) and resolutions of the order of 10 to 20 μm.

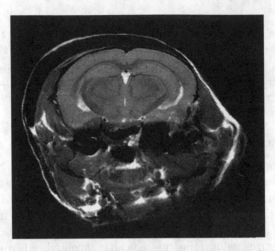

FIGURE 7.1 MR image of a live mouse at 750 MHz (17.6 T) obtained in 8:41 minutes and with a resolution of $0.78 \times 0.78 \times 0.5$ mm. (Image courtesy of Xeve Silver. With permission.)

Although spatial resolution is clearly an issue, image contrast is also important because it determines the ability to discriminate different tissue types or signal changes. Nearly all contrast mechanisms employed in MR (e.g., T_1, T_2, and diffusion) result in reduced SNR with increased contrast, and spatial resolution may have to be reduced to compensate. At certain magnetic fields and RF coil values, the image contrast, spatial resolution, and acquisition time can be traded with respect to each other, depending on the priority required with regard to the information content of the data set. This will be reflected in the large range of applications and imaging protocols cited in the rest of this chapter. Also of major concern in high resolution and microscopic MR studies on *in vivo* samples is the presence of motion artefacts and limitations imposed by sample stability, especially on sick animals (see Section 7.2).

7.1.4 ONGOING DEVELOPMENTS

Several exciting and novel technological developments have begun to impact MR studies of rodent nervous systems. These are briefly listed here, although full discussions are beyond the scope of this chapter:

- Increases in magnetic field strength
- Improvements in RF coil technology
  - Phased array coils[7,8]
  - Lower temperature RF coils[9]
  - Multicoil arrays for multiple animals within a single magnet[10]
- Improved physiological monitoring and gating[11]
- Targeted ("smart") contrast agents[12]

7.1.5 SUMMARY OF OVERVIEW

The use of high magnetic fields and optimized RF coils facilitates the generation of MR images of rodents at microscopic spatial resolutions (<100 μm). The resolution achieved depends in part on the magnetic field strength, but is mainly dictated by the size of the sample and RF coil and the data acquisition time, ranging from <100 μm or less on whole rats in a few minutes to ~10 μm on small pieces (<5 mm) of tissue in hours. The spatial and temporal resolution obtained may then be traded for image contrast.

Often, the spatial resolution may be nonisotropic, with one dimension (slice width) greater than the other two (in-plane resolution in the final image). Nonisotropic imaging improves the SNR and can be traded for temporal resolution with varying impact on image clarity, especially when the sample has some degree of two-dimensional symmetry. Together, the spatial and temporal resolution and the image contrast ultimately determine the utility of the technique. Several ongoing technical developments will gradually improve MR microscopy over the next few years.

7.2 NORMAL RODENT BRAIN AND SPINAL CORD ANATOMY

The scientific drive to optimize visualization of rodent brain anatomy by MR microscopy has persisted and even escalated over the last two decades for several reasons. First, the rodent always has been and continues to be the most widely used species in neuroscience research. Second, the increasing availability of genetically engineered mouse models of human disease has been another major instigator. Thirdly, MR technology has improved to the point where good quality data can now be obtained from small animals.

The scientist's need for noninvasive imaging tools suitable to visualize rodent structural anatomy at any given time point and longitudinally during progression of disease processes and/or development has driven the MR microscopy field into refining hardware and software for this purpose. In the following sections we will review *in vivo* and *in vitro* MR microscopy experiments pertaining to the rodent brain and spinal cord. Because experimental requirements for *in vivo* microscopy are very different from those encountered *in vitro*, we will discuss them separately.

7.2.1 *In Vivo* MR Microscopy: General Considerations

MR microscopy of live small animals such as rats and mice is technically challenging and requires a multidisciplinary team of experienced investigators for successful outcome. Physiological monitoring and MR imaging parameters must be considered and planned carefully for *in vivo* experiments (see Table 7.1). For survival protocols, it is generally desirable to adhere to noninvasive monitoring and limit scan times so as not to prolong anesthesia exposure. Certain *in vivo* protocols require strict hemodynamic control and invasive blood pressure monitoring that add complexity to the experimental set-up.

TABLE 7.1
Experimental Considerations for Live Animal MRI Microscopy Studies

Factor	Considerations	Importance	Refs.
Anesthesia	Choice of agent	Anesthetics such as halothane or isoflurane may interfere with data output, e.g., during functional activation studies	86–88
	Need for mechanical ventilation?	Prolonged exposure to anesthesia is likely to require mechanical ventilation to avoid loss of airway	
	Repetitive administration?	Need for intravenous or intraperitoneal access during prolonged imaging protocols	89
Motion	Scan-synchronous ventilation, cardiac gating, immobilization devices (stereotaxic frames, head holders)	*In vivo* MR microscopy of heart, lungs and intraabdominal organs requires a combination of scan-synchronous ventilation, cardiac gating and/or specialized pulse sequences	13,14,90–93
Total scan time	Pulse sequence design, spatial resolution, smaller RF coil	Most *in vivo* MR microscopy studies involve <1 hour scan time; in some instances, 7-hour scan times are feasible	94
RF coil design	Position of animal; position of head in stereotaxic device; physiological monitoring equipment	Prone position is thought to transmit more respiratory motion; bird-cage RF coil designs can be difficult to reconcile with bulky head-holders and physiological equipment	
Physiological parameters to be monitored	ECG, heart rate, respiratory rate, body temperature, end tital CO_2, inspiratory O_2 and/or anesthetic gas concentration, blood pressure, EEG	As a minimum, heart rate, respiratory rate, and body temperature should be monitored	

Maintaining normal body temperatures of the rodents during imaging is obviously essential for all *in vivo* studies and is especially important for stroke studies unless hypothermia is a required experimental condition. Typically, heated air vented through the magnet bore or warm-water circulating heating blankets wrapped around the animals are used to maintain normothermia during imaging. Hedlund and coworkers designed refined MR-compatible breathing valves for mechanical respiratory control and gas delivery for rodents.[13,14]

7.2.2 *In Vivo* Appearance of Rodent Brain and Spinal Cord Anatomy

It is important to remember that the term "anatomy" can be defined at different optical resolutions. Gross anatomy structures are large enough to be examined without the help of magnifying devices, while microscopic anatomy concerns structural units that can only be seen under a light microscope. Finally, cytology deals with cells and their contents. MR microscopy can provide information at all three optical resolutions but under different physical and chemical conditions. For example, MR microscopy performed *in vivo* in an intact animal consistently displays gross and only limited microscopic anatomy. *In vitro* MR microscopy of tissue samples or whole isolated organs routinely reveals gross and microscopic structures (see Section 7.2.4).

Hansen and coworkers[15] were the first to publish *in vivo* images of the rat brain at a spatial resolution range of $0.33 \times 0.33 \times 8.4$ mm^3. Since then, technological advances in MR microscopy have made it possible to routinely visualize a wide variety of larger structures and organisms *in vivo*. Figure 7.2 shows how the mouse cerebellum and forebrain (including the olfactory bulbs) can be displayed using a three-dimensional MR microscopy data set acquired *in vivo* at a spatial resolution of $58 \times 58 \times 469$ μm^3. Figure 7.3 shows another three-dimensional MR microscopy data set acquired *in vivo* that visualizes rat cervical spinal cord. Only the spinal cord has been volume rendered and is seen surrounded by its vertebral column and the neck musculature. Sufficient spatial resolution and SNR to visualize structures in the microscopic range come with a price related to acquisition time. The three-dimensional MR microscopy data set presented in Figure 7.3 required 7 hours of scan time.

Numerous investigators have successfully imaged the gross anatomical features of the rodent brain and spinal cord *in vivo* using MR microscopy, but microscopic anatomic information is inadequately represented as shown in Table 7.2. *Microscopic* refers to visualization of structures such as cells, clusters of cells, cell layers, axons, arterioles, and capillaries small enough to be seen only with a light microscope. Figure 7.4 is a histologically processed mouse brain section of cerebellar Purkinje cells. While individual 30- to 50 micro-meter diameter Purkinje cells can be clearly recognized in the histologically processed image (a), they cannot be identified on the (b) and (c) MR microscopy images. Failure of Purkinje cells to appear on MR microscopy images in this case is due to a combined lack of SNR and CNR and associated insufficient spatial resolution.

In some instances, however, certain microscopic structures will appear *in vivo*. Johnson and coworkers[16] successfully demonstrated the granule cell layers in rats at a spatial resolution of 0.016 mm^3. Munasinghe[17] revealed the hippocampus sulcus of the mouse at a spatial resolution of 0.018 mm^3. The granule cell layer of the mouse dentate gyrus can also be made to appear *in vivo* at a spatial resolution of 0.0016 mm^3 as shown in Figure 7.5, although not consistently.

Diffusion MR signals offer the potential of generating nerve fiber maps in the brain and spinal cord in the microscopy domain both *in vivo* and *in vitro*. The anisotropy of water translational diffusion is used to visualize structures in the central nervous system and provides the basis for a new method of visualizing nerve fiber

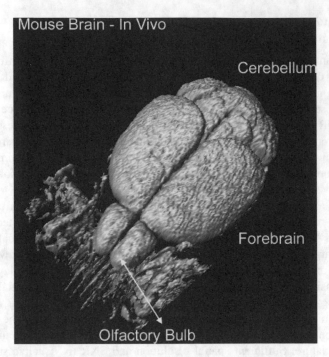

FIGURE 7.2 Three-dimensional MR microscopy data set of a C57BL6/J mouse brain acquired *in vivo* at a spatial resolution of 0.0016 mm³. The MR data are surface rendered and emphasize the brain (the skull is not displayed). Gross anatomical structures such as olfactory bulbs, forebrain, and cerebellum are easily identified.

tracts. Initial results are encouraging and suggest that this approach to fiber mapping may be applied to a wide range of studies in living organisms.

Basser and colleagues[18-22] discussed general methods of acquiring and processing the complete diffusion tensor of NMR-measured translational self-diffusion. They showed that directly measured diffusion tensors could be recast in a rotationally invariant form and reduced to parametric images that represent the average rate of diffusion (tensor trace) and diffusion anisotropy (relationship of eigenvalues). They further demonstrated how the diffusion ellipsoid (eigenvalues and eigenvectors) could be related to the laboratory reference frame. Parametric imaging methodology[18] is now used to characterize normal tissue and pathologies such as ischemia. The development of diffusion tensor acquisition, processing, and analysis methods also provides the framework for procedures for fiber tract mapping.[23-26]

Makris et al.[25] visualized human brain fiber bundles by color coding the direction (eigenvector of largest eigenvalue) of the largest component of the diffusion tensor (largest eigenvalue). Mori and colleagues produced the first three-dimensional rendering of fiber tracts using diffusion tensor images of white matter regions in excised fixed rat brain,[26] then extended this work to fiber tract mapping of rat brain *in vivo*.[27]

Exogenously applied contrast agents have also been used to enhance the appearance of microscopic pathways in the rodent brain *in vivo*. A dilution of $MnCl_2$ was administered into the olfactory epithelia in living anesthetized rats via the nares

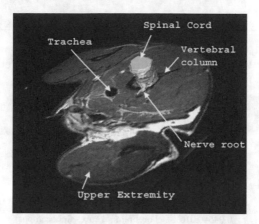

FIGURE 7.3 T_2-weighted three-dimensional MR microscopy data set acquired on a 7.1 T MR instrument (http://wwwcivm.mc.duke.edu/) *in vivo* from the cervical spinal cord of a 160-gm Fisher rat. The spatial resolution of the data set is 0.0038 mm³ and required 7.7 hrs of scan time (TR = 850 ms; TE = 30 ms; 256 × 256 × 128 pixels; NA = 1). Data acquisition was performed with scan-synchronous ventilation and cardiac gating. The spinal cord and nerve root are surface rendered and shown surrounded by the vertebral column and paravertebral/neck musculature. Other relevant gross anatomical structures are indicated.

and/or directly into the aqueous humors of the eyes.[28] Twenty-four hours later, Mn^{2+} highlighted the olfactory pathway and optic tracts that were otherwise not apparent on T_1-weighted MR microscopy images.

7.2.3 *In Vitro* MR Microscopy: Concepts and Practical Considerations

MR microscopy of tissue specimens has been referred to as MR histology[29] and virtual neuropathology.[30] The general idea behind this concept is to use T_1, T_2, $T_{1}\rho$, or diffusion contrast to stain the tissue structures instead of using chemicals as in conventional histology. Developing MR microscopy for this purpose is considered advantageous because it would save time and offer two-and three-dimensional visualization of microstructures.

MR microscopy images acquired *in vitro* on tissue specimens typically have superior SNR, spatial resolution, and CNR compared to *in vivo* acquisitions for a number of reasons. First, nonviable tissue specimens can be scanned for very long periods (>10 to 20 hours) and provide more overall SNR that can be converted into increased spatial resolution. Second, the tissue specimens do not move during imaging. This enhances SNR compared to *in vivo* imaging (in some cases, however, the tissue specimens can be exposed to micro motion inflicted by the very strong magnetic field gradients active during imaging). Third, formalin fixation used to preserve the tissue will often enhance CNR in the MR microscopy images for unknown reasons. Finally, tissue specimens can be fitted into smaller RF coils which will also improve SNR for a given imaging sequence.

TABLE 7.2
Overview of *In Vivo* Anatomic MR Microscopy Studies Performed on Rodents

Species	Spatial Resolution mm^3	Anatomical Structures	Year	Refs.
Sprague-Dawley rats	0.915	Forebrain; no substructures	1980	15
Fisher 344 rats	0.0185	Forebrain: cortex, hippocampus, thalamus, ventricles, mesencephalon, pons	1986	95
Fisher 344 rats	0.045–0.016	Forebrain: cortex, hippocampus (granule cell layer?), corpus callosum, ventricles, thalamus; hindbrain: pons, cerebellum; pituitary	1987	16
Sprague-Dawley rats	0.0216	Forebrain: olfactory bulbs; eye	1987	96
	0.018	Forebrain: cortex, hippocampus, corpus callosum, thalamus, ventricles	1988	97
A/J mice	0.003	Forebrain: cortex, hippocampus, hippocampus sulcus, corpus callosum, vessels	1990	98
Rats	0.16	Forebrain: cortex, hippocampus, thalamus, ventricles, basal ganglia	1990	68
Gerbils	0.11	Forebrain: cortex, thalamus, ventricles	1992	99
TO mice	0.018	Forebrain: cortex, hippocampus (hippocampus sulcus?), corpus callosum, ventricles, thalamus; hindbrain: cerebellum	1995	17
Fisher rats	0.003	Spinal cord: medulla spinalis, gray and white matter, nerve ganglia, nerve root, peripheral nerve	1998	94
SJL mice	0.0033	Forebrain: olfactory system, ventricles, hippocampus, thalamus; hindbrain: cerebellum	1998	100
C57BL6/J mice	0.0016 0.0016	Forebrain: olfactory bulbs, cortex, basal ganglia, ventricles, hippocampus; hindbrain: cerebellum	2001	43

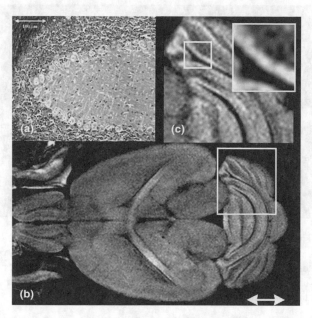

FIGURE 7.4 A histologically processed C57BL6/J mouse brain section at the cerebellum level. (a) A diffusion-weighted MR microscopy image of a C57Bl6/J mouse brain acquired *in vivo* at an in-plane spatial resolution of 58 × 58 μm (slice thickness: 469 μm). (b) Part of the cerebellum. (c) Enlarged part of cerebellum. While individual Purkinje cells are apparent in (a), they are not visible on the *in vivo* MR microscopy images due to a combined lack of CNR and SNR and insufficient spatial resolution. MR microscopy data acquired from the Duke University Center for *In Vivo* Microscopy.

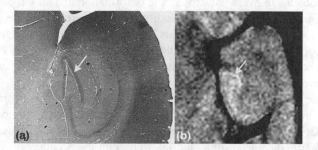

FIGURE 7.5 Hematoxylin and eosin stained C56Bl6/J mouse brain section at the level of the ventral hippocampus. (a) Corresponding diffusion-weighted *in vivo* MR microscopy image acquired at a spatial resolution of 0.0016 mm³. (b) The granule cell layer appears as a faint bright line in the diffusion-weighted image (arrow). MR microscopy data acquired from the Duke University Center for *In Vivo* Microscopy. See Color Figure 7.5 following page 210.

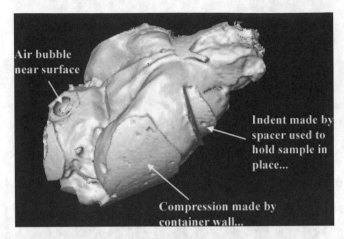

FIGURE 7.6 Three-dimensional MR microscopy data set of a formalin-perfusion fixed mouse brain acquired at a spatial resolution of 0.00011 mm^3 (9.4 T). The surface-rendered format clearly illustrates the positioning artifacts: (1) surface deformation, (2) indent made by spacer used to hold sample in position during imaging, and (3) air bubble. MR microscopy data acquired from the Duke University Center for *In Vivo* Microscopy.

When performing MR microscopy on tissue specimens, certain procedures are recommended. For long scan times, it is important that a specimen not dry out as this will impair image quality and interfere with data interpretation. Dehydration can be prevented by using embedding media such as 1% gelling agar,[31,32] 10% formalin,[33,34] perfluoropolyethers,[33,35,36] and fluorocarbons.[37] Gelling agars and perfluoropolyethers offer only limited protection (12 to 36 hours) against specimen dehydration and are not recommended for general storage purposes. Specimens should be returned to their original storage media, e.g., formalin, after imaging.

Other problems to overcome are sample deformation and air bubble contamination during imaging (see Figure 7.6). Both artefacts severely interfere with general image quality and data interpretation. This issue is of particular importance if surface registration or surface analysis algorithms are to be used on the data. Sample deformation occurs when samples are fitted into RF coils that are too small (smaller RF coils provide better SNR).

For whole brain studies, some investigators circumvented the deformation problem by imaging the brain encased in the skull[38]; others used solidified agars. The presence of air bubbles within a specimen or near the specimen surface during imaging can ruin an entire data acquisition and interfere with the accuracy of interpretation. Air bubble entrapment within specimens might occur during cardiac perfusion fixation procedures if air enters the myocardium and/or is present in the fixation fluid. It can be partially avoided by preheating the fixative to body temperature.

7.2.4 ANATOMY STUDIES

We implied that *in vitro* MR microscopy offers better conditions for display of microscopic anatomy compared to *in vivo* studies because images acquired *in vitro*

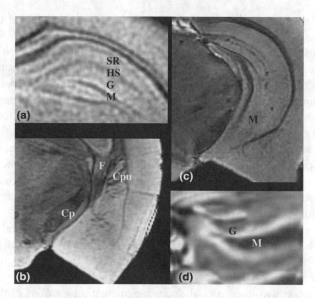

FIGURE 7.7 MR microscopy images acquired from formalin perfusion fixed C57BL6/J mouse brains (a) and perfusion fixed with formalin and Gd-DTPA (b, c, and d). (a) Diffusion-weighted MR microscopy image from the dorsal hippocampus acquired at a spatial resolution of 0.00012 mm³ (9.4 T). MR microscopy data acquired from the Duke Center for *In Vivo* Microscopy. The other images show details from a T_2*-weighted contrast-enhanced MR microscopy data set acquired at the same spatial resolution. SR = stratum radiatum; HS = hippocampal sulcus; G = granule cell layer; M = mossy fiber pathway; F = fimbria; Cpu = caudate putamen; Cp = cerebral peduncle, basal.

typically provide increased spatial resolution (due to more overall SNR) and enhanced CNR (as a possible consequence of formalin fixation). Additionally, para-magnetic contrast agents can be added to the perfusion fixation media to further improve tissue discrimination in MR images when intrinsic CNRs between structures are lacking.[29,32,35,39,40] Figure 7.7 shows an MR microscopy images from various C57BL6/J mouse perfusions fixed with 10% formalin and with contrast-enhanced 10% formalin. Note the variety of microscopic structural units in the mouse brain that can be displayed under these combined conditions of optimized SNR, spatial resolution, and CNR enhancement.

Several contrast agents have been used to enhance CNR in MR microscopy images acquired *in vitro*. Smith et al. were the first to use albumin coupled to DTPA-Gd dissolved in 1% gelatin to augment anatomical visualization in mouse embryos.[32] Using this technique, Smith and colleagues completed a digital atlas that contains MRIs of normal mouse embryos from 9.5 days after conception to new-borns.[41] The addition of gelatin to the macromolecular contrast agent fixation media allowed for better than normal image contrast due to intravascular retention of the contrast agent.[32] Without it, the contrast/formalin solution would have diffused out of the intravascular compartment and reduced the CNR.[35] Johnson and coworkers referred to the use of contrast agents for *in vitro* MR microscopy as *active staining*.[42]

In vitro MR microscopy is currently used to produce anatomical three-dimensional atlas templates of the rodent brain — templates that will eventually be developed into functional and extendable databases. Scientists in the NIH-supported multi-institute Brain Molecular Anatomy Project are creating interoperable databases capable of extracting, storing, fitting, and displaying anatomy and spatially distributed gene expression patterns of the rodent brain. MR microscopy is perfectly suited for this purpose because it is nondestructive and inherently three-dimensional and can visualize a large enough number of structures in the rodent brain to be anatomically informative and useful as a mapping template. Several investigators are working on producing the optimal three-dimensional rodent brain anatomical atlas template. Ghosh et al.[38] published a three-dimensional digital MR microscopy atlas of a neonate mouse lemur and a C57BL6/J mouse brain atlas initiative is underway (http://www.loni.ucla.edu/MAP).

Another detailed brain atlas website of the developing mouse brain (http://mouseatlas.caltech.edu/13.5dpc/) has recently been produced by Dhenain, Ruffins, and Jacobs of the Biological Imaging Center at CalTech.[37] Their atlas also offers users access to three-dimensional rendered models of labeled segmented structures produced from single two-dimensional slices (segmentation routines can be reviewed on a two-dimensional viewer).

7.3 ANATOMICAL PHENOTYPING OF TRANSGENIC MOUSE MODELS BY MR MICROSCOPY

In recent years, we have seen an enormous increase in genetically engineered mouse models. For example, the Jackson Laboratory of Bar Harbor, Maine advertises more than 1200 mouse models on its website (http://www.jax.org). The transgenic mouse models, targeted mutations (knockouts), and chemically induced mutational models add to our knowledge about genotypic and phenotypic changes that lead to disease. This information ultimately will help improve disease detection in humans. For example, diagnostic criteria can be defined more accurately in terms of molecular abnormalities characteristic of a specific disorder. Another important contribution of genetically engineered mouse models of human disease is the ability to test new experimental therapies.

The increase in animal models is accompanied by a concomitant need for noninvasive imaging technologies that can track (1) the phenotypic effects of a given genetic manipulation and (2) the effects of therapeutic intervention. For example, when scientists produce a genetic manipulation with the hope of creating a particular disease model, it is always necessary to document the presence of the desired phenotype for the disease in the genetically engineered mice. It can be very time consuming to use conventional histological methods to verify a particular pathology and at the same time determine whether the anatomy of the rest of the organs is normal. Several investigators suggested the use of MR microscopy for this purpose.[35,42,43]

The phenotypic descriptor attached to each mouse model in the Jackson Laboratory database is incomplete because the data are not yet available or the desired clinical phenotype is not there. For example, in the section on behavioral and learning defects, a description of the B6CBA-TgN(HDexon1)61Gpb strain (a transgenic model of the 5′ end of the human Huntington's disease (HD) gene carrying (CAG)115-(CAG)150 repeat expansions) includes this morphological phenotype statement: "Neuronal intranuclear inclusions which contain both the huntingtin and ubiquitin proteins" (http://jaxmice.jax.org/html/infosearch/ pricelistframeset.html). However, no information is available about other essential clinical HD pathological features such as atrophy of the caudate nucleus, putamen, and globus pallidus.

Information for the transgenic mouse model C57BL/6-TgN(SOD1)3Cje intended to express human SOD1 includes no morphological information (*http://jaxmice.jax.org/jaxmice-cgi/jaxmicedb.cgi?objtype = pricedetail&stock = 002629*). More complete details of morphology would be extremely valuable for investigators for obvious reasons. First, for the HD transgenic mouse models and many other neurodegenerative transgenic strains, it will be important to ascertain that these particular mice will have identical features to those found in humans afflicted with HD, e.g., brain atrophy. This is especially important if therapeutic intervention is to be tested in these models.

MR microscopy has already been used to anatomically phenotype a variety of body organs in knockout and transgenic mice.[36,42,44–47] Smith was the first to use MR microscopy to analyze the hearts and outflow tracts of Cx43 knockout mice and transgenic mice overexpressing the Cx43 gap junction gene, CMV43.[34] The anatomical detail reported in this study is extraordinary, considering the fact that the mouse embryo hearts are <1.5 mm wide.

Investigators have just begun to implement MR microscopy as a tool to phenotype genetically engineered mice models of neurological disease. Enlarged ventricles were reported in a transgenic mouse model of aspartylglucosaminuria[45] and the AnkyrinB knockout mouse.[36] The literature is still sparse on this topic, probably because the logistics of using MR microscopy efficiently for this purpose still must be worked out. The fact that gross and microscopic anatomy can be visualized in a mouse organ or entire body does not necessarily mean that valuable quantitative information can be extracted. New software must be developed and/or current software must be modified to efficiently meet the demands of this new field. The large volumes of three-dimensional MR microscopy data that will become available will require development, testing, and application of automated algorithms for registration, alignment, warping, segmentation, etc. Several computational initiatives are underway to meet this demand.

7.4 MR MICROSCOPY VISUALIZATION OF PATHOLOGY IN RODENTS

We already discussed the use of MR microscopy for the visualization of normal rodent neuroanatomy. This section will review abnormal anatomy and pathology of the rodent brain.

7.4.1 BRAIN ATROPHY

One of the hallmarks of neurodegenerative diseases in the human brain is the development of atrophy. Global or focal brain atrophy develops over time in Alzheimer's disease,[48] Huntington's disease, and Parkinson's disease.[49] Development of brain atrophy over time in C57BL6/J mouse brains has been tracked by MR microscopy.[43] Development of forebrain atrophy was documented by measuring ventricle volume increases on diffusion-weighted MR microscopy images before and 30 days after exposure to transient forebrain ischemia.

Until now, only preliminary reports of development of brain atrophy in genetically engineered mouse models of Alzheimer's disease (AD) were available.[50,51] They suggest that brain atrophy does not develop over time in the PDAPP transgenic AD mouse model[51] or in the PS-APP transgenic AD mouse model.[50] The ventricle systems in PDAPP mice appear highly abnormal compared to systems in normal control mice.[51] More data on MRI characterizations of genetically engineered mouse models of AD will undoubtedly appear in the literature and clarify the utility of these models for studying equivalent clinical conditions in humans.

7.4.2 HYDROCEPHALUS

Hydrocephalus is a condition characterized by increased volume of cerebrospinal fluid (CSF) inside the head. Transgenic mouse models of hydrocephalus exist and the presence of dilated ventricles and/or outflow obstructions have been demonstrated in mouse brains by means of MR microscopy.[36,45] The stenosis of the aqueduct was demonstrated in neonatal perfusion-fixed mouse brains using three-dimensional visualization software.[36]

7.5 SPINAL CORD MR MICROSCOPY

Most MR studies of the rodent spinal cord involved examination of spinal cord injuries with the long term goal of using MR to assess the degree of injury and therapeutic response noninvasively. Therapies range from drug intervention to surgical procedures and tissue transplantation.

7.5.1 PATHOGENESIS OF SPINAL CORD INJURY

The evolution of spinal cord injury resulting from mechanical trauma is a complex process that can be separated into acute and late phases to emphasize important differences in pathophysiological events that occur in the course of an injury. In the acute phase, hemorrhage and edema develop in the central gray matter within a few minutes and lead to the onset of hemorrhagic necrosis after a few hours. A lesion plateau is reached exponentially after about 24 hours. Secondary damage continues from 24 to 72 hours.

Microscopic findings in the acute phase include hemorrhages, mechanical axonal disruption, and direct mechanical injury of neuronal cell bodies. Secondary damage involves hemorrhagic necrosis, infiltration of inflammatory cells, edema, diffuse axonal injury, and myelin degeneration. The repair phase (weeks to months after injury) is dominated by gliosis and/or syrinx formation (for more detail see De Girolami[52]).

The combination of tissue structure and content changes following spinal cord injury makes MRI a natural candidate for noninvasive tracking of damage and therapeutic response. Scientists have started exploring its potential clinically in humans and experimentally in rodents. Small animal MR microscopy studies on the rodent spinal cord are more technically challenging *in vivo* than rodent brain studies. Several obstacles must be overcome to assure optimal data acquisition in the small animal spinal cord including (1) ensuring good SNR on the small and difficult-to-access spinal cord, and (2) minimizing motion artefacts. Much of the MR microscopy in the area of spinal cord injury has been (and still is) performed on larger animals (with larger spinal cords), such as cats. However as MR and SNR technologies improve (higher magnetic fields and implantable RF coils),[53,54] studies of spinal cord injuries in rats will be more prevalent.

Many research groups have already carried out extensive studies focusing on various spinal cord injury models and approaches to minimizing or repairing injuries. Most notable are the works of D.B. Hackney et al. of the University of Pennsylvania[55] and P.A. Narayana et al. of the University of Texas.[56]

7.5.2 MR MICROSCOPY STUDIES OF SMALL ANIMAL SPINAL CORD INJURIES

A great deal has been done to demonstrate the utility of MR methods and the feasibility of applying them to significant spinal cord injury studies. Work to date has explored the ability of MR techniques to characterize and monitor such injuries using standard (T_1 and T_2) methods,[57–61] magnetization transfer contrast,[55,62] and diffusion-weighted MR[63–69] with extension to diffusion tensor MRI.[70–73] All methods demonstrated potential to assess spinal cord injuries. Some appear to have greater utility than others for assessing functional information. Figure 7.8 shows an example of differentiation of a spinal cord injury.

While MRI techniques clearly can detect injuries, their diagnostic potential for accurately determining *type* and *degree* of injury is currently under investigation. This ability is especially important in order to correctly interpret responses to treatment for which some kind of functional information is likely to be necessary. With this goal in mind, Schwartz et al. demonstrated that cystic lesions could be detected using ADC maps before the the lesions were observed on conventional T_1- and T_2-weighted images.[66] During the first 6 hours following a contusive compression injury in rat spinal cord, Bilgen et al. noted that the hemorrhagic lesion expanded both laterally and longitudinally in a predictable fashion that was accurately modeled as an exponential process in time and space.[56]

Diffusion tensor techniques are particularly interesting because they clearly delineate the fiber structure in the spinal cord and may have great potential for evaluating therapies aimed at cord repair. However these data, although of high quality *ex vivo*, are difficult and time consuming to obtain *in vivo* and may have limited utility in the spine.

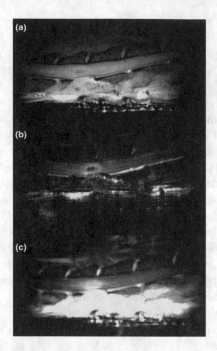

FIGURE 7.8 MR images of a 250-gm Sprague-Dawley rat spine with a moderate contusion injury imaged on the day of the injury. Images acquired *in vivo* at a spatial resolution of 0.012 mm³. (a) T_1-weighted scan showing dark central region of hemorrhage. (b) T_2-weighted scan highlighting dark central region of hemorrhage surrounded by enhanced signal from edema. (c) T_1-weighted image after contrast administration via tail vein showing enhancing lesion in the center of the cord indicating disrupted blood–spinal cord barrier (maximum signal enhancement observed at ~50 minutes). Images acquired from the Center for Structural Imaging at University of Florida.

MR contrast agents (e.g., Gd chelates) have also been used to study animal models of spinal cord injury.[74,75] In a longitudinal study of injury evolution in rats,[75] the region of spinal cord injury showed maximum contrast agent enhancement on the day of injury. A steady decrease was observed in measurements made a week later, indicating that the disrupted blood–spine-barrier is gradually restored after approximately 4 weeks. In addition, the length of the lesion, assessed as the region of contrast enhancement, also decreased steadily.[75]

Bilgen et al. examined the evolution of moderate contusion spinal cord injury in rats with high spatial and temporal resolution using Gd-DTPA enhanced T_1-weighted MRI and correlated the results with behavior outcome.[74] As in the earlier study by Runge et al.,[75] they observed maximum enhancement on the day of injury with gradually decreasing enhancement during injury evolution in all rats for the entire 42-day study. They also found a linear correlation of enhancing lesion volume with behavior at each time point.[74] About 21 days following injury, they also observed local areas of Gd-DTPA enhancement in normal-appearing and injured white matter that they confirmed, in histological examination of excised tissue, corresponded to revasculization. These studies show that MR contrast agents have the potential to provide functional information about the spinal cord which may be of great utility in assessing pharmaceutical interventions.

7.5.3 OTHER SPINAL CORD PATHOLOGIES

Diffusion tensor MR was used to examine the development of a glioma engrafted in a rat spinal cord and provided a good comparison with histology studies.[76] Accompanied by great excitement (and controversy) is the feasibility of using fetal tissue transplantation into humans for spinal cord repair. Recent success has been reported,[77] demonstrating that at least tissue can be transplanted safely into patients with syringomyelia. Implanted fetal tissue has also been reliably detected when implanted in cat spinal cords.[78] Analogous experiments in rats are in progress and future developments in stem cell research are expected to impact spinal injury repairs.

7.6 PERFUSED BRAIN SLICING AND ORIGINS OF MR SIGNALS

Rodent models of the nervous system are accessible by MR imaging and microscopy. They provide a wealth of information, means of investigating the origins and pathogeneses of multiple disease states, and noninvasive monitoring of therapies and other interventions. MR methods provide unprecedented anatomical detail and ongoing developments promise additional improvements. However, as in the clinical MR arena, the preclinical MR signals are still used for the main part in a qualitative fashion.

Signal changes are useful but they only reflect pathology in a qualitative manner, primarily because the origins of MR signals in tissues are complex and poorly understood. The resolution achievable with MR microscopy is still large compared to the heterogeneity of tissues at the microscopic scale. Additionally, on the timescale of the MR measurements, water moves among tissue microcompartments, averaging out signal distributions in most MR measures such as T_1 and T_2. Attempts to use T_1 and T_2 quantitatively have met only with limited success.

MR systems with strong high quality gradient sets that facilitate accurate and stable measurements of the diffusion coefficient of water have been developed. This led to exciting developments in imaging diffusion anisotropy in tissues, in particular related to fiber track mapping as briefly described in Section 7.2. Researchers observed that when high b values (high diffusion weightings) are used, the diffusion curves are multiexponential,[79,80] implying that multiple water compartments contribute to the signal. This created some speculation about the origins of these compartments. Although *in vivo* experiments are possible, motion, sample control, and the relatively large sizes of the animal models make data collection problematic. *Ex vivo* experiments also show multiexponential diffusion behavior, but there is little confidence that these measures will be the same *in vivo*, and perturbation studies on *ex vivo* samples have become problematic.

An established physiological tissue model, the isolated perfused brain slice, has recently been addressed using MR imaging.[81] Single (2 to 500 μm thick) isolated brain slices can be imaged in a perfusion chamber that maintains the tissue physiologically. Figure 7.9 shows an image of such a brain slice. The tissue may then be

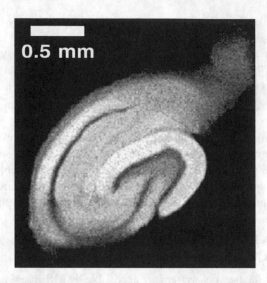

FIGURE 7.9 MR microimage of an isolated hipocampal rat brain slice. This high resolution (15 × 15 × 300 µm) image was collected in 14 hours at 600 MHz to provide structural detail. Lower resolution images (30 to 50 µm in-plane) can be collected in minutes to facilitate meaningful physiological studies (for example, with pharmacological perturbations). Images acquired from the Center for Structural Imaging at University of Florida.

manipulated, for example with hypo- and hypertonic perturbations,[81] membrane channel blocking with ouabain,[82] and excitotoxic intervention.[83]

Simplistic preliminary studies with biexponential mathematical models indicate that the changes observed in the multiexponential curves may directly reflect changes in the intra- and extracellular compartmentation in the tissue, thus reflecting the tissue microstructure.[82] Further studies are underway with more sophisticated models that include exchange[84,85] with extension to facilitate more than two compartments. Nevertheless, the exciting possibility of understanding tissue compartmentation and how it changes in disease states may improve the quantitative capabilities of MR, which in turn may improve its diagnostic and clinical potential. The feasibility of similar studies on human brain slices has been demonstrated recently (private communication), and produced results similar to those obtained with rat brain tissue. This reinforces the relevance of the animal models for these studies and demonstrates the possibility of similar measurements on human brains in clinical settings.

7.7 CONCLUSIONS

We hope that this chapter has emphasized the broad range of structural applications of MR microscopy to the rodent nervous system. This review is by no means exhaustive, but has concentrated on the major applications presently being explored. These applications continue to diversify and expand as MR technology and bioengineering techniques improve.

The drive for higher field strength and improved gradient and RF technologies is likely to continue in the near future and eventually allow improved MRI sensitivity and flexibility. Just as important, however, are continuing improvements in the development of relevant animal models for experimentation, particularly recent developments in genetic engineering. These developments, coupled with improved understanding of the origins of MR signals in tissues and how they change with disease states, therapies, and other interventions, will provide unprecedented amounts of *ex vivo* and *in vivo* details about tissue structure and function.

Developments in MR microscopy parallel similar progress in the area of human MR. Although the focus is on increasing field strength, limits related to cost and potential bioeffects will likely limit human studies to shorter timescales. The information provided by rodent models is essential if the human data is to be understood and optimally interpreted and utilized. Most exciting for the future are emerging developments in multimodality studies in humans and animal models that will provide complementary information to strengthen the utility of the investigative procedures and the usefulness of animal models for experimentation from a basic science standpoint and for improving patient care.

Several multimodality imaging centers have evolved and they foster strong synergy among investigators conventionally focused on a single modality. So far, this has proved healthy by encouraging interactions among scientists in many disciplines and leading to new ideas. The potential of MR microscopy, impressive as it is even now, will continue to grow in the foreseeable future.

REFERENCES

1. Mansfield, P. and P.G. Morris, *NMR Imaging in Biomedicine*, Academic Press, New York, 1982.
2. Haacke, E.M. et al., *Magnetic Resonance Imaging: Physical Principles and Sequence Design*, John Wiley & Sons, New York, 1999.
3. Smith, R. and R. Lange, *Understanding Magnetic Resonance Imaging*, CRC Press, Boca Raon, FL, 1998.
4. Callaghan, P.T., *Principles of Nuclear Magnetic Resonance Microscopy*, Clarendon Press, Oxford, 1991.
5. Stark, D.D. and W.G. Bradley, Magnetic Resonance Imaging, 3rd ed., C.V. Mosby, St. Louis, 1999.
6. Edelman, R., N. Hesselink, and M. Zlatatkin, *Clinical Magnetic Resonance Imaging*, 2nd ed., Harcourt Brace, Orlando, FL, 1996.
7. Roemer, P.B. et al., The NMR phased array, *Mag. Res. Med.*, 16, 192, 1990.
8. Beck, B. and S.J. Blackband, Phased array imaging on a 4.7 T/33 cm animal research system, *Rev. Sci. Instruments*, 72, 4292, 2001.
9. Hurlston, S.E. et al., A high temperature superconducting Helmholtz probe for microscopy at 9.4 T, *Mag. Res. Med.*, 41, 1032, 1999.
10. Bock, N.A., N.B. Konyer, and R.M. Henkelman, Multiple mouse MRI, in *Proc. 9th Annl. Meg. Int. Soc. Mag. Res. Med.*, 2001.
11. Brau, A.C. et al., Fiberoptic stethoscope: a cardiac monitoring and gating system for magnetic resonance microscopy, *Mag. Res. Med.*, 47, 314, 2002.
12. Bell, J.D. and S.D. Taylor-Robinson, Assessing gene expression *in vivo*: magnetic resonance imaging and spectroscopy, *Gene Ther.*, 7, 1259, 2000.

13. Hedlund, L.W. et al., MR-compatible ventilator for small animals: computer-controlled ventilation for proton and noble gas imaging, *Mag. Res. Imaging*, 18, 753, 2000.

14. Hedlund, L.W. et al., Mixing oxygen with hyperpolarized [3]He for small animal lung studies, *NMR Biomed.*, 13, 202, 2000.

15. Hansen, G. et al., *In vivo* imaging of the rat anatomy with nuclear magnetic resonance, *Radiology*, 136, 695, 1980.

16. Johnson, G.A., M.B. Thomson, and B.P. Drayer, Three-dimensional MRI microscopy of the normal rat brain, *Mag. Res. Med.*, 4, 351, 1987.

17. Munasinghe, J.P. et al., Magnetic resonance imaging of the normal mouse brain: comparison with histologic sections, *Lab. Animal Sci.*, 45, 674, 1995.

18. Basser, P.J., Inferring microstructural features and the physiological state of tissues from diffusion-weighted images, *NMR Biomed.*, 8, 333, 1995.

19. Basser, P.J. and C. Pierpaoli, A simplified method to measure the diffusion tensor from seven MR images, *Mag. Res. Med.*, 39, 928, 1998.

20. Mattiello, J., P.J. Basser, and D. LeBihan, Analytical expressions for the b matrix in NMR diffusion imaging and spectroscopy, *J. Mag. Res. Imaging*, A108, 131, 1994.

21. Pierpaoli, C. et al., Diffusion tensor MR imaging of the human brain, *Radiology,* 201, 637, 1996.

22. Shrager, R.I. and P.J. Basser, Anisotropically weighted MRI, *Mag. Res. Med.*, 40, 160, 1998.

23. Conturo, T. et al., Tracking neuronal fiber pathways in the living human brain, *Proc. Natl. Acad. Sci. U.S.A.*, 96, 10422, 1999.

24. Jones, D.D., A. Simmons, and S.C.R. Williams, Noninvasive assessment of axonal fiber connectivity in the human brain via diffusion tensor MRI, *Mag. Res. Med.*, 42, 37, 1999.

25. Makris, N. et al., Morphometry of *in vivo* human white matter association pathways with diffusion-weighted magnetic resonance imaging, *Ann. Neurol.*, 42, 951, 1999.

26. Mori, S. et al., Three-dimensional tracking of axonal projections in the brain by magnetic resonance imaging, *Ann. Neurol.*, 45, 265, 1999.

27. Xue, R. et al., *In vivo* three-dimensional reconstruction of rat brain axonal projections by diffusion tensor imaging, *Mag. Res. Med.*, 42, 1123, 1999.

28. Pautler, P.G., A.C. Silva, and A.P. Koretsky, *In vivo* neuronal tract tracing using manganese-enhanced magnetic resonance imaging, *Mag. Res. Med.*, 70, 740, 1998.

29. Johnson, G.A. et al., Histology by magnetic resonance microscopy, *Mag. Res. Q.*, 9, 1, 1993.

30. Lester, D.S. et al., Virtual neuropathology: three-dimensional visualization of lesions due to toxic insult, *Toxicol. Pathol.*, 28, 100, 2000.

31. Jacobs, R.E. and S.E. Fraser, Imaging neuronal development with magnetic resonance imaging (NMR) microscopy, *J. Neurosci. Methods*, 54, 198, 1994.

32. Smith, B.R. et al., Magnetic resonance microscopy of mouse embryos, *Proc. Natl. Acad. Sci. U.S.A.,* 91, 3530, 1994.

33. Smith, B.R. et al., Time-course imaging of rat embryos *in utero* with magnetic resonance microscopy, *Mag. Res. Med.*, 39, 673, 1998.

34. Smith, B.R., Magnetic resonance microscopy in cardiac development, *Microscopy Res. Tech.*, 52, 323, 2001.

35. Benveniste, H. et al., Magnetic resonance microscopy of the C57BL mouse brain, *Neuroimage*, 1, 601, 2000.

36. Scotland, P. et al., Nervous system defects of AnkyrinB (-/-) mice suggest functional overlap between the cell adhesion molecule L1 and 440-kD AnkyrinB in premyelinated axons, *J. Cell Biol.*, 143, 1305, 1998.
37. Dhenain, M., S.W. Ruffins, and R.E. Jacobs, Three-dimensional digital mouse atlas using high-resolution MRI, *Dev. Biol.*, 232, 458, 2001.
38. Ghosh, P. et al., Mouse lemur microscopic MRI brain atlas, *Neuroimage*, 1, 345, 1994.
39. Mellin, A.F. et al., Three-dimensional magnetic resonance microangiography of rat neurovasculature, *Mag. Res. Med.*, 32, 199, 1994.
40. Smith, B.R. et al., Magnetic resonance microscopy of embryos, *Comp. Med. Imaging Graphics,* 20, 483, 1996.
41. Smith, B.R., D.S. Huff, and G.A. Johnson, Magnetic resonance imaging of embryos: an internet resource for the study of embryonic development, *Comp. Med. Imaging Graphics,* 23, 33, 1999.
42. Johnson, G.A. et al., Morphologic phenotyping with MR microscopy: the visible mouse, *Radiology*, 222, 789, 2002.
43. McDaniel, B. et al., Tracking brain volume changes in C57BL/6J and ApoE-deficient mice in a model of neurodegeneration: a 5-week longitudinal micro-MRI study, *Neuroimage*, 14,1244, 2001.
44. Lanens, D. et al., *In vitro* NMR microimaging of the spinal cord of chronic relapsing EAE rats, *Mag. Res. Imaging*, 12, 469, 1994.
45. Tenhunen, K. et al., Monitoring the CNS pathology in aspartylglucosaminuria mice, *J. Neuropathol. Exp. Neurol.*, 57, 1154, 1998.
46. Meyding-Lamade, U. et al., Herpes simplex virus encephalitis: cranial magnetic resonance imaging and neuropathology in a mouse model, *Neurosci. Lett.*, 248, 13, 1998.
47. Ahrens, E.T. et al., MR Microscopy of transgenic mice that spontaneously acquire experimental allergic encephalomyelitis, *Mag. Res. Med.*, 40, 1998.
48. Esiri, M.M. et al., Ageing and dementia, in *Greenfield's Neuropathology*, Graham, D.I. and P.L. Lantos, Eds., Arnold, London, 1997.
49. Lowe, J., G. Lennox, and P.N. Leigh, Disorders of movement and system degenerations, in *Greenfield's Neuropathology*, Graham, D.I. and P.L. Lantos, Eds., Arnold, London, 1997.
50. Helpern, J.A. et al., *In vivo* detection of neuropathology in an animal model of Alzheimer's disease by magnetic resonance imaging, *Soc. Neurosci. Abstr.*, Program 572.14, 2001.
51. Zhang, L. et al., Tracking of pathology in PDAPP mice by MRI: a two-year longitudinal study, *Soc. Neurosci. Abstr.*, Program 572.14, 2001.
52. De Girolami, U., M.P. Frosch, and E.P. Richardson, Jr., Regional neuropathology: diseases of the spinal cord and vertebral column, in *Greenfield's Neuropathology*, Graham, D.I. and P.L. Lantos, Eds., Arnold, London, 1997.
53. Bilgen, M., R. Abbe, and P.A. Narayana, *In vivo* magnetic resonance microscopy of rat spinal cord at 7 T using implantable RF coils, *Mag. Res. Med.*, 46, 1250, 2001.
54. Silver, X. et al., *In vivo* 1H magnetic resonance imaging and spectroscopy of the rat spinal cord using an inductively-coupled chronically implanted RF coil, *Mag. Res. Med.*, 46, 1216, 2001.
55. McGowan, J.C. et al., Characterization of experimental spinal cord injury with magnetization transfer ratio histograms. *J. Mag. Res. Imaging*, 12, 247, 2000.
56. Bilgen, M. et al., Spatial and temporal evolution of hemorrhage in the hyperacute phase of experimental spinal cord injury: *in vivo* magnetic resonance imaging, *Mag. Res. Med.*, 43, 594, 2000.

57. Metz, G.A. et al., Validation of the weight-drop contusion model in rats: a comparative study of human spinal cord injury, *J. Neurotrauma*, 17, 1, 2000.

58. Franconi, F. et al., *In vivo* quantitative microimaging of rat spinal cord at 7 T, *Mag. Res. Med.*, 44, 893, 2000.

59. Ohta, K. et al., Experimental study on MRI evaluation of the course of cervical spinal cord injury, *Spinal Cord*, 37, 580, 1999.

60. Narayana, P.A. et al., Does loss of gray and white matter contrast in injured spinal cord signify secondary injury? *In vivo* longitudinal MRI studies, *Mag. Res. Med.*, 41, 315, 1999.

61. Fukuoka, M. et al., Magnetic resonance imaging of experimental subacute spinal cord compression, *Spine*, 23, 1540, 1998.

62. Gareau, P.J., L.C. Weaver, and G.A. Dekaban, *In vivo* magnetization transfer measurements of experimental spinal cord injury in the rat, *Mag. Res. Med.*, 45, 159, 2001.

63. Nevo, U. et al., Diffusion anisotropy MRI for quantitative assessment of recovery in injured rat spinal cord, *Mag. Res. Med.*, 45, 1, 2001.

64. Inglis, B.A. et al., Diffusion anisotropy in excised normal rat spinal cord measured by NMR microscopy, *Mag. Res. Imaging,* 15, 441, 1997.

65. Assaf, Y., A. Mayk, and Y. Cohen, Displacement imaging of spinal cord using q-space diffusion-weighted MRI, *Mag. Res. Med.*, 44, 713, 2000.

66. Schwartz, E.D. et al., Diffusion-weighted MR imaging in a rat model of syringomyelia after excitotoxic spinal cord injury, *Am. J. Neuroradiol.*, 20, 1422, 1999.

67. Benveniste, H. et al., *In vivo* diffusion-weighted magnetic resonance microscopy of rat spinal cord: effect of ischemia and intrathecal hyperbaric 5% lidocaine, *Reg. Anesth. Pain Med.*, 24, 311, 1999.

68. Ford, C.C. et al., Magnetic resonance imaging of experimental demyelinating lesions, *Mag. Res. Med.,* 14, 461, 1990.

69. Ford, J.C. et al., A method for *in vivo* high resolution MRI of rat spinal cord injury, *Mag. Res. Med.*, 31, 218, 1994.

70. Beck, B. et al., Progress in high field MRI at the University of Florida, *Magma*, 13, 152, 2002.

71. Fenyes, D.A. and P.A. Narayana, *In vivo* diffusion tensor imaging of rat spinal cord with echo planar imaging, *Mag. Res. Med.*, 42, 300, 1999.

72. Inglis, B.A. et al., Visualization of neural tissue water compartments using biexponential diffusion tensor MRI, *Mag. Res. Med.*, 45, 580, 2001.

73. Gulani, V. et al., A multiple echo pulse sequence for diffusion tensor imaging and its application in excised rat spinal cords, *Mag. Res. Med.*, 38, 868, 1997.

74. Bilgen, M., R. Abbe, and P.A. Narayana, Dynamic contrast-enhanced MRI of experimental spinal cord injury: *in vivo* serial studies, *Mag. Res. Med.,* 45, 614, 2001.

75. Runge, V.M. et al., Evaluation of temporal eveoluation of acute spinal cord injury, *Invest. Radiol.*, 32, 105, 1997.

76. Inglis, B.A. et al., Diffusion tensor MR imaging and comparative histology of glioma engrafted in the rat spinal cord, *Am. J. Neuroradiol.*, 20, 713, 1999.

77. Wirth, E.D. et al., Feasibility and safety of neural tissue transplantation in patients with syringomyelia, *J. Neurotrauma*, 18, 911, 2001.

78. Wirth, E.D. et al., *In vivo* magnetic resonance imaging of fetal cat neural tissue transplants in the adult cat spinal cord, *J. Neurosurg.*, 76, 261, 1992.

79. Henkelman, R.M. et al., Anisotropy of NMR properties of tissues, *Mag. Res. Med.*, 32, 592, 1994.

80. Niendorf, T. et al., Biexponential diffusion attenuation in various states of brain tissue: implications for diffusion-weighted imaging, *Mag. Res. Med.*, 36, 847, 1996.

81. Blackband, S.J. et al., MR microscopy of perfused brain slices, *Mag. Res. Med.*, 38, 1012, 1997.

82. Buckley, D.L. et al., The effect of ouabain on water diffusion in the rat hippocampal slice measured by high resolution NMR imaging, *Mag. Res. Med.*, 41, 137, 1999.

83. Bui, J.D. et al., Nuclear magnetic resonance imaging measurements of water diffusion in the perfused hippocampal slice during N-methyl-D-aspartate-induced excitotoxicity, *Neuroscience*, 93, 487, 1999.

84. Stanisz, G.J. et al., Water dynamics in human blood via combined measurements of T_2 relaxation and diffusion in the presence of gadolinium, *Mag. Res. Med.*, 39, 223, 1998.

85. Stanisz, G.J. et al., An analytical model of restricted diffusion in bovine optic nerve, *Mag. Res. Med.*, 37, 103, 1997.

86. Yang, X., F. Hyder, and R.G. Shulman, Activation of single whisker barrel in rat brain localized by functional magnetic resonance imaging, *Proc. Natl. Acad. Sci. U.S.A.*, 93, 475, 1996.

87. Prichard, J.W. et al., Diffusion-weighted NMR imaging changes caused by electrical activation of the brain, *NMR Biomed.*, 8, 359, 1995.

88. Gyngell, M.L. et al., Variation of functional MRI signal in response to frequency of somatosensory stimulation in α-chloralose anesthetized rats, *Mag. Res. Med.*, 36, 13, 1996.

89. Wood, A.K.W. et al., Prolonged general anesthesia in MR studies of rats, *Acad. Radiol.*, 8, 1136, 2001.

90. Fayad, Z.A. et al., Noninvasive *in vivo* high resolution magnetic resonance imaging of atherosclerotic lesions in genetically engineered mice, *Circulation*, 98, 1541, 1998.

91. Hedlund, L.W. et al., A ventilator for magnetic resonance imaging, *Invest. Radiol.*, 21, 18, 1986.

92. Wiesmann, F. et al., Dobutamine stress magnetic resonance microimaging in mice: acute changes of cardiac geometry and function in normal and failing murine hearts, *Circ. Res.*, 88, 563, 2001.

93. Ruff, J. et al., Magnetic resonance imaging of coronary arteries and heart valves in a living mouse: techniques and preliminary results, *J. Mag. Res.* 146, 290, 2000.

94. Benveniste, H. et al., Spinal cord neural anatomy in rats examined by *in vivo* magnetic resonance microscopy, *Reg. Anesth. Pain Med.*, 23, 589, 1998.

95. Johnson, G.A. et al., Nuclear magnetic resonance imaging at microscopic resolution, *J. Mag. Res.*, 68, 129, 1986.

96. Rudin, M., MR microscopy on rats *in vivo* at 4.7 T using surface coils, *Mag. Res. Med.*, 5, 443, 1987.

97. Martin, M. et al., The center-tapped slotted tube autotransformer resonator: a coil for use with a high-resolution small animal imaging system, *Mag. Res. Med.*, 8, 171, 1988.

98. Ogawa, S. et al., Oxygenation-sensitive contrast in magnetic resonance image of rodent brain at high magnetic fields, *Mag. Res. Med.*, 14, 68, 1990.

99. Busza, A.L. et al., Diffusion-weighted imaging studies of cerebral ischemia in gerbils: potential relevance to energy failure, *Stroke*, 23, 1602, 1992.

100. Xu, S. et al., Study of relapsing remitting experimental allergic encephalomyelitis SJL mouse model using MION-46L enhanced *in vivo* MRI: early histopathological correlation, *J. Neurosci. Res.*, 52, 549, 1998.

8 Magnetic Resonance Spectroscopy: Principles and Applications

Stephen R. Williams and Nicola R. Sibson

CONTENTS

8.1 INTRODUCTION

Nuclear magnetic resonance spectroscopy (NMR/MRS) is the most sensitive and specific technique for determining chemical and macromolecular structures and conformations. Although nuclear magnetic resonance was discovered in the mid 1940s, it did not create a major impact in chemistry until the 1960s through improvements in magnets, computers and the introduction of Fourier transform (FT) methods. Although it was used in some early studies of biological systems, applications in biology developed from studies by Moon and Richards on red blood cells in 1973 and by Hoult et al. on skeletal muscle in 1974.[1] MRS offered the promise of measuring biochemical compounds in intact biological tissue noninvasively and the ability to follow dynamic changes over time. As this chapter demonstrates, this promise has been realized — most effectively in the brain where it has offered new insights into disease and improved our understanding of metabolic processes and metabolic compartmentation.

This chapter will briefly introduce the physical basis of MRS and describe the compounds that can be detected in brain spectra and their importance. Applications in the measurement of metabolic fluxes and steady state metabolite measurements will be discussed with an emphasis on neurotransmitter metabolism and the characterization of disease. An exhaustive review of the field would require a whole book.[2] We have chosen specific areas in which we have an interest to serve as examples of the uses of NMR spectroscopy.

8.2   BASIC PHYSICS OF SPECTROSCOPY AND IMAGING

All modern biomedical MR equipment is at least technically capable of spectroscopy. Since imaging has already been introduced, it is appropriate to explain how the techniques differ. Table 8.1 lists the most important differences between imaging and spectroscopy.

These differences are due to the fact that spectroscopy detects compounds at much lower concentrations than water (water is present at several thousand times the concentration of metabolites) and that frequencies need to be measured to a precision of 0.1 parts per million or less. The low signal strength in spectroscopy means that spatial resolution cannot match that of imaging. The necessity to measure small frequency differences demands good magnetic field homogeneity and stability.

8.2.1   CHEMICAL SHIFT

The frequency differences among protons in different chemical environments (or other NMR active nuclei such as ^{19}F, ^{31}P, ^{15}N, ^{13}C) are due to slight differences between the magnetic field at the nucleus and the applied field because of the shielding provided by electrons. As the electron distribution is affected by even subtle changes in molecular structure, any changes are reflected by small shifts in NMR frequency. This phenomenon is known as the chemical shift (σ) and it is expressed in dimensionless ppm units:

$$\sigma = (\nu - \nu_0)/\nu_0 \times 10^6$$

where ν is the resonance frequency of the proton of interest, and ν_0 is the frequency of a reference compound set at 0 ppm.

Since $\nu_0 = \gamma B_0$, the chemical shift of a given nucleus with respect to a reference is independent of field strength, although the absolute frequency will not be. The

TABLE 8.1
Comparison of MR Imaging and Spectroscopy

Property	Imaging	Spectroscopy
What is measured?	Water	Metabolites
How is the MR signal treated?	Spatial encoding of frequency	Chemical encoding of frequency[a]
"Read" gradient (during acquisition)	Yes	No[b]
Use of gradients	Spatial encoding	Spatial localization[c]
Spatial resolution	High (mm)	Low (cm)
Signal-to-noise	High	Low
Magnet field strength	Any (0.05 T or more)	Mid-high (1.5 T or more)
Field homogeneity required	Poor–reasonable[d]	Excellent[d]
Quality of eddy current compensation required	Poor–good[e]	Good–very good[e]
Acquisition bandwidth	10–450 kHz	1 kHz or less[f]

[a] NMR-active nuclei in different molecules and different parts of the same nuclei generally resonate at slightly different frequencies (chemical shift).

[b] Some specialized spectroscopic imaging sequences acquire data in the presence of a read gradient to provide one dimension of spatial encoding. Chemical shift encoding (at relatively low resolution) is accomplished in the evolution phase of the sequence, before detection of the signal.

[c] This is true for single voxel spectroscopy. In conventional spectroscopic imaging, phase encoding gradients are used along one to three axes to encode spectra spatially.

[d] Conventional imaging places few requirements on magnet homogeneity. Adjacent pixels 1 to 2 mm apart are typically separated by >40 Hz in frequency. However, in spectroscopy, frequency differences of a few Hertz must be measured and the magnet needs to achieve homogeneity over large volumes (approaching that of the whole brain for chemical shift imaging). Echo planar imaging (epi) is much more prone to inhomogeneity-related distortion than conventional imaging, and whole brain epi has homogeneity requirements approaching those of spectroscopy.

[e] Eddy currents induce oscillations in the magnetic field that severely affect spectroscopy performed at short echo times. The biochemical information obtained from short echo times is much richer but requires good gradient performance to achieve that. Although conventional imaging is largely tolerant of eddy currents, they become more serious issues in epi. The magnet and gradient performance needed to undertake epi-based functional imaging is equivalent or superior to that needed for the most demanding spectroscopy experiments.

[f] A bandwidth of 1 kHz is adequate for ^{1}H MRS at 1.5 T. Higher fields and/or other nuclei require larger bandwidths.

X axis of an MR spectrum is the chemical shift in ppm. Figure 8.1 illustrates chemical shift.

8.2.2   ACQUIRING SPECTRA

In this section the principles of acquisition methods are described. Readers should refer to the specialist literature for more explanation. Two factors are essential for successful *in vivo* ^{1}H MRS: (1) the signal must be properly localized without contamination from outside the prescribed area and (2) the dominant water signal

Chemical Shift

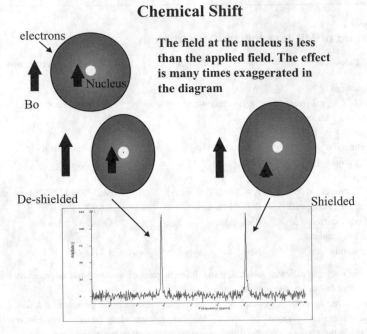

FIGURE 8.1 Chemical shift. The field at the nucleus is less than the applied field because of the shielding effects of electrons. The magnitude of this effect is a few parts per million for ^1H (greater for other nuclei; 200 ppm for ^{13}C) and is exaggerated in the diagram. The bottom panel indicates spectra from deshielded and shielded nuclei. Shielded nuclei resonate at low frequency. By convention, frequency increases to the left in MR spectra.

must be suppressed (even though recent specialized applications that do not use water suppression have been described). Other nuclei present no need to suppress a dominant signal, but signal-to-noise and spectroscopic resolution become important factors. Localization is achieved by frequency selective excitation in the presence of a magnetic field gradient.

Unlike imaging in which slice selection is usually in one dimension only, three orthogonal slices are typical for spectroscopy (Figure 8.2). Common methods such as STEAM and PRESS are explained elsewhere[1,2] and can be used for human and animal studies after appropriate adaptation. Localization is sometimes unnecessary in animal studies if the exact anatomical location of the signals is unimportant and if the large lipid signal from the scalp does not interfere with metabolite measurements. Nonlocalized experiments are much simpler to undertake, and signal-to-noise is improved by increased detection volume. In most clinical studies, the standard head imaging coil is used for excitation and detection of signals. This is straightforward to implement, gives uniform coverage of the brain, and can be integrated within standard clinical imaging protocols.

Water suppression is necessary because the large concentration difference between water and metabolites makes detection of the latter difficult. *In vivo* water suppression is carried out usually by methods that effectively destroy the water signal

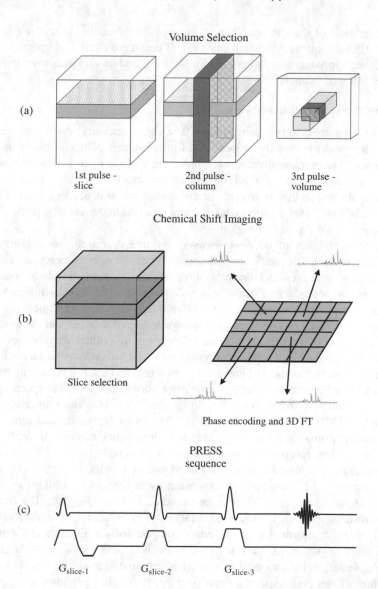

FIGURE 8.2 Localization methods. (a) volume selection. A small cube can be selected within a larger cube, by ensuring that coherent signal is only collected from the volume that experienced all three RF excitations. This volume is at the intersection of the three slices and can be positioned at will. (b) chemical shift imaging (spectroscopic imaging). This is a hybrid technique, incorporating elements of volume selection and imaging. After excitation (and optional volume selection), the spectrum is phase encoded in two dimensions prior to acquisition. A grid of spectra can be extracted from the slice. In comparison to single voxel spectra, a minimum of n^2 acquisitions are required (where n is the number of phase encode steps in each direction). (c) PRESS sequence. A slice is excited by a slice-selective 90° pulse. The magnetization is then refocused by two orthogonal 180° pulses. Crusher gradients ensure that only the spin-echo signal excited by all three pulses is collected.

prior to excitation of the spectrum. The commonest method in clinical use is the so-called CHESS sequence[3,4] implemented on all commercial clinical spectroscopy systems. Other approaches are often used for nonlocalized measurements in animals and for ^{1}H MRS of extracts.[2-5]

8.2.3 SPECTROSCOPIC QUANTIFICATION

MRS is an inherently quantitative technique. The signal intensity of a resonance (or area under the peak) is directly proportional to the number of nuclei resonating at that frequency. However, the situation is complicated by three factors. Proportionality constants are not the same for all signals in the spectra; the signal cannot be absolutely calibrated so that an internal or external standard is needed; and the area or amplitude of low signal-to-noise peaks cannot be measured precisely, particularly if the baseline is not flat in that region.

Accurate measurement of peak areas is relatively straightforward in well resolved spectra with flat baselines. All commercial MR spectrometers and third party processing packages include integration routines that are simple to use and give accurate and reproducible measurements. However, even signals in high resolution spectra (e.g., from extracts) can be difficult to quantify where lines overlap.

Deconvolution methods, in which the spectra are fitted to a number of independent lines, are needed to extract information from individual metabolites (see Figure 8.3). Varying levels of sophistication can be applied to deconvolution methods, from simple manual adjustment of line width, frequency, and intensity of components, to more automated approaches incorporating prior knowledge about the spectra. The two most common approaches to spectral fitting used for *in vivo* analyses are the LC model[6] and AMARES,[7] which fit data in the frequency (spectral) and time (free induction decay) domains, respectively. Manually driven methods may be preferable for analyzing a few spectra, but most analyses will benefit from the extra effort required to set up automated and prior knowledge-based methods.

Quantification of *in vitro* spectra does not present the same problems in terms of overlap, signal-to-noise, or baseline encountered with *in vivo* data. If a limited number of resonances must be measured, analysis of even large data sets is straightforward. If no prior information about certain compounds is available and the entire spectrum must be surveyed, measuring all individual peaks in all spectra is not feasible. However, techniques of data reduction, automated analysis, and statistical classification of the entire spectrum can be used.[8-10] These methods can treat the spectrum as a pattern without any knowledge of individual resonances or they can extract regions from differing spectra to identify metabolites that are responsible for or modulated by the process under investigation.

8.3 METABOLITES: THEIR SPECTRA AND BIOLOGICAL SIGNIFICANCE

A fundamental problem encountered when studying brain biochemistry is the relative inaccessibility to conventional methods of investigation. Most biochemical studies of the brain were performed with tissue and cell cultures *in vitro*; then the relevance of the findings had to be associated to the situation *in vivo*. While the biochemical

Deconvolution of Human Brain Spectrum
(Time Domain Fit)

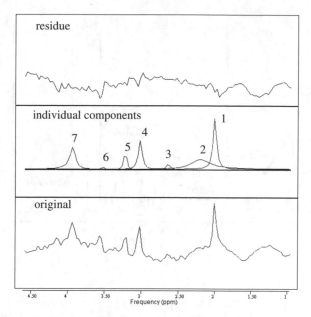

FIGURE 8.3 Deconvolution. The bottom panel shows a 1.5-T human brain spectrum analyzed using the AMARES routine in the JAVA MRUI package (van Ormondt, D., http://carbon.uab.es/mrui/) Prior knowledge of relative frequencies, line widths, phases, and starting values is used to fit the data in the time domain and the results are presented as spectra. The middle panel shows the fitted lines. The top panel shows the residual. The routine only fits peaks for which prior knowledge is supplied. The fitted peaks are 1, NAA; 2, Glx; 3, NAA; 4, PCr + Cr; 5, Cho; 6, Ino; 7, PCr + Cr (see Figure 8.4 legend).

pathways of energy metabolism in the brain are similar to those of other tissues, the very high oxidative demands of the brain and the existence of the blood–brain barrier influence the way the brain handles substrates. As a consequence, the extrapolation of metabolic function in the brain from the situation *in vitro* to that *in vivo* is fraught with difficulties. A more integrated systems level approach is needed.

MRS offers opportunities to meet this need through noninvasive measurements of steady state metabolite levels and cerebral metabolic fluxes *in vivo*. While the sensitive ^{1}H and ^{31}P MRS techniques provide valuable information on changes in cerebral metabolite concentrations under normal and pathological conditions, the low natural abundance nuclei, ^{13}C and ^{15}N, are especially useful for measuring metabolic fluxes using isotopically enriched precursors.

An MR spectrum provides a noninvasive assay of metabolites in various media from human or animal brain *in vivo* through brain slices, tissue extracts, and pure cell preparations. ^{1}H, ^{31}P, ^{13}C, and ^{15}N nuclei are all MR-detectable and allow access to a large number of important neurochemicals. Figure 8.4 shows spectra from a number of different brain preparations and nuclei.

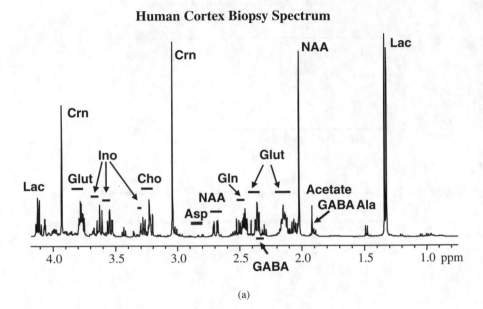

(a)

FIGURE 8.4 A range of samples of brain spectra. (a) 11.7 T human biopsy. Sample of normal appearing human cortex removed at surgery, frozen and extracted with perchloric acid. Because of the high field and excellent resolution, more metabolites are detectable than in clinical 1.5 T spectra of human brain. (b) 11.7 T cell extracts. Samples from extracted primary cultures of neural cell types. Metabolic differences are apparent in the different cell types. (c) 9.4 T rat brain *in vivo*. This spectrum demonstrates that resolution and sensitivity *in vivo* can approach those of extract spectra, with the use of high field magnets and appropriate pulse sequences and shimming. (From Tkac, I. et al., *Mag. Res. Med.,* 41, 649, 1999. With permission from Wiley-Liss Inc., a subsidiary of John Wiley & Sons.) (d) human spectra at 1.5 T. This spectrum is representative of spectra that can be obtained on a modern 1.5-T scanner, with minimal user input to optimize measurement. Spectroscopy can easily be appended to an imaging procedure without lengthy set-up measures. (e) ^{31}P brain slice. Rat brain slices were superfused in an 8.5-T magnet. The brain energy status, pH, and free Mg^{2+} concentration can all be measured. The spectra are stable for many hours and allow control of oxygenation and substrate delivery together with pharmacological challenges. (f) 9.4 T ^{13}C rat brain. At high field, the detection of a number of compounds using a low sensitivity nucleus such as ^{13}C becomes a practical possibility. This spectrum is from rat brain following an infusion of ^{13}C labelled glucose. (From Choi, I.Y. et al., *Mag. Res. Med.,* 44, 387, 2000. With permission from Wiley-Liss, Inc., a subsidiary of John Wiley & Sons. Ace – acetate; Ala – alanine; Asp – aspartate; Cho – choline-containing compounds; Cr – creatine; GABA – γ-aminobutyric acid; Glc – glucose; Gln – glutamine; Glu/Glut – glutamate; Glx – glutamate + glutamine; Ins – inositol; Lac – lactate; Lys, Arg – lysine and arginine; MM – macromolecules; NAA – N-acetylaspartate; NAAG – N-acetylaspartylglutamate; PCr – phosphocreatine; PDE – phosphodiesters; P_i – inorganic phosphate; PME – phosphomonoesters; Suc – succinate; Tau – taurine; Val, Leu, Ile – valine, leucine, and isoleucine.

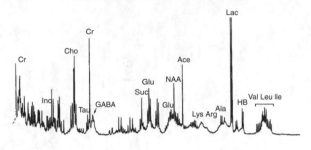

Spectra of Cell Culture Extracts

CEREBELLAR GRANULE NEURONS

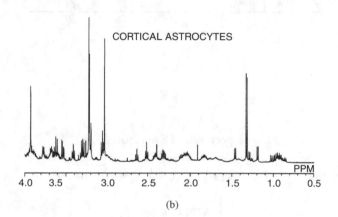

CORTICAL ASTROCYTES

(b)

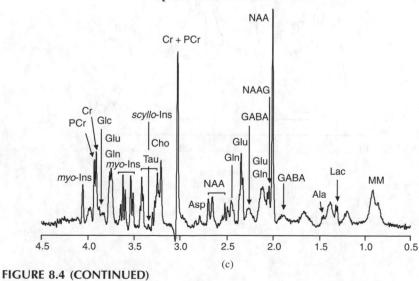

^{1}**H Spectrum of Rat Brain** *in vivo*

(c)

FIGURE 8.4 (CONTINUED)

Human Brain Spectrum

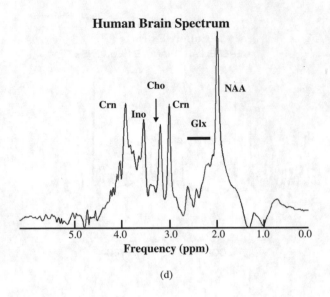

(d)

Spectrum of Superfused Brain Slices

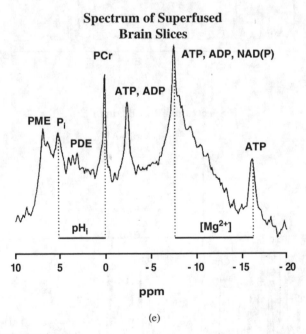

(e)

FIGURE 8.4 (CONTINUED)

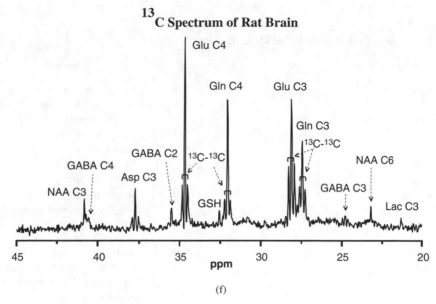

(f)

FIGURE 8.4 (CONTINUED)

In vivo, MRS can be used to detect most metabolites present in tissue at concentrations of 1 mMol/kg or greater. In ^{1}H spectroscopy, where the number of compounds that can be detected is large and the frequency range is small, special techniques are required to detect small buried signals (e.g., from GABA) in the same region of the spectrum as more intense resonances (e.g., from glutamate). Other nuclei are less sensitive, but the increased frequency range and reduced overlap mean detection limits are similar, although longer spectroscopic acquisitions and/or decreased spatial resolution will usually be needed. Low natural abundance nuclei (^{13}C, ^{15}N) require enrichment, but can be used to follow specific metabolic pathways.

Many more compounds can be detected in tissue or cell extracts, where higher magnetic fields and better spectroscopic resolution allow improved sensitivity and resolution of closely separated signals. Such studies lack the real-time dynamic nature of *in vivo* spectroscopy and the ability to follow time courses in single subjects, but with appropriate design they are still powerful methods to measure steady state metabolite concentrations and probe pathways and fluxes. *In vivo* measurement is the only option for studying processes in human brains, except in situations where surgical biopsy material is available.

Table 8.2 lists some neurochemicals that can be measured in the brain *in vivo*. The table gives a brief indication of the biological importance of these compounds and their significance in MRS studies. In addition to compounds that can be detected *in vivo*, a large number of other metabolites can be detected in extracts by ^{1}H MRS. They include branched chain and aromatic amino acids, β-hydroxybutyrate, hypotaurine, succinate, and acetate. Most neuroscientists will find at least some of these molecules relevant to their interests. The table indicates areas in which MRS has impacted our understanding of neurochemistry, human pathology, and disease

TABLE 8.2
Compounds Detectable by MRS in the Brain

Compound	^{1}H	^{31}P	^{13}C/^{15}N	Relevance
Alanine	+	−	+	Nitrogen/protein metabolism; elevated in hyperammonemia
Aspartate	+	−	+	Neurotransmitter
Creatine[a]	+	−	−	Energy metabolite
GABA[b]	+	−	+	Neurotransmitter
Glucose	+	−	+	Energy substrate
Glutamate[c]	+	−	+	Neurotransmitter
Glutamine[c]	+	−	+	Neurotransmitter recycling. Elevated in hyperammonaemia
Glutathione[b]	+	−	−	Anti-oxidant
Glycine[d]	+	−	−	Neuromodulator
Glycogen	+	−	+	Energy substrate
Lactate	+	−	+	Anaerobic metabolism; elevated in ischemic disease, high grade tumors
Macro-molecules	+	−	−	Affect accurate metabolite quantification.
myo-Inositol[e]	+	−	−	Osmolyte, cell signaling precursor. Decreased in hepatic encephalopathy
N-acetylaspartate[f] (NAA)	+	−	+	Neuronal marker
N-acetylaspartylglutamate[f] (NAAG)	+	−	−	NAA/glutamate metabolite and precursor
Phenylalanine[g]	+	−	−	Elevated in phenylketourea
Phosphocholine[h,i]	+	+	−	Cell proliferation, cancer marker, membrane metabolite
Phosphocreatine[a]	+	+	−	Energy metabolite
Phosphodiesters[h,j]	+	+	−	Cell proliferation, cancer marker, membrane metabolite
Scyllo-Inositol	+	−	−	
Taurine	+	−	−	Neuromodulator, osmolyte
ADP[k]	−	+	−	Energy metabolite
ATP	*in vitro*	+	−	Energy metabolite
Lipid/phospholipid	+	+	+	Elevated in high grade tumors
Phosphoethanolamine[i]	*in vitro*	+	−	Cell proliferation, cancer marker, membrane metabolite
H$^+$ ion[l]	−	+	−	Regulator of metabolism
Inorganic phosphate	−	+	−	Energy metabolite
Mg^{2+} ion[m]		+		Regulator of metabolism and neurotransmission

continued

TABLE 8.2 (CONTINUED)
Compounds Detectable by MRS in the Brain

Note: This table lists compounds that can be measured *in vivo* by MRS and which nuclei can be used (+). *I.V.* means a metabolite only detected *in vitro* by ^{1}H MRS. ^{13}C/^{15}N detection is after enrichment with an appropriate substrate except in special circumstances.

[a] Creatine and phosphocreatine cannot usually be distinguished by ^{1}H MRS *in vivo*.

[b] GABA and glutathione usually require editing for detection *in vivo*.

[c] Glutamate and glutamine cannot be distinguished by ^{1}H MRS *in vivo* at 1.5 T,

[d] In normal brain, detection is difficult because of overlap with *myo*-inositol.

[e] Inositol monophosphate can be detected following lithium treatment by ^{31}P MRS.

[f] NAA and NAAG usually cannot be distinguished by ^{1}H MRS *in vivo*.

[g] Phenylalanine detection requires large volumes and long acquisition times.

[h] Phosphocholine and glycerophosphocholine cannot be separated by ^{1}H MRS *in vivo*.

[i] A range of phosphomonoesters, in addition to phosphocholine and phosphoethanolamine can be measured by ^{31}P MRS *in vitro*.

[j] Phosphodiesters, glycerophosphocholine, and glycerophosphoethanolamine can be distinguished by ^{31}P MRS *in vivo* and *in vitro*.

[k] ADP concentration *in vivo* can be calculated from creatine kinase equilibrium. ADP can be measured directly *in vitro* by ^{31}P MRS.

[l] pH is determined from the chemical shift of the inorganic phosphate resonance.

[m] Mg^{2+} ion can be measured from the chemical shift of ATP resonances although the measurement is not very precise. Ca^{2+} can be measured in brain slice preparations by ^{19}F MRS after loading with a fluorinated indicator (F-BAPTA).

management. MRS detects compounds involved in a wide range of cellular processes, including neurotransmission; metabolism of energy, nitrogen, amino acids, and lipids; and metabolic regulation. The concentrations of many metabolites change during the course of disease or therapy. MRS can aid diagnosis and patient management and improve our understanding of metabolic disregulation in disease.

8.3.1 INTERPRETATION OF STEADY STATE CHANGES IN METABOLITES

The functions of most of the metabolites listed in Table 8.2 are at least partially understood and much of the information would probably be available without MRS. However, the roles and importances of some of them such as N-acetylaspartate (NAA), choline-containing compounds (Cho), and *myo*-inositol (mI) have only been fully appreciated as a result of MRS studies. Better understood chemicals such as ATP, glucose, and lactate now can now be measured noninvasively and repeatedly in human disease and in animal models. We will describe how the major metabolites detected by ^{1}H and ^{13}C MRS change in disease and how the changes are interpreted.

8.3.1.1 N-acetylaspartate, Creatine, and Choline-Containing Compounds

These compounds give rise to the three most intense signals in normal brains and are the only ones that usually can be detected at long echo times (TE >120 ms).

N-acetylaspartate (NAA) is present predominantly in neurons,[11–13] and is also expressed in cells of oligodendrocyte lineage.[12,14] No evidence indicates astrocytes contain any NAA, so it is generally used as a marker of neuronal/axonal integrity. NAA is reduced or undetectable in certain brain diseases[15] including most tumors, multiple sclerosis lesions,[16,17] stroke infarcts,[18,19] epilepsy,[20] and psychiatric disorders.[21] Early studies suggested loss of NAA was irreversible and associated with loss of neuronal cells. Studies of multiple sclerosis and mitochondrial disorders indicate that decreases in NAA can be reversed.[22] A loss of NAA can be interpreted as a dysfunction of neurons rather than a simple neuronal loss based on biochemical evidence that NAA is synthesized in mitochondria and that its synthesis is disrupted in damaged mitochondria.[23]

Phosphocreatine (PCr) is one of the major signals detected by ^{31}P MRS, and plays an important role in maintaining ATP during acute hypoxia/ischemia and in facilitating transport of ATP equivalents within the cytosol. It has been used in experimental studies to characterize energy failure in ischemic injury.[24] It has proven a valuable prognostic indicator of outcomes in neonates who suffer hypoxic/ischemic insults at birth.[25,26] The creatine signal at 3.03 ppm in ^{1}H spectroscopy is the sum of signals from creatine (Crn) and PCr. The ^{1}H resonance does not change acutely during disruptions to energy metabolism, but it is reduced chronically in necrotic regions and in certain brain tumors.[27] The two components of creatine can be measured separately *in vivo* by using the increased frequency difference between the CH_2 resonances (0.02 ppm compared to 0.001 for the CH_3 signals) and working at a high field with excellent resolution.[28] The creatine signal is often used as a reference to calculate metabolite ratios such as NAA/creatine or choline/creatine. These ratios have been shown to change in a number of diseases (e.g., temporal lobe epilepsy[20]), but the use of ratios, although valuable in certain circumstances, can be misleading.

The signal assigned to choline-containing compounds (Cho) is predominantly from the glycerophosphocholine and phosphocholine intermediates of membrane metabolic pathways. The Cho signal is elevated in brain tumors[15] and is a defining characteristic of brain tumor spectra. High resolution studies of cell line extracts and human tumor biopsy specimens suggest reversal of the relative amounts of glycerophosphocholine and phosphocholine when cells undergo malignant transformation.[29,30]

8.3.1.2 Lactate

Lactate is elevated acutely following hypoxia/ischemia. It has been used extensively in experimental studies as an early marker of acute stroke,[24] and has been shown to be elevated chronically in human stroke. It has been suggested that measurement of lactate in clinical stroke may help as a prognostic indicator, although the evidence of that is conflicting.[18,31] Lactate is also often elevated clinically in tumors.[32] Measurements of signals in the lactate region (that often includes mobile lipid in necrotic tumors) can aid classification of tumor type and grade.[10,33]

8.3.1.3 Glutamate, Glutamine, and Other Amino Acids

Glutamate is the most concentrated organic molecule in the brain (10 to 15 mmol/l), but it is not detectable by ^{1}H MRS at long echo times (TE >120 ms) because of its complex spectrum that undergoes phase modulation with echo time, leading to signal cancellation as the echo time is prolonged. At short echo times (TE <30 ms), signals from glutamate and glutamine are readily detectable[34] and are modulated in disease. Chronic hepatic encephalopathy has been shown by ^{1}H MRS to be associated with increased glutamine and decreased mI in the brain.[5,35] The burden of clinical disease correlates well with spectroscopic measurements of glutamine and mI, and may prove to be good indicators of disease progression and treatment.

Other amino acids such as γ-aminobutyrate (GABA), alanine, and aspartate that are present at lower concentrations can be detected *in vivo* with specialized techniques such as spectral editing,[36,37] at very high fields,[28] or *in vitro* in cell or tissue extracts. ^{1}H MRS has been used to measure elevated GABA in the brains of epilepsy patients undergoing treatment with GABA-raising drugs.[38] Seizure control appears closely linked to cerebral GABA concentration. This suggests that MRS measurements may be valuable pharmacologically in a variety of areas including *in vivo* pharmacokinetics, dose ranging studies, and dose targeting in individual patients. Alanine is elevated in cultures of meningiomas and meningeal cells.[39] It has also been detected in human meningiomas *in vivo* and in tissue extracts of meningeal tumors.[40]

8.3.1.4 Glucose and Inositol

Glucose, *myo*-inositol, and *scyllo*-inositol can be detected *in vivo* using short echo time spectroscopy.[41,42] The importance of glucose homeostasis barely needs mention, and the use of kinetic measurements of glucose labelling is discussed in Section 8.3.2. *Myo*-inositol has been suggested as a marker of astrocytes,[43] although careful inspection of the spectra from neuronal cells revealed its presence in neurons.[12] *Myo*-inositol appears to function as an osmoregulator and its decrease in hepatic encephalopathy is thought to reflect osmotic disturbances in glial cells. Measurement of *myo*-inositol may be useful in monitoring osmotically stressed patients whose treatment must be judged finely in order to be effective without causing damage.[44]

8.3.2 Metabolic Fluxes

One major advantage of MRS for studying metabolic rates is that reaction kinetics can be measured noninvasively. Studies can now address various aspects of energy metabolism (including oxidative and nonoxidative glucose consumption, ATP turnover, and creatine kinase flux) and certain neurotransmitter fluxes (glutamate, GABA) intrinsically linked to neuronal activity. *Neuronal activity* describes a spectrum of energy-requiring processes that include neurotransmitter release, uptake, and recycling, vesicular recycling, and action potential propagation, restoration, and maintenance of membrane potentials.

The energetic cost of neuronal activity and the fraction of total cerebral energy consumption it represents have long been sources of scientific interest and debate. The relationship of neuronal activity and energy metabolism has implications for the interpretation of functional neuroimaging (including fMRI; see Chapter 4) that rely on implied relationships between measured parameters (glucose consumption, oxygen consumption, or blood flow) and neuronal activity. The MRS techniques

TABLE 8.3
Properties of Nuclei Used in Metabolic Flux Studies

Nucleus	Resonance frequency at 7 T (MHz)	Natural Abundance (%)	Relative Sensitivity[a]	Chemical Shift Range[b] (ppm)
^{1}H	299.5	99.99	100	~8
^{13}C	75.3	1.11	1.6	~250
^{15}N	30.4	0.37	0.1	~400
^{31}P	121.2	100.00	6.6	~30

[a] Same number of nuclei at constant field.
[b] For biological compounds.

discussed in this chapter answer some of these key biochemical questions that have remained elusive for decades. This section covers recent developments in MRS *in vivo* for the measurement of energy metabolism, neurotransmitter fluxes, and the relationship of neuronal activity and energetics.

8.3.2.1   Methods

8.3.2.1.1   *^{13}C Magnetic Resonance Spectroscopy*

The natural abundance of the ^{13}C isotope is only ~1.1%; it has much less intrinsic sensitivity than ^{1}H MRS (see Table 8.3). This makes ^{13}C MRS ideal for measuring metabolic rates. Since the normal concentration of ^{13}C-labelled metabolites is extremely low, it is possible to infuse enriched substrates into a subject and detect incorporation of the ^{13}C isotope into brain metabolites as they become enriched. Metabolic rates can be determined from these isotope incorporation curves via metabolic modelling. These experiments followed the same principle as ^{14}C labelling studies dating back many years, with two distinct advantages: (1) ^{13}C is a nonradioactive, stable isotope, and (2) the well resolved signals obtained with MRS can be attributed to specific carbon positions within a molecule. The positioning allows differentiation of biochemical pathways and allows investigation of metabolic compartmentation.

The main disadvantage of ^{13}C MRS is its intrinsically low sensitivity. Rather than the trace amounts of ^{14}C required, the ^{13}C nucleus must be present in more substantial concentrations. This has cost implications since ^{13}C-labelled substrates are expensive and relatively large quantities are required, particularly for human studies. However, the ^{13}C MRS signal can be enhanced by certain methods including proton decoupling, nuclear Overhauser effect (NOE), and polarization transfer (discussed extensively elsewhere). The wide chemical shift range and narrow line widths of ^{13}C (Table 8.3) signals yield good spectral resolution and this compensates somewhat for its poor sensitivity.

Theoretically, a wide range of metabolites are detectable by ^{13}C MRS, but the detectability depends on a number of factors including metabolite concentrations in the brain, relative rates of pathways bringing labelled and unlabelled carbon into the metabolite pool, and the desired temporal resolution. The same factors limit the range of metabolic fluxes that can be successfully quantified by this method, particularly *in vivo*, when experiment duration is limited. Nonetheless, ^{13}C MRS has been used successfully *in vitro* and *in vivo* to study brain metabolic flux, enzyme activity, and metabolic regulation.

Enhanced sensitivity may be achieved by indirectly detecting ^{13}C-labelled molecules through the protons coupled to the ^{13}C nucleus. This ^{1}H–^{13}C MRS method utilizes the greater sensitivity of ^{1}H MRS. Rothman et al. first demonstrated the effectiveness of this approach to studies of brain metabolism *in vivo*.[45] Since then numerous studies of tissue metabolism have taken advantage of the additional information that spectral editing techniques can provide.

8.3.2.1.2 ^{15}N Magnetic Resonance Spectroscopy

Nitrogen MRS can, in principle, be studied with ^{14}N or ^{15}N. ^{14}N is 99.6% abundant, but the characteristics of the nucleus tend to lead to rapid relaxation and very broad signals. Although ^{15}N has a much lower natural abundance (0.37%; Table 8.3) the signals obtained are much sharper and, consequently, ^{15}N has much greater applicability. In a similar manner to ^{13}C, ^{15}N has a wide chemical shift range (Table 8.3), and when combined with the narrow line width of ^{15}N, it yields high spectral resolution. Its sensitivity is considerably lower even than that of ^{13}C (Table 8.3), however, as for ^{13}C MRS, proton decoupling can substantially increase the sensitivity of the detected signal. The low natural abundance of ^{15}N allows selective observation of ^{15}N-enriched metabolites during infusion of ^{15}N-labelled precursors in a similar manner to the ^{13}C isotope incorporation experiments.

As with the ^{1}H-^{13}C MRS method described above, the sensitivity of ^{15}N detection can be considerably enhanced by indirect detection through coupled protons. The technique is called heteronuclear multiple quantum coherence (HMQC) transfer MRS.[2,46] This technique permits selective detection of protons spin-coupled to ^{15}N, provided the proton is nonlabile under physiological conditions. Consequently, [5-^{15}N]glutamine is detectable by this method, but the amine protons of glutamate and GABA are undetectable at physiological pH owing to their rapid exchange with water. Possibly as a result of the limited number of biologically relevant metabolites that can be studied by this method, the ^{1}H–^{15}N HMQC technique first described *in vivo* by Kanamori et al.[46] has only been used to measure metabolic fluxes *in vivo* in a limited number of cases.

8.3.2.1.3 ^{31}P Magnetic Resonance Spectroscopy

The nucleus used most extensively for metabolic studies is the high natural abundance phosphorus nucleus, ^{31}P, and the earliest studies date back about 25 years. Although ^{31}P MRS is less sensitive than ^{1}H MRS (Table 8.3), and has a narrower chemical shift range than ^{13}C and ^{15}N, the dominant signals are ATP, phosphocreatine, and inorganic phosphate (Pi), all of which are central to cerebral energy metabolism. The importance of the metabolites cannot be doubted. Their vital role in all aspects of cellular function produced evolutionary mechanisms that preserve their concentrations in all but the most pathological states.[47–49] In addition to the very stable steady state concentrations,[50] the creatine kinase exchange flux can also be measured via ^{31}P-magnetization transfer, although this technique is at best an indirect and imprecise indicator of metabolic activity. These applications of ^{31}P MRS are reviewed extensively elsewhere.[1,2]

8.3.2.2 MRS Measurements of Energy Metabolism

Glucose is the primary substrate for brain energy metabolism *in vivo*.[51] Each glucose molecule undergoes nonoxidative (anaerobic) glycolysis to yield two molecules of pyruvate. The pyruvate is oxidized to CO_2 via the tricarboxylic acid (TCA) or Krebs cycle. The oxidative steps of glucose metabolism contribute 36 of a total of 38 high energy ATP molecules generated during metabolism of a single glucose molecule; the remaining two come from the glycolytic pathway. About 15% of the glucose undergoing glycolysis is converted to lactate and does not enter the TCA cycle, although this may be balanced by corresponding uptake and oxidative metabolism of ketone bodies.

Glutamate is the major excitatory neurotransmitter in the mammalian brain and GABA is the primary inhibitory transmitter. In contrast, glutamine is synaptically inert, yet plays a key role in metabolizing both neurotransmitters. The brain pools of glutamate, GABA, and glutamine are localized within glutamatergic neurons, GABA-ergic neurons, and astrocytes, respectively, under nonpathological conditions. It is likely that these cell populations differ in their energetic requirements and metabolic rates. The localization of key enzymes involved in glutamate, GABA, and glutamine metabolism in specific cell types underlies the ability of MRS to study separate neuroenergetic requirements of these cell populations. This section discusses how ^{13}C MRS can measure pathways of energy metabolism in the cerebral cortex.

The general approach adopted to measure metabolic rates by ^{13}C MRS is to intravenously infuse a ^{13}C-labelled substrate (e.g., glucose, acetate) that easily passes through the blood–brain barrier and is metabolized inside the brain. Over time, a variety of metabolite pools in the brain become enriched with ^{13}C, and they can be detected by ^{13}C MRS. Studies in humans[52–55] demonstrated that several key cerebral metabolites coupled to brain energy metabolism including glutamate, glutamine, GABA, aspartate, and NAA can be detected using ^{13}C MRS (see Figure 8.4). The development of metabolic models[54–59] that describe the flux of ^{13}C label through the cerebral metabolite pools as a series of coupled differential equations allowed determination of absolute metabolic rates from the time courses of isotopic labelling in the brain during infusion of ^{13}C-labelled precursors.

The most common isotopic precursor for ^{13}C and ^{1}H-^{13}C MRS studies is [1-^{13}C]glucose. The first MRS measurements of metabolic fluxes in the brain were of TCA cycle and glucose oxidation rates, using ^{1}H-^{13}C MRS to follow the flow of ^{13}C isotope from [1-^{13}C]glucose into glutamate.[60] Figure 8.5(a) illustrates the flow of ^{13}C label from a [1-^{13}C]glucose precursor to [4-^{13}C]glutamate. The [1-^{13}C]glucose is metabolized to pyruvate by the glycolytic pathway that labels pyruvate at C-3. The label is then transferred to the TCA cycle by the sequential actions of pyruvate dehydrogenase (PDH) and citrate synthase. When the label reaches α-ketoglutarate (C-4), it is transferred to the large neuronal glutamate pool by high activity exchange reactions of amino acid transaminases and mitochondrial and cytosolic transporters.

^{13}C Labeling of Amino Acids

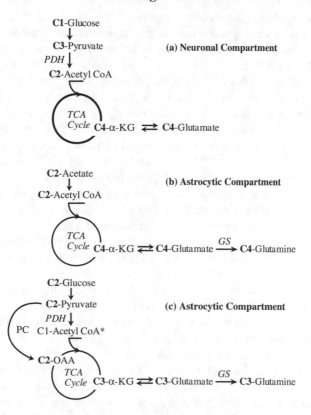

FIGURE 8.5 The flow of ^{13}C label from isotopic precursors into brain amino acids. [1-^{13}C]glucose is metabolized to [3-^{13}C]pyruvate by the glycolytic pathway. Label is subsequently transferred to the TCA cycle by the pyruvate dehydrogenase pathway. The α-ketoglutarate (α-KG) pool is in rapid exchange with the glutamate pool via the amino acid transaminases and mitochondrial/cytosolic transporters. Although these pathways are active in neurons and astrocytes, the flux of label from [1-^{13}C]glucose to [4-^{13}C]glutamate measured by ^{13}C MRS is taken to reflect primarily the neuronal compartment owing to the small size (and hence low sensitivity) of the astrocytic glutamate pool. [2-^{13}C]acetate is metabolized to acetyl CoA and enters the astrocytic TCA cycle. The label passes into the astrocytic glutamate pool and subsequently into glutamine where it is first observed by ^{13}C MRS. Acetate is exclusively used in the brain by astrocytes. This label flux reflects metabolism solely in the astrocytic compartment. [2-^{13}C]glucose metabolized via the astrocytic-specific pathway of pyruvate carboxylase brings label into the C-3 position of α-KG, and subsequently the small astrocytic glutamate pool and glutamine (scrambling of label in the TCA cycle also results in C-2 enrichment of these metabolites). [2-^{13}C]glucose metabolized via the PDH pathway (in neurons and astrocytes) results in labelling of acetyl CoA at C-1, which does not contribute to labelling in the C-3 or C-2 positions of glutamate and glutamine. Thus, as with [2-^{13}C]acetate, label flux into these positions reflects metabolism solely in the astrocytic compartment.

The large glutamate pool was first identified in ^{14}C tracer studies.[61] Based on kinetic and immunohistochemical staining studies, it is believed to correspond to the glutamate pools in glutamatergic neurons.[57,62,63] Thus, the flux of ^{13}C isotope from [1-^{13}C]glucose into glutamate enables quantitative determination of the neuronal TCA cycle rate.[54–57,64] Since glucose is the primary fuel for neuronal oxidation, TCA cycle measurements may be converted to measurements of glucose oxidation using known stoichiometries.[56,57] This measurement of neuronal glucose oxidation is believed to reflect metabolism mainly in glutamatergic neurons, since it is associated with the large glutamate pool localized to this neuronal population.[61]

The rate of neuronal glucose oxidation was determined in several studies from ^{13}C and ^{1}H–^{13}C MRS measurements of cortical glutamate labelling during infusion of [1-^{13}C]glucose in animals[56,58–60,65–70] and humans.[52–55,57,71,72] Comparison of the rates of neuronal glucose oxidation (0.25 to 0.5 mmol/min/g) measured in these studies with conventional arteriovenous difference and PET measurements of total glucose consumption indicates that the majority (60 to 90%) of total glucose oxidation is associated with glutamatergic neurons in rat and human brains. The large percentage of cortical synapses that are glutamatergic and the high electrical activity of glutamatergic pyramidal cells[73,74] may explain why such a large fraction of total glucose oxidation is associated with glutamatergic neurons.

The caveat to the interpretation of the glutamate labelling measurement is that glutamate is present in all brain cells including GABAergic neurons and astrocytes, albeit in lower concentrations than in glutamatergic neurons. It is thought that over 30% of the synapses in the cerebral cortex may be GABAergic.[74–76] Most of the brain GABA pool is localized to GABAergic neurons under normal conditions. GABA is synthesized from glutamate in GABAergic neurons by glutamic acid decarboxylase (GAD). By following the flux of ^{13}C label from [1-^{13}C]glucose into the GABA pool, it is possible to obtain an estimate of oxidative glucose metabolism in GABAergic neurons.[64] The time course of label flux into the GABA pool was determined by *in vitro* MRS analysis of cortical extracts from rats infused with [1-^{13}C]glucose.[77–79] Calculation of the relative rates of glucose oxidation in the glutamate and GABA pools suggests that the rate of glucose oxidation in GABAergic neurons is 10 to 20% of total neuronal glucose oxidation.[78]

A long term controversy of brain metabolism studies has been the rate of glucose oxidation in astrocytes. Early estimates range from 10 to over 50% of total glucose oxidation.[51] MRS may be used to measure the rate of astrocytic glucose oxidation based on the localization of glutamine synthetase to astrocytes.[80] As a result, the rate of the astrocytic TCA cycle may be calculated based on the labelling of glutamine from astrocytic glutamate. However, it is difficult to obtain this metabolic rate with the common [1-^{13}C]glucose precursor since the label enters glutamate in neurons and astrocytes via the PDH reaction. Due to the differences in pool sizes (neuronal glutamate $\approx$ 10 mM; astrocytic glutamate <1 mM), the labelling observed *in vivo* is dominated by the neuronal compartment. The label subsequently entering glutamine is largely derived from the neuronal glutamate pool and reflects pathways other than the astrocytic TCA cycle. A solution is to use alternatively labelled isotopic precursors that yield data specific to astrocytic metabolism.

The use of alternative precursors to [1-^{13}C]glucose in combination with ^{13}C and ^{1}H–^{13}C MRS has been common practice *in vitro* and *ex vivo* for years[81] and provides a unique approach to studying metabolic compartmentation. One isotopic precursor that is used extensively, often in combination with [1-^{13}C]glucose to investigate differences between neuronal and glial metabolism, is [2-^{13}C]acetate. Acetate is used exclusively in the brain by astrocytes, due to a lack of acetate transporters on neurons.[82] With [2-^{13}C]acetate, the ^{13}C label enters the astrocytic TCA cycle via acetyl CoA, passes into the astrocytic glutamate pool, and subsequently into glutamine. See Figure 8.5(b). Comparison of labelling patterns following infusion of [1-^{13}C]glucose and [2-^{13}C]acetate has yielded valuable information about cellular compartmentation and neuronal glial interactions.[83–90] Few measurements of absolute metabolic rates have been reported. In a recent review the ratio of neuronal to total glucose oxidation was estimated at ~70%.[91] This result is similar to the findings of the *in vivo* studies described above.

Despite the long standing use of alternative isotopic precursors *in vitro*, they have been utilized extensively *in vivo* only recently. One study of human cerebral cortex used [2-^{13}C]acetate to determine the rate of astrocytic glucose oxidation (~15% of total glucose oxidation).[92] Similar *in vivo* studies in rats used [2-^{13}C]glucose as the isotopic precursor.[59,93] Although [2-^{13}C]glucose will be metabolized by astrocytes and neurons, it acts as an astrocyte-specific precursor as a consequence of the anaplerotic pyruvate carboxylase pathway, which is localized exclusively to astrocytes in the adult brain. Via this pathway, label from [2-^{13}C]glucose is brought into the C-3 and C-2 positions of the small astrocytic glutamate pool,[43,59,93,94] while label flux through the neuronal and astrocytic PDH pathways does not contribute to labelling in these positions. See Figure 8.5(c). The ^{13}C label is first observed in glutamine (C-3 and C-2), due to the small size (low sensitivity) of the astrocytic glutamate and TCA cycle intermediate pools, and this labelling flux can be used to obtain measurements of astrocytic metabolism.

8.3.2.3 MRS Measurements of Neurotransmitter Fluxes

The metabolism of glutamatergic neurons, GABAergic neurons, and astrocytes is coupled by neurotransmitter cycles. The cycles are intended to enable rapid removal of neurotransmitters from the synaptic cleft while preventing depletion of the nerve terminal glutamate and GABA pools by synaptic release. Glutamate released from nerve terminals is taken up by surrounding astrocytes.[95–97] Glutamate is converted to glutamine within the astrocytes and subsequently released, taken up by the neurons, and converted back to glutamate, thereby completing the cycle. See Figure 8.6(a).

GABA released into the synaptic cleft is thought to participate in a neuronal–astrocytic cycle. GABA released synaptically and taken up by astrocytes is converted, via the sequential actions of the GABA transaminase and succinic semialdehyde dehydrogenase to the TCA cycle intermediate succinate. Subsequently, the molecule passes through the TCA cycle to glutamate, and is converted to glutamine. The glutamine is released from the astrocyte and taken up again by the GABAergic neuron for conversion to glutamate and subsequent GABA resynthesis.

The glutamate/glutamine cycle

(a)

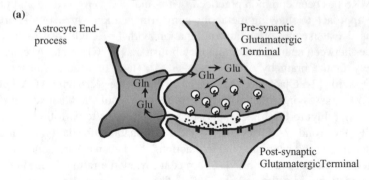

(b)

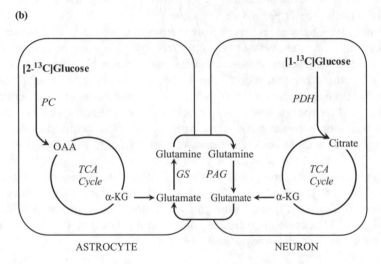

FIGURE 8.6 (a): The glutamate–glutamine cycle. Glutamate released from nerve terminals is taken up by surrounding astrocytes and converted to glutamine by glutamine synthetase. The glutamine is subsequently released for uptake by neurons and glutamate resynthesis via the phosphate-activated glutaminase pathway. (b): The principle of using different isotopic precursors to validate the glutamate–glutamine cycle. The use of [1-^{13}C]glucose as the isotopic precursor leads to labelling of MRS-visible metabolites by predominantly neuronal pathways, such that the label is first observed in neuronal glutamate. If glutamate–glutamine cycling exists, the label will appear in the astrocytic glutamine pool. In contrast, [2-^{13}C]glucose can be utilized as an astrocyte-specific precursor. Due to the small size of the astrocytic glutamate pool, the isotopic label is first observed in glutamine. If glutamate–glutamine cycling is significant, the label would be expected to appear subsequently in neuronal glutamate.

A wealth of *in vitro* evidence confirms the existence of such cycles, particularly the glutamate–glutamine cycle. The evidence came from enzyme localization studies, isotope labelling studies in cells and brain slices, and immunohistochemical studies of the cellular distribution of glutamate and glutamine.[98] Before the development of *in vivo* ^{13}C MRS techniques, no available methodology allowed these cycles to be demonstrated *in vivo*. *In vitro* measurements of the glutamate–glutamine cycle were unable to determine the magnitude of the pathway. The next section discusses how MRS can be used to measure neurotransmitter cycle fluxes *in vivo*.

The ^{13}C label from [1-^{13}C]glucose rapidly labels the large neuronal pool of glutamate. The subsequent release of glutamate and uptake and conversion to glutamine in astrocytes should permit the label to enter the astrocytic glutamine via glutamine synthetase. Early ^{13}C MRS studies of human occipital and parietal cortex showed clearly that glutamine is labelled rapidly from [1-^{13}C]glucose in human cerebral cortex[52,57] (Figure 8.7). It was suggested that ^{13}C MRS labelling time courses of glutamate and glutamine could be used to calculate the rate of the glutamate–glutamine cycle. However, this measurement is dependent on the absence of other significant fluxes through the glutamine synthetase pathways in astrocytes that may contribute to the labelling observed in glutamine. Glutamine synthesis may act as a detoxification pathway for blood-borne ammonia entering the brain.[99] In order to validate the measurements of cycling via this method, it was important to determine the contribution of ammonia detoxification to the total rate of glutamine synthesis. ^{13}C MRS studies of different levels of plasma ammonia in rats showed that the contribution is <10% under normal physiological conditions.[58,100]

One approach to validating MRS measurements of the glutamate–glutamine cycle is measuring the rate of cycling under conditions that alter neuronal glutamate neurotransmitter release. Neuronal glutamate release increases with increased action potential propagation and neuronal depolarization. If the rate of cycling measured by ^{13}C MRS truly reflects synaptic glutamate release, the calculated rate of this pathway should correlate with brain electrical activity. To test this, ^{13}C MRS was used to measure the rates of neuronal glucose oxidation and the glutamate–glutamine cycle in rat cerebral cortices at three levels of electrocortical activity: isoelectric EEG induced by high dose pentobarbital anaesthesia and two milder levels of anesthesia.[70] Under isoelectric conditions at which minimal glutamate release takes place, almost no glutamine synthesis was measured (0.04 mmol/min/g). Above isoelectricity, the cycling rate increased with higher electrical activity. These findings indicate that ^{13}C MRS measurement of glutamine synthesis primarily reflects the glutamate–glutamine cycle and neuronal synaptic activity.

The rate of the glutamate–glutamine cycle found was of a similar order of magnitude (0.2 to 0.4 mmol/min/g) to the rate of oxidative glucose consumption measured by ^{13}C MRS, as described. Thus, this work also demonstrates that the glutamate–glutamine cycle is a major metabolic pathway in the mammalian cortex and highlights the importance of astrocytes in maintaining synaptic glutamate homeostasis. ^{13}C MRS has also been used to measure the rate of cycling in the human occipital and parietal cortex.[53-55] Those studies yielded similar rates (0.26 to 0.32 mmol/min/g) to the rat cortices.

Subsequent studies using isotopically labelled precursors that enter the metabolic pathways of the brain specifically via different cell types verified the above findings. In contrast to the [1-^{13}C]glucose studies in which the label first enters the MRS-visible metabolites by neuronal pathways, [2-^{13}C]glucose can be utilized as an astrocyte-specific precursor, as discussed above. Since the TCA cycle intermediate pools in astrocytes are very small, the isotopic label is first observed in glutamine. If the cycling of labelled glutamine from the astrocyte to the neuron is significant (as

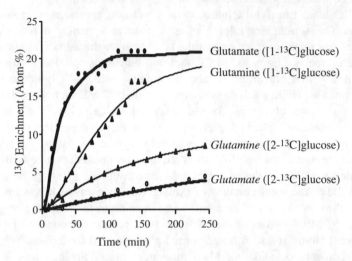

^{13}C enrichment of glutamate and glutamine

FIGURE 8.7 Glutamate and glutamine ^{13}C enrichment during infusion of different isotopic precursors, acquired under hyperammonemic conditions. The graph demonstrates reversal of the product–precursor relationship between glutamate and glutamine labelling. ^{13}C enrichment data acquired from rat cortex during infusion of [1-^{13}C]glucose, together with fits obtained via metabolic modelling. Label first appears in [4-^{13}C]glutamate (●) and subsequently in [4-^{13}C]glutamine (▲). ^{13}C enrichment data acquired from rat cortex during infusion of [2-^{13}C]glucose, together with fits obtained via metabolic modelling. Label first appears in [3-^{13}C]glutamine (△) and, subsequently, in [3-^{13}C]glutamate (○).

predicted by the glutamate–glutamine cycle), label would be expected to appear subsequently in neuronal glutamate (Figure 8.6(b)). Labelling of neuronal glutamate has been demonstrated using [2-^{13}C]glucose in rat brain.[59]

Spectra acquired during [1-^{13}C]- and [2-^{13}C]glucose infusions, respectively, demonstrate more rapid labelling of glutamate than glutamine in the [1-^{13}C]glucose experiment; in the [2-^{13}C]glucose experiment, glutamine labelling precedes that of glutamate. This reversal of the precursor–product relationship can be seen clearly in the isotopic labelling curves from the two experiments shown in Figure 8.7. The absolute rates of cycling measured using the different isotopic precursors are in close agreement. Preliminary experiments in humans and rats infused with [2-^{13}C]acetate yielded results that are consistent with the [1-^{13}C]- and [2-^{13}C]glucose studies.

^{15}N MRS can be used to measure glutamine synthesis through label incorporation from ^{15}N-labelled ammonia into the amide position of cerebral glutamine.[101–104] The rates of glutamine synthesis obtained in these studies varied somewhat. This can be explained largely by the fact that different metabolic models were used to fit the data. If the same metabolic model is used to fit the ^{13}C MRS data described above and ^{15}N MRS data obtained under similar experimental conditions, the rates of glutamate–glutamine cycling obtained from MRS studies agree closely.[104] This is a test of the metabolic model used to analyze data obtained in these metabolic MRS studies. It is unlikely that a model will accurately fit data obtained from several independent experimental approaches if it does not reasonably reflect the metabolic situation. In fact, the same metabolic model has been shown to fit data obtained using ^{13}C MRS and multiple ^{13}C-labelled isotopic precursors ([1-^{13}C]glucose, [2-^{13}C]glucose, and [2-^{13}C]acetate) and data obtained from ^{15}N MRS studies.[64]

In addition to measurements of glutamine synthesis, ^{15}N MRS can be used to estimate flux through two other enzymatic pathways that are closely related to the glutamate–glutamine cycle: glutamate dehydrogenase (GDH) and phosphate-activated deaminase (PAG). GDH catalyzes the reversible formation of glutamate from α-ketoglutarate and ammonia. By following the flux of label from ^{15}N-labelled ammonia into the amine position of cerebral glutamate–glutamine, the rate of GDH reaction in the direction of reductive amination can be determined.[105] PAG, a predominantly neuronal enzyme, catalyzes the hydrolysis of glutamine to glutamate, and forms the opposite leg of the glutamate–glutamine cycle to the glutamine synthetase pathway (see Figure 8.6). The rate of this pathway may be determined by first prelabelling the brain glutamine pool with ^{15}N through infusion of ^{15}N-labelled ammonia as discussed above. If further glutamine synthesis is inhibited with methionine sulfoximine, the subsequent decrease in the [5-^{15}N]glutamine signal yields an estimate of PAG activity.[106]

A preliminary study demonstrated the ability to use isotopic labelling strategies, similar to those developed to measure the glutamate–glutamine cycle, to measure the rate of the GABA–glutamate cycle. This strategy in combination with the manipulation of GABA levels pharmacologically or through transgenic methods may provide significant insight into the way regulation of GABA concentration affects GABAergic function. The rate of GABA synthesis in GABAergic neurons was determined from the ^{13}C labelling kinetics of GABA, glutamate, and glutamine in two recent *ex vivo* ^{13}C MRS studies.[107,108]

8.3.2.4 Energetic Requirements of Neurotransmission

Neuronal activity requires energy that is provided almost exclusively by glucose oxidation.[51] Since the brain has virtually no energy reserves, a continuous vascular supply of glucose and oxygen is mandatory to sustain neuronal activity. This supply is regulated locally and dynamically to meet the increased energetic demands of functional activation. Functional imaging utilizes this association between increased neuronal activity and energetic demand by measuring changes in blood flow, glucose utilization, or oxygen metabolism and delivery.[109] The implicit assumption of functional imaging methodologies is that changes in one or more of these parameters accurately reflect changes in neuronal activity. Despite the increasing use of these imaging tools in basic and clinical applications, the neurobiological processes responsible for the imaging signals measured are still unknown. Recent advances suggest that glutamate release may trigger vascular and metabolic responses via different signalling processes. Thus, glutamate may serve as a key coordinator of all the physiological responses that underlie the signal changes observed in brain imaging.

^{13}C MRS provides a means by which the relationship of glutamatergic neurotransmission and energy metabolism can be tested *in vivo*. This was achieved in the rat

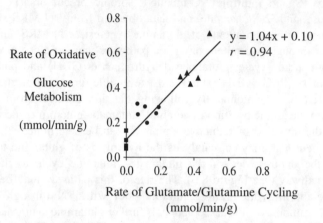

FIGURE 8.8 The stoichiometric relationship between oxidative glucose consumption and glutamate–glutamine cycling. ^{13}C MRS data acquired at different levels of neuronal activity (achieved with graded anesthesia) yielded rates of oxidative glucose consumption and glutamate–glutamine cycling. The equation of the regression line shown is y = 1.04x + 0.10, with a Pearson product-moment correlation coefficient (r) of 0.94. The units of the x and y axes are the same. Hence these two metabolic rates increase with a 1:1 molar stoichiometry above a basal level. The basal level of energy metabolism was measured at isoelectric EEG (i.e., no cycling/neurotransmission) and reflects energetic requirements of the brain that are unrelated to neuronal activity.

brain by using ^{13}C MRS to simultaneously measure the rates of glutamate–glutamine cycling and neuronal glucose oxidation in the cerebral cortex at different levels of neuronal activity.[70] Electrocortical activity was varied by using differing levels of anaesthesia. When plotted as a graph of oxidative glucose consumption against glutamate–glutamine cycling rate, a linear relationship was obtained (Figure 8.8). The relationship between oxidative glucose metabolism and glutamate–glutamine cycling demonstrates two important points: (1) a molar (1:1) stoichiometry between these two rates above a basal level of energy metabolism (isoelectric EEG), and (2) the basal level of glucose consumption unrelated to synaptic activity is only 15 to 20% of resting levels. The first point implies that the energy requirements of pre- and postsynaptic events related to neuronal firing and synaptic transmission may be met by the oxidative metabolism of one mole of glucose for every mole of glutamate released synaptically. These studies were unable to assign fractions of energy utilization to each individual process (action potential propagation, restoration and maintenance of membrane potentials, vesicle recycling, and glutamate cycling), although recent theoretical calculations have begun to address this issue.[49] This clear stoichiometric relationship is also supportive of the concept that glutamate release may be a means by which energy metabolism can be regulated in line with neuronal activity.

The second finding of a low basal metabolic rate measured under isoelectric conditions is in close agreement with recent theoretical calculations of the energetic expenditures of the brain.[49] It represents a departure from the conventional view that most energy consumption in the brain subserves "housekeeping" functions instead of those involved in neuronal activity and synaptic transmission. Importantly, measurements of these metabolic rates in human brains[54,55] are consistent with those obtained from rat brain, and are in accord with the linear relationship described. To date, no study of the human brain under different levels of neuronal activity has been performed, so it is not possible to confirm that a similar linear relationship between neurotransmission and energy metabolism exists in humans.

The implications of these ^{13}C MRS studies for the interpretation of functional imaging signal changes can be most readily understood by converting the measured rates of glucose oxidation to fractions of total glucose consumption in the brain. We find that glucose oxidation by glutamatergic neurons comprises 75 to 80% of the total energy consumption of the brain, while the astrocytic and GABAergic neuron consumptions are estimated to be 10 to 15% and 10%, respectively. The energy requirements of glutamatergic neurons potentially explain a large part of the glucose consumption of the resting awake human brain. These findings may provide a mechanism for converting energy changes measured in human brain activation studies into a specific neuronal process, in this case excitatory glutamate release.

8.4 FUTURE DIRECTIONS

Applying MRS to the study of neurotransmitter and energy metabolism in the brain provided several new insights into the relationship of metabolism and function. Contrary to the previous view of separate metabolic and neurotransmitter pools of glutamate, glutamate release and recycling were shown to represent major metabolic pathways. One important consequence is that steady state measurements of neurotransmitter levels may reflect alterations in regional brain activity through feedback between neurotransmitter release and resynthesis. MRS studies of GABA metabolism in rodent and human brains suggest an important role of the metabolic pool of GABA in inhibitory function.[36,110,111] The 1:1 coupling of neurotransmission and neuroenergetics (above isoelectricity) links functional imaging and specific neuronal processes.

The further development of new labelling strategies such as [2-^{13}C]acetate and higher sensitivity MRS measurements should allow more accurate determination of the metabolic contributions of different cell populations (including those not involved in glutamate–GABA metabolism, e.g., dopaminergic and serotinergic activities). The higher sensitivity available using inverse MRS methods and the development of ultra-high field magnets for human studies should make measurements of the rate of glucose oxidation in GABAergic neurons possible.

One issue still to be addressed is the comparison of the ^{13}C MRS measurements with direct measurements of neuronal glutamate release and electrical activity. Correlation of the MRS glutamate–glutamine cycle with indirect measures of neuronal glutamate release such as microdialysis and nerve terminal labelling would be a first step toward direct measurement of bulk glutamate release. The recording of local field potentials during fMRI activation studies has been reported.[112] Similar experiments combining measurements of neuronal signalling with ^{13}C MRS measurements of glutamate–glutamine cycling are future goals. In addition, the stoichiometry between neuronal glucose oxidation and the glutamate–glutamine cycle remains to be measured under conditions of sensory stimulation in different brain regions (e.g., subcortical) and in the human brain over a range of neuronal activation levels.

Undoubtedly, with continuing development and refinement, the MRS techniques described in this section will provide ever more powerful methods of investigating neurochemistry *in vivo*. While the possibility is challenging, it is not inconceivable that these techniques, particularly ^{13}C MRS, will ultimately be available in clinical settings. A number of studies used ^{13}C MRS to demonstrate abnormalities in *ex vivo* extracts from animal models of brain injury or disease, including hyperammonemia,[113,114] focal cerebral ischemia,[115,116] cerebral glioma,[117] epilepsy,[118] and hypoxia.[119]

Several studies demonstrated the application of ^{13}C and ^{15}N MRS to investigations of hyperammonemic rat brains *in vivo*.[58,59,101–106] Although ^{13}C MRS finds greater utility in studying the human brain, the clinical feasibility and diagnostic potential of these measurements remain to be proven. Nonetheless, ^{13}C MRS has been performed on a routine 1.5 T clinical scanner in a hospital environment, and preliminary data demonstrating abnormalities in glucose, glutamate, and glutamine metabolism from a range of neurological disorders have been reported.[120,121] Allthough no attempts were made to derive metabolic flux rates in these preliminary studies, the data obtained and differences observed between patients and controls were highly encouraging. We have little doubt that quantitative metabolic measurements by the MRS techniques described in this chapter will ultimately be used to diagnose and monitor metabolic abnormalities and alterations in neurotransmission in human brain disorders. Such studies may provide significant contributions to our understanding of human neuropathophysiology.

REFERENCES

1. Gadian, D.G., *Nuclear Magnetic Resonance and its Application to Living Systems*, 2nd ed., Oxford University Press, London, 1995.
2. de Graaf, R.A., *In Vivo NMR Spectroscopy*, John Wiley & Sons, Chichester, 1998.
3. Haase, A. et al., ^{1}H NMR chemical shift selective (CHESS) imaging, *Phys. Med. Biol.*, 30, 341, 1985.
4. van Zijl, P.C.M. and Moonen, C.T.W., Highly effective water suppression schemes for *in vivo* localized spectroscopy (DRYSTEAM), *J. Mag. Res.*, 88, 28, 1990.
5. Williams, S.R., Cerebral amino acids studied by nuclear magnetic resonance spectroscopy *in vivo*, *Prog. Nucl. Mag. Res.Spectroscopy*, 34, 301, 1999.
6. Provencher, S.W., Estimation of metabolite concentrations from localized *in vivo* proton NMR spectra, *Magn. Res.Med.*, 30, 672, 1993.
7. van Ormondt, D., Advanced signal processing for medical magnetic resonance imaging and spectroscopy, http://carbon.uab.es/mrui/.
8. Holmes, E. et al., Development of a model for classification of toxin-induced lesions using ^{1}H NMR spectroscopy of urine combined with pattern recognition, *NMR Biomed.*, 11, 235, 1998.

9. Beckwith-Hall, B.M. et al., Nuclear magnetic resonance spectroscopic and principal components analysis investigations into biochemical effects of three model hepato-toxins, *Chem. Res. Toxicol.*, 11, 260, 1998.

10. Tate, A.R. et al., Toward a method for automated classification of ^{1}H MRS spectra from brain tumours, *NMR Biomed.*, 11, 177, 1998.

11. Koller, K.J., Zaczek, R., and Coyle, J.T., N-acetyl-aspartyl-glutamate: regional levels in rat brain and the effects of brain lesions as determined by a new HPLC method, *J. Neurochem.*, 43, 1136, 1984.

12. Urenjak, J. et al., Specific expression of N-acetylaspartate in neurons, oligodendrocyte type-2 astrocytes and immature oligodendrocytes *in vitro*, *J. Neurochem.*, 59, 55, 1992.

13. Ebisu, T. et al., N-acetylaspartate as an *in vivo* marker of neuronal viability in kainate-induced status epilepticus: [1]H magnetic resonance spectroscopic imaging, *J. Cereb. Blood Flow Metabol.*, 14, 373, 1994.

14. Bhakoo, K.K. and Pearce, D., *In vitro* expression of N-acetyl aspartate by oligo-dendrocytes: implications for proton magnetic resonance spectroscopy signal *in vivo*, *J. Neurochem.*, 74, 254, 2000.

15. Howe, F.A. et al., Proton spectroscopy *in vivo*, *Mag.Res.Q.*, 9, 31, 1993.

16. Matthews, P.M. et al., Proton magnetic resonance spectroscopy for metabolic char-acterization of plaques in multiple sclerosis, *Neurology*, 41, 1251, 1991.

17. Davie, C.A. et al., Serial proton magnetic resonance spectroscopy in acute multiple sclerosis lesions, *Brain*, 117, 49, 1994.

18. Gillard, J.H. et al., Proton MR spectroscopy in acute middle cerebral artery stroke, *Am. J. Neuroradiol.*, 17, 873, 1996.

19. Saunders, D.E. et al., Continuing ischemic damage after acute middle cerebral artery infarction in humans demonstrated by short-echo proton spectroscopy, *Stroke*, 26, 1007, 1995.

20. Cross, J. H. et al., Proton magnetic resonance spectroscopy in children with temporal lobe epilepsy, *Ann. Neurol.*, 39, 107, 1996.

21. Kegeles, L.S. et al., Hippocampal pathology in schizophrenia: magnetic resonance imaging and spectroscopy studies, *Psychiatr. Res.*, 98, 163, 2000.

22. De Stefano, N., Matthews, P.M., and Arnold, D.L., Reversible decreases in N-acety-laspartate after acute brain injury, *Mag.Res.Med.*, 34, 721, 1995.

23. Bates, T.E. et al., Inhibition of N-acetylaspartate production: implications for ^{1}H MRS studies *in vivo*, *Neuroreport*, 7, 1397, 1996.

24. Crockard, H.A. et al., Acute cerebral ischemia: concurrent changes in cerebral blood flow, energy metabolites, pH, and lactate measured with hydrogen clearance and ^{31}P and ^{1}H NMR spectroscopy. I. Changes during ischemia, *J. Cereb. Blood Flow Metabol.*, 7, 394, 1987.

25. Lorek, A. et al., Secondary energy failure after acute cerebral hypoxia–ischemia in newborn pigs, *Pediatr. Res.*, 35, 274, 1994.

26. Reynolds, E.O. et al., New noninvasive methods for assessing brain oxygenation and haemodynamics, *Br. Med. Bull.*, 44, 1052, 1988.

27. Florian, C.L. et al., Characteristic metabolic profiles revealed by ^{1}H NMR spectros-copy for three types of human brain and nervous system tumours, *NMR Biomed.*, 8, 253, 1995.

28. Tkac, I. et al., *In vivo* ^{1}H NMR spectroscopy of rat brain at 1 ms echo time, *Mag. Res. Med.*, 41, 649, 1999.

29. Usenius, J.P. et al., Choline-containing compounds in human astrocytomas studied by ^{1}H NMR spectroscopy *in vivo* and *in vitro*, *J. Neurochem.*, 63, 1538, 1994.

30. Bhakoo, K.K. et al., Immortalization and transformation are associated with specific alterations in choline metabolism, *Cancer Res.*, 56, 4630, 1996.

31. Wardlaw, J.M. et al., Studies of acute ischemic stroke with proton magnetic resonance spectroscopy: relation between time from onset, neurological deficit, metabolite abnormalities in the infarct, blood flow, and clinical outcome, *Stroke*, 29, 1618, 1998.

32. Negendank, W., Studies of human tumors by MRS: a review, *NMR Biomed.*, 5, 303, 1992.

33. Preul, M.C. et al., Accurate, noninvasive diagnosis of human brain tumors by using proton magnetic resonance spectroscopy, *Nature Med.*, 2, 323, 1996.

34. Frahm, J. and Hanefeld, F., Localized proton magnetic spectroscopy of cerebral metabolites, *Neuropediatrics*, 27, 64, 1996.

35. Kreis, R. et al., Metabolic disorders of the brain in chronic hepatic encephalopathy detected with H-1 MR spectroscopy, *Radiology*, 182, 19, 1992.

36. Preece, N.E. et al., Nuclear magnetic resonance detection of increased cortical GABA in the vigabatrin- treated rat *in vivo*, *Epilepsia*, 35, 431, 1994.

37. Behar, K.L. and Boehm, D., NMR measurement of GABA *in vivo* following gabac-uline administration, *J. Cereb. Blood Flow Metabol.*, 11, 783, 1991.

38. Petroff, O.A.C. et al., Low brain GABA levels are associated with poor seizure control in patients with complex partial epilepsy, *Proc. Annl. Mtg. Intl. Soc. Mag. Res. Med.*, 131, 1996.

39. Florian, C.L. et al., Cell-type specific fingerprinting of meningioma and meningeal cells by ^{1}H NMR spectroscopy, *Cancer Res.*, 55, 420, 1995.

40. Gill, S.S. et al., Proton NMR spectroscopy of intracranial tumours: *in vivo* and *in vitro* studies, *J. Comput. Assist. Tomogr.*, 14, 497, 1990.

41. Gyngell, M.L. et al., Cerebral glucose is detectable by localized ^{1}H NMR spectroscopy in normal rat brain *in vivo*, *Mag. Res. Med.*, 19, 489, 1991.

42. Michaelis, T. et al., Identification of scyllo-inositol in proton NMR spectra of human brain *in vivo*, *NMR Biomed.*, 6, 105, 1993.

43. Brand, A., Richter-Landsberg, C., and Leibfritz, D., Multinuclear NMR studies on the energy metabolism of glial and neuronal cells, *Dev. Neurosci.*, 15, 289, 1993.

44. Videen, J.S. et al., Human cerebral osmolytes during chronic hyponatremia: a proton magnetic resonance spectroscopy study, *J. Clin. Invest.*, 95, 788, 1995.

45. Rothman, D.L. et al., [1]H-observe/^{13}C-decouple spectroscopic measurements of lactate and glutamate in the rat brain *in vivo*, *Proc. Natl. Acad .Sci. U.S.A.*, 82, 1633, 1985.

46. Kanamori, K., Ross, B.D., and Tropp, J., Selective, *in vivo* observation of [5-15N]glutamine amide protons in rat brain by 1H–15N heteronuclear multiple quantum-coherence transfer NMR, *J. Mag. Res.*, 107, 107, 1995.

47. Williams, S.R., Energy supply for the maintenance of brain function, in *Neurosurgery: The Scientific Basis of Clinical Practice*, 3rd ed., Crockard, H.A. et al., Eds., Blackwell Scientific, Oxford, 2000, p. 99.

48. Erecinska, M. and Silver, I.A., ATP and brain function, *J. Cereb. Blood Flow Metabol.* 9, 166, 1989.

49. Attwell, D. and Laughlin, S.B., An energy budget for signaling in the grey matter of the brain, *J. Cereb. Blood Flow Metabol.*, 21, 1133, 2001.

50. Balaban, R.S., Regulation of oxidative phosphorylation in the mammalian cell, *Am. J. Physiol.*, 258, C377, 1990.

51. Siesjo, B., *Brain Energy Metabolism*, John Wiley & Sons, New York, 1978.

52. Gruetter, R. et al., Localized 13C NMR spectroscopy in the human brain of amino acid labelling from d-[1-13C]glucose, *J. Neurochem.*, 63, 1377, 1994.

53. Gruetter, R. et al., Localized *in vivo* ^{13}C NMR of glutamate metabolism in the human brain: initial results at 4 T, *Dev. Neurosci.*, 20, 380, 1998.
54. Gruetter, R., Seaquist, E.R., and Ugurbil, K., A mathematical model of compartmentalized neurotransmitter metabolism in the human brain, *Am. J. Physiol. Endocrinol. Metabol.*, 281, E100, 2001.
55. Shen, J. et al., Determination of the rate of the glutamate/glutamine cycle in the human brain by *in vivo* ^{13}C NMR, *Proc. Natl. Acad. Sci. U.S.A.,* 96, 8235, 1999.
56. Mason, G.F. et al., NMR determination of the TCA cycle rate and α-ketoglutarate/glutamate exchange rate in rat brain, *J. Cereb. Blood Flow Metabol.*, 12, 434, 1992.
57. Mason, G.F. et al., Simultaneous determination of the rates of the TCA cycle, glucose utilization, α-ketoglutarate/glutamate exchange, and glutamine synthesis in human brain by NMR, *J. Cereb. Blood Flow Metabol.*, 15, 12, 1995.
58. Sibson, N.R. et al., *In vivo* ^{13}C NMR measurements of cerebral glutamine synthesis as evidence for glutamate–glutamine cycling, *Proc. Natl. Acad. Sci. U.S.A.*, 94, 2699, 1997.
59. Sibson, N.R. et al., *In vivo* ^{13}C NMR measurement of neurotransmitter glutamate cycling, anaplerosis and TCA cycle flux in rat brain during [2-^{13}C]glucose infusion, *J. Neurochem.*, 76, 975, 2001.
60. Fitzpatrick, S.M. et al., The flux from glucose to glutamate in the rat brain *in vivo* as determined by ^{1}H-observed, ^{13}C-edited NMR spectroscopy, *J. Cereb. Blood Flow Metabol.*, 10, 170, 1990.
61. van den Berg, C.J. and Garfinkel, D., A simulation study of brain compartments: metabolism of glutamate and related substances in mouse brain, *Biochem. J.*, 123, 211, 1971.
62. Ottersen, O.P. et al., Metabolic compartmentation of glutamate and glutamine: morphological evidence obtained by quantitative immunocytochemistry in rat cerebellum, *Neuroscience*, 46, 519, 1992.
63. Conti, F. and Minelli, A., Glutamate immunoreactivity in rat cerebral cortex is reversibly abolished by 6-diazo-5-oxo-l-norleucine (don), an inhibitor of phosphate-activated glutaminase, *J. Histochem. Cytochem.*, 42, 717, 1994.
64. Rothman, D.L. et al., *In vivo* nuclear magnetic resonance spectroscopy studies of the relationship between the glutamate–glutamine neurotransmitter cycle and functional neuroenergetics, *Philos. Trans. R. Soc. Lond. B. Biol. Sci.*, 354, 1165, 1999.
65. van Zijl, P.C. et al., *In vivo* proton spectroscopy and spectroscopic imaging of [1-^{13}C]-glucose and its metabolic products, *Mag. Res. Med.*, 30, 544, 1993.
66. van Zijl, P.C. et al., Determination of cerebral glucose transport and metabolic kinetics by dynamic MR spectroscopy, *Am. J. Physiol.*, 273, E1216, 1997.
67. Hyder, F. et al., Increased tricarboxylic acid cycle flux in rat brain during forepaw stimulation detected with ^{1}H[^{13}C]NMR, *Proc. Natl. Acad. Sci. U.S.A.*, 93, 7612, 1996.
68. Hyder, F. et al., Oxidative glucose metabolism in rat brain during single forepaw stimulation: a spatially localized ^{1}H[^{13}C] nuclear magnetic resonance study, *J. Cereb. Blood Flow Metabol.*, 17, 1040, 1997.
69. Hyder, F. et al., *In vivo* carbon-edited detection with proton echo-planar spectroscopic imaging (ICED PEPSI): [3,4-$^{(13)}$CH(2)]glutamate/glutamine tomography in rat brain, *Mag. Res. Med.*, 42, 997, 1999.
70. Sibson, N.R. et al., Stoichiometric coupling of brain glucose metabolism and glutamatergic neuronal activity, *Proc. Natl. Acad. Sci. U.S.A.*, 95, 316, 1998.

71. Mason, G.F. et al., Measurement of the tricarboxylic acid cycle rate in human grey and white matter *in vivo* by ^{1}H-[^{13}C] magnetic resonance spectroscopy at 4.1 T, *J. Cereb. Blood Flow Metabol.*, 19, 1179, 1999.

72. Pan, J.W. et al., Spectroscopic imaging of glutamate C4 turnover in human brain, *Mag.Res.Med.*, 44, 673, 2000.

73. Nowak, L.G., Sanchez-Vives, M.V., and McCormick, D.A., Influence of low and high frequency inputs on spike timing in visual cortical neurons, *Cereb. Cortex*, 7, 487, 1997.

74. Shephard, G.M., *The Synaptic Organization of the Brain*, Oxford University Press, Oxford, 1994.

75. Roberts, E., Failure of GABAergic inhibition: a key to local and global seizures, *Adv. Neurol.*, 44, 319, 1986.

76. Roberts, E., The establishment of GABA as a neurotransmitter, in *GABA and Benzodiazepine Receptors*, Squires, R., Ed., CRC Press, Boca Raton, FL, 1988.

77. Shank, R.P., Leo, G.C., and Zielke, H.R., Cerebral metabolic compartmentation as revealed by nuclear magnetic resonance analysis of d-[1-^{13}C] glucose metabolism, *J. Neurochem.*, 61, 315, 1993.

78. Manor, D. et al., The rate of turnover of cortical GABA from [1-^{13}C]glucose is reduced in rats treated with the GABA–transaminase inhibitor vigabatrin (γ-vinyl GABA), *Neurochem. Res.*, 21, 1031, 1996.

79. Brainard, J.R., Kyner, E., and Rosenberg, G.A., ^{13}C nuclear magnetic resonance evidence for γ-aminobutyric acid formation via pyruvate carboxylase in rat brain: a metabolic basis for compartmentation, *J. Neurochem.*, 53, 1285, 1989.

80. Martinez-Hernandez, A., Bell, K.P., and Norenberg, M.D., Glutamine synthetase: glial localization in brain, *Science*, 195, 1356, 1977.

81. Bachelard, H., Landmarks in the application of ^{13}C magnetic resonance spectroscopy to studies of neuronal/glial relationships, *Dev. Neurosci.*, 20, 277, 1998.

82. Waniewski, R.A. and Martin, D.L., Preferential utilization of acetate by astrocytes is attributable to transport, *J. Neurosci.*, 18, 5225, 1998.

83. Bachelard, H. et al., High-field MRS studies in brain slices, *Mag. Res. Imaging*, 13, 1223, 1995.

84. Badar-Goffer, R.S. et al., Neuronal–glial metabolism under depolarizing conditions: a ^{13}C NMR study, *Biochem. J.*, 282, 225, 1992.

85. Brand, A., Richter-Landsberg, C., and Leibfritz, D., Metabolism of acetate in rat brain neurons, astrocytes and cocultures: metabolic interactions between neurons and glia cells monitored by NMR spectroscopy, *Cell. Mol. Biol.*, 43, 645, 1997.

86. Cerdan, S., Kunnecke, B., and Seelig, J., Cerebral metabolism of [1,2-^{13}C2]acetate as detected by *in vivo* and *in vitro* ^{13}C NMR, *J. Biol. Chem.*, 265, 12916, 1990.

87. Hassel, B. and Sonnewald, U., Glial formation of pyruvate and lactate from TCA cycle intermediates: implications for the inactivation of transmitter amino acids? *J. Neurochem.*, 65, 2227, 1995.

88. Hassel, B., Sonnewald, U., and Fonnum, F., Glial–neuronal interactions as studied by cerebral metabolism of [2-^{13}C] acetate and [1-^{13}C]glucose: an *ex vivo* ^{13}C NMR spectroscopy study, *J. Neurol.*, 64, 2773, 1995.

89. Haberg, A. et al., *In vivo* injection of [1-^{13}C]glucose and [1,2-^{13}C]acetate combined with *ex vivo* ^{13}C nuclear magnetic resonance spectroscopy: a novel approach to the study of middle cerebral artery occlusion in the rat, *J. Cereb. Blood Flow Metabol.*, 18, 1223, 1998.

90. Sonnewald, U. et al., NMR spectroscopic studies of ^{13}C acetate and ^{13}C glucose metabolism in neocortical astrocytes: evidence for mitochondrial heterogeneity, *Dev. Neurosci.*, 15, 351, 1993.

91. Cruz, F. and Cerdan, S., Quantitative ^{13}C NMR studies of metabolic compartmentation in the adult mammalian brain, *NMR Biomed.*, 12, 451, 1999.

92. Lebon, V. et al., Measurement of astrocytic TCA cycle flux in humans using ^{13}C labelled acetate., *Proc. Int. Soc. Mag.Res. Med.*, 1, 1053, 2001.

93. Kanamatsu, T. and Tsukada, Y., Effects of ammonia on the anaplerotic pathway and amino acid metabolism in the brain: an *ex vivo* ^{13}C NMR spectroscopic study of rats after administering [2-^{13}C]glucose with or without ammonium acetate, *Brain Res.*, 841, 1999.

94. Taylor, A. et al., Approaches to studies on neuronal/glial relationships by ^{13}C MRS analysis, *Dev. Neurol.*, 18, 434, 1996.

95. Bergles, D.E., Diamond, J.S., and Jahr, C.E., Clearance of glutamate inside the synapse and beyond, *Curr. Opin. Neurobiol.*, 9, 293, 1999.

96. Bergles, D.E. and Jahr, C.E., Glial contribution to glutamate uptake at Schaffer collateral commissural synapses in the hippocampus, *J. Neurosci.*, 18, 7709, 1998.

97. Rothstein, J.D. et al., Knockout of glutamate transporters reveals a major role for astroglial transport in excitotoxicity and clearance of glutamate, *Neuron*, 16, 675, 1996.

98. Erecinska, M. and Silver, I.A., Metabolism and role of glutamate in mammalian brain, *Progr. Neurobiol.*, 35, 245, 1990.

99. Cooper, A.J.L. and Plum, F., Biochemistry and physiology of brain ammonia, *Physiol. Rev.* 67, 440, 1987.

100. Sibson, N.R. et al., Functional energy metabolism: *in vivo* ^{13}C NMR spectroscopy evidence for coupling of cerebral glucose consumption and glutamatergic neuronal activity, *Dev. Neurosci.*, 20, 321, 1998.

101. Kanamori, K. et al., Severity of hyperammonemic encephalopathy correlates with brain ammonia level and saturation of glutamine synthetase *in vivo*, *J. Neurochem.*, 67, 1584, 1996.

102. Kanamori, K. and Ross, B.D., ^{15}N NMR Measurement of the *in vivo* rate of glutamine synthesis and utilization at steady state in the brain of the hyperammonaemic rat, *Biochem. J.*, 293, 461, 1993.

103. Kanamori, K., Parivar, F., and Ross, B.D., A ^{15}N NMR study of *in vivo* cerebral glutamine synthesis in hyperammonemic rats, *NMR Biomed.*, 6, 21, 1993.

104. Shen, J. et al., ^{15}N NMR spectroscopy studies of ammonia transport and glutamine synthesis in the hyperammonemic rat brain, *Dev. Neurosci.*, 20, 434, 1998.

105. Kanamori, K. and Ross, B.D., Steady-state *in vivo* glutamate dehydrogenase activity in rat brain measured by ^{15}N NMR, *J. Biol. Chem.*, 270, 24805, 1995.

106. Kanamori, K. and Ross, B.D., *In vivo* activity of glutaminase in the brain of hyperammonaemic rats measured by ^{15}N nuclear magnetic resonance, *Biochem. J.*, 305, 329, 1995.

107. Mason, G.F. et al., Decrease in GABA synthesis rate in rat cortex following GABA–transaminase inhibition correlates with the decrease in gad(67) protein, *Brain Res.*, 914, 81, 2001.

108. Hassel, B. et al., Quantification of the GABA shunt and the importance of the GABA shunt versus the 2-oxoglutarate dehydrogenase pathway in GABAergic neurons, *J. Neurochem.*, 71, 1511, 1998.

109. Raichle, M.E., Behind the scenes of functional brain imaging: a historical and physiological perspective, *Proc. Natl. Acad. Sci. U.S.A.*, 95, 765, 1998.

110. Mattson, R.H. et al., Vigabatrin: effect on brain GABA levels measured by nuclear magnetic resonance spectroscopy, *Acta Neurol. Scand. Suppl.*, 162, 27, 1995.
111. Rothman, D.L. et al., Localized ^{1}H NMR measurements of γ-aminobutyric acid in human brain *in vivo*, *Proc. Natl. Acad. Sci. U.S.A.*, 90, 5662, 1993.
112. Logothetis, N.K. et al., Neurophysiological investigation of the basis of the fMRI signal, *Nature*, 412, 150, 2001.
113. Kanamori, K. et al., A ^{15}N NMR study of isolated brain in portacaval-shunted rats after acute hyperammonemia, *Biochim. Biophys. Acta*, 5, 270, 1991.
114. Lapidot, A. and Gopher, A., Quantitation of metabolic compartmentation in hyperammonemic brain by natural abundance ^{13}C NMR detection of [13]C–[15]N coupling patterns and isotopic shifts, *Eur. J. Biochem.*, 243, 597, 1997.
115. Pascual, J.M. et al., Glutamate, glutamine, and GABA as substrates for the neuronal and glial compartments after focal cerebral ischemia in rats, *Stroke*, 29, 1048, 1998.
116. Haberg, A. et al., *In vivo* injection of [1-^{13}C]glucose and [1,2-^{13}C]acetate combined with *ex vivo* [13]C nuclear magnetic resonance spectroscopy: a novel approach to the study of middle cerebral artery occlusion in the rat, *J. Cereb. Blood Flow Metabol.*, 18, 1223, 1998.
117. Bouzier, A.K. et al., [1-[(13)]C]glucose metabolism in the tumoral and nontumoral cerebral tissue of a glioma-bearing rat, *J. Neurochem.*, 72, 2445, 1999.
118. Muller, B. et al., Amino acid neurotransmitter metabolism in neurons and glia following kainate injection in rats, *Neurosci. Lett.*, 279, 169, 2000.
119. Chateil, J. et al., Metabolism of [1-^{13}C]glucose and [2-^{13}C]acetate in the hypoxic rat brain, *Neurochem. Int.*, 38, 399, 2001.
120. Bluml, S., Moreno-Torres, A., and Ross, B.D., [1-^{13}C]glucose MRS in chronic hepatic encephalopathy in man, *Mag. Res. Med.*, 45, 981, 2001.
121. Bluml, S. et al., 1-[(13)]C glucose magnetic resonance spectroscopy of pediatric and adult brain disorders, *NMR Biomed.*, 14, 19, 2001.

9 Small Animal Imaging with Positron Emission Tomography

Simon R. Cherry and Harley I. Kornblum

CONTENTS

9.1 INTRODUCTION

Recent years have seen a large increase in the number of investigators studying brain pathology and neural repair. Many basic neuroscience studies are now devoted to the study of disease models as well as the means to repair injury, disease, or degeneration. Additionally, numerous studies are designed to "create" a pathologic state by disrupting genes of interest. These types of studies require the neuroscientist to be able to discern changes in brain function or structure as a result of both the pathologic state as well as alterations due to therapeutic interventions. Such information can often only be obtained by sacrifice of the animal and histologic or biochemical observation of the brain. Obviously, this approach has its limitations. First, the use of histologic outcomes precludes the longitudinal studies of individual animals. Changes that may occur as a result of an intervention have to be inferred by examining populations prior to and at different times following intervention. The groups then must be statistically compared to each other. While often useful, these types of studies require the use of extremely large numbers of animals. Furthermore, this type of investigation would tend to underestimate the significance of variation between animals, potentially missing distinctions between groups of responders and nonresponders. Ideally, one would like to have the ability to make repeated observations in individual animals. The ability to make repeated observations would not only allow for the investigator to more accurately assess interanimal variability, it would also allow for a direct analysis of change over time due to a given intervention as well as enhance the ability to make both short term and long term observations.

Another key advantage of *in vivo* imaging is the ability to perform multiple types of studies in the same animal. For example, one might wish to correlate behavior, structure, and neurochemical observations as the result of an intervention or gene mutation. These types of correlative studies would gain an enormous degree of power if all observations were made in the same animal. Such an ability is particularly advantageous in cases where an enormous amount of time, effort, and money are invested in individual animals such as animals that have had lesions placed followed by therapeutic transplantation of stem cells. Nonconsumptive methods of study are particularly suitable for the investigation of knockout and transgenic mice where the numbers of animals may be severely limited and there is a high motivation to obtain the maximal amount of information from an individual animal.

Positron emission tomography (PET) has been used for a number of years in the study of the function and neurochemistry in the human and nonhuman primate brain.[1] PET is a noninvasive and extremely safe imaging modality that allows for repeated observations in an individual. The adaptation of PET to repeatedly and noninvasively image small animals represents a unique opportunity to explore neuroplasticity and neuropathology in living rodents. This chapter will describe the basic physical principles underlying PET imaging, review some of the work that has successfully utilized PET in rodent brain imaging, and will indicate future directions for rodent research with PET.

9.2 BASIC PRINCIPLES OF POSITRON EMISSION TOMOGRAPHY IMAGING

PET is a radiotracer imaging technique that utilizes small amounts of a compound or biomolecule of interest labeled with radioactive atoms. The radiation emitted as the radioactive label decays is picked up by a series of external detectors and the resulting information is used to compute images that show the distribution of the radioactive tracer in the subject. PET can essentially be thought of as a noninvasive version of autoradiography, with inferior spatial resolution, but with the advantages that the pharmacokinetics of the tracer can be measured in a single experiment and repeat studies can be performed on the same subject.

9.2.1 Positron-Emitting Radionuclides and Tracers

PET imaging makes exclusive use of radionuclides that decay by positron emission. Table 9.1 lists commonly used positron-emitting radionuclides. Some of the radionuclides are isotopes of biologically ubiquitous elements such as carbon, nitrogen, and oxygen, enabling radioactively labeled tracers of small organic molecules to be produced by direct isotopic substitution, for example, by replacing a stable carbon-12 atom with a positron-emitting carbon-11 atom. In this case the radioactive tracer has the same biodistribution, kinetics, and target specificity as the unlabeled native compound. Unfortunately, the half-lives of these biologically relevant positron-emitting radionuclides are rather short, ranging from 2 minutes for oxygen-15 to 20 minutes for carbon-11.

Centers that use these radionuclides must synthesize them on site in a compact biomedical cyclotron.[2] Once the radionuclide is produced, rapid synthetic pathways are needed to produce the radiolabeled product and it must then be immediately injected into the subject; the time between production and injection typically is no more than 4 to 6 half-lives. With carbon-11, this amounts to only about 2 hours from production of radionuclide to injection of radiotracer. Despite these challenges, several hundred carbon-11 labeled compounds have been reported in the literature[3] and carbon-11 remains the radionuclide of choice for radiolabeling neuroreceptor ligands and drugs. Several hundred academic centers (2001 figures) now have direct access to short-lived radionuclides through their own biomedical cyclotron facilities.

Some of the longer-lived positron-emitting radionuclides listed on Table 9.1 can be produced in the same biomedical cyclotrons but also have long enough half-lives that enable them to be distributed from regional or national facilities. The most popular of these radionuclides is fluorine-18 which has a 110-minute half-life. Fluorine-18 can substitute readily for hydrogen atoms or hydroxyl groups in small molecules. Its longer half-life permits pursuit of more complex synthetic pathways and opens up the possibility of performing PET studies without an on-site cyclotron.

The substitution of fluorine for hydrogen creates labeled analog tracers that are likely to differ in their kinetic properties and target affinities compared with the unlabeled compound, although sometimes this alteration leads to improved imaging properties. Largely driven by the clinical demand for the tracer ^{18}F-fluorodeoxyglucose (FDG), a glucose analog used for clinical PET studies of metabolism in oncology, neurology, and cardiology, fluorine-18 and FDG are widely available in Northern America, Europe, and Japan. Interest is growing in much longer half-life positron-emitting radionuclides such as copper-64 (half-life 12.6 hours) and iodine-124 (half-life 4.2 days). A range of interesting labeled compounds can be created by iodination, and the radiometals offer possibilities in creating labeled chelates of larger biomolecules such as peptides and antibodies. Again, the longer half-lives permit these tracers to be produced without an on-site cyclotron.

The wide range of positron-emitting radionuclides that are available and their biological relevance offer virtually unlimited possibilities for creating labeled tracers that can be imaged by PET. Thousands of PET tracers have been reported in the literature.[3] They were designed to explore a variety of biological processes and molecular targets, ranging from tissue perfusion and substrate metabolism to receptor targets, enzyme kinetics, and most recently, gene expression.[4] Like all other radionuclide assays, PET is exquisitely sensitive because of the very low background of natural radioactivity and the relatively high likelihood of detection of a single radioactive decay. Also, PET tracers generally have high specific activities (on the order of 10^3 Ci/mmol with fluorine-18 and carbon-11). Therefore, most PET experiments require the injection of micrograms or less of the compound of interest to obtain an image, resulting in nanomolar or lower concentrations *in vivo*. At these concentrations, the measurements usually are in the tracer regime, far removed from levels at which pharmacological effects might become a concern. The exceptions are studies of easily saturated receptor systems in mice and rats, where care needs to be exercised in determining the mass of the tracer injected and the saturation levels of the receptors of interest.[5]

9.2.2 PHYSICS OF PET IMAGING

The radiolabeled tracer is administered to the subject, most commonly by intravenous injection. Typical injected doses are in the range of $\sim 10^2$ (mice) to $\sim 10^3$ (rats) μCi in small animal studies. When the radioactive atom incorporated in a particular molecule decays, it ejects a positron that quickly loses its kinetic energy by interacting with nearby electrons in tissue. After the positron loses most of its energy, it combines with an electron and undergoes annihilation. The masses of the electron and positron are converted into energy emitted in the form of high energy photons (Figure 9.1). To conserve momentum and energy, two photons are emitted 180° apart, and each carries away 511 keV of energy.

The energy of these photons falls in the γ-ray region of the electromagnetic spectrum (roughly 10-fold higher energy than x-rays used in diagnostic imaging) and they have a fairly high probability of escaping from the body. This unique back-to-back emission of photons forms the basis for the localization of the tracer, because simultaneous detection (also known as coincidence detection) of the two annihilation photons defines a line along which the annihilation must have occurred. Since the distance from the point of emission to the site of annihilation is generally short ($\sim 10^{-2}$ to 10^{-1} cm), this line also passes very close to the location of the decaying atom (and hence the labeled molecule) in the body.

The decay properties of positron-emitting radionuclides also produce two spatial resolution limitations related to the physics of positron emission. First, the PET scanner detects the location of the annihilation, not the location of the radioactive atom attached to the molecule of interest. This error is known as the positron range and varies from radionuclide to radionuclide because some radionuclides emit more energetic positrons than others (see Table 9.1). More energetic positrons will travel further before annihilation, leading to larger positron range errors. Mean positron range can vary from tenths of a millimeter for low energy radionuclides such as

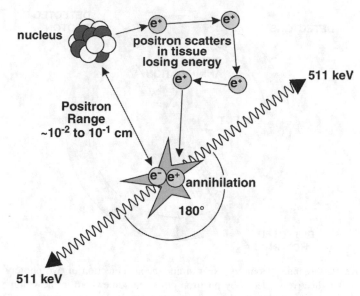

FIGURE 9.1 Basic physics of positron emission followed by annihilation that results in the emission of two back-to-back high energy photons that are recorded by external scintillation detectors.

TABLE 9.1
Partial List of Positron-Emitting Radionuclides and Their Half-Lives and Maximum Positron Energy

Radionuclide	Half-life	β^+ fraction	Maximum energy
C-11	20.4 min.	0.99	960 keV
N-13	9.96 min.	1.00	1.19 MeV
O-15	123 sec.	1.00	1.72 MeV
F-18	110 min.	0.97	635 keV
Cu-62	9.74 min.	0.98	2.94 MeV
Cu-64	12.7 hr.	0.19	580 keV
Ga-68	68.3 min.	0.88	1.9 MeV
Br-76	16.1 hr.	0.56	3.7 MeV
Rb-82	78 sec.	0.95	3.35 MeV
I-124	4.18 days	0.22	1.5 MeV

Source: Lide, D.R., *Handbook of Chemistry and Physics*, 71st ed., CRC Press, Boca Raton, FL, 1990.

fluorine-18 and carbon-11, to several millimeters for high energy radionuclides such as bromine-76 and iodine-124.

The second limitation is that emission of the annihilation photons is not exactly back-to-back, but in fact has some distribution around 180°. The error this causes depends on the diameter of the detector ring, and for small animal imaging is on the order of 0.25 to 0.5 mm. The combined effect of these two factors suggests that

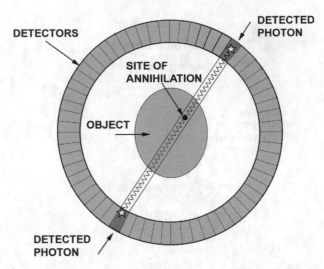

FIGURE 9.2 PET scanner geometry. Near simultaneous detection of two photons in a pair of detectors is indicative of decay by positron emission somewhere in the volume between the two detectors. Large numbers of such events are recorded and the methods of computed tomography are used to reconstruct a cross-sectional image in which the image intensity is proportional to the radionuclide concentration.

it will be very challenging to obtain spatial resolution better than 500 μm using PET even with a low energy positron emitter such as fluorine-18. Another limitation is that simultaneous imaging of multiple tracers is not possible.

9.2.3 PET Scanners

A PET scanner typically consists of rings of scintillation detectors placed around the subject, with each detector linked electronically in coincidence with detectors on the opposite side of the ring (Figure 9.2). Valid events occur when two detectors record a signal almost simultaneously (within a few nanoseconds of each other). A large number of annihilation events are detected in a PET scan (typically 10^6 to 10^8); the number of events recorded by a particular detector pair is proportional to the integrated radioactivity along the line joining the two detectors. Mathematical reconstruction algorithms are then used to compute tomographic images in which the intensity in any image voxel (volumetric pixel) is ideally directly proportional to the radioactivity (and hence the concentration of the labeled molecule) contained within that voxel. A range of reconstruction techniques are available, from simple Fourier-based methods (e.g., filtered backprojection) to more complex statistically based iterative methods that can contain sophisticated models of the entire imaging system and the data formation process.

A modern PET scanner (Figure 9.3A) may consist of as many as 10,000 to 20,000 individual scintillator detector elements capable of producing images with a resolution as high as 3 to 6 mm in human brains and 1 to 2 mm in mouse and rat brains. Most PET scanners are designed to image the entire brain simultaneously and produce a stack of contiguous two-dimensional image slices or a three-dimensional image

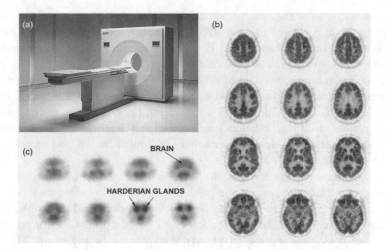

FIGURE 9.3 (a): Clinical PET scanner (ECAT Exact HR+, CTI/Siemens, Knoxville, TN). [^{18}F]-FDG images of a human brain (b) and rat brain (c) acquired on this system. Image resolution is about 4 mm. In the human brain, many structures can be clearly resolved, but the resolution is not sufficient for structures in the much smaller rat brain.

volume. The temporal resolution can be as high as a few seconds, and imaging the changing distribution of a radiolabeled tracer over a period of minutes to hours is routine. This dynamic data can then be fed into tracer kinetic models[6] to quantitatively measure the rates of specific biologic processes or assess binding characteristics of the tracer to the target of interest.

To obtain fully quantitative PET images that reflect the concentration of radio-labeled tracer in a particular region of interest over time, a number of corrections must be applied,[7] including corrections for photon attenuation (roughly a 50% correction in rats) and photon scatter. A class of events known as random coincidences, in which photons from two unrelated decays happen to strike opposing detectors within a few nanoseconds of each other, must also be corrected for.[8] If a time sequence of images is taken, it is necessary to correct for physical decay of the radionuclide, and finally the scanner must be calibrated against a source of known radioactivity concentration to achieve absolute quantification.

9.2.4 FACTORS DETERMINING IMAGE QUALITY

The three performance characteristics of a PET scanner that largely determine image quality are spatial resolution, system sensitivity, and count-rate performance. Spatial resolution relates to the ability to visualize and discriminate between the structures of interest. It is largely dominated by the resolution of the detectors. In general, the smaller the detector elements, the better the spatial resolution, although once the detectors start to approach a few millimeters in size, other effects such as scatter of the photons between detectors, positron range, and noncolinearity result in diminishing returns.

The system sensitivity of a PET scanner relates to the fraction of the emitted annihilation photon pairs that it detects. Sensitivity is important as it determines the signal-to-noise level of the reconstructed image. Large numbers of events must be detected to produce images of high statistical quality, and the number of detected events is often a limiting factor. This is particularly true in rapid dynamic studies, where information may only be collected for a few seconds or minutes at each time point. This depends on the square of efficiency of the detectors (both photons must be detected to obtain a valid event) and the availability of enough detectors to capture events. Sensitivity is maximized by using scintillators capable of stopping the 511-keV photons with high efficiency and completely surrounding the subject with a tight ring of detectors. Maximal sensitivity is limited by the cost of using large numbers of detectors.

The count-rate performance of the scanner is related to the linearity of the counting rate with the activity in the field of view. If no counting rate limitations exist, doubling the radioactivity in the field of view should lead to doubling of the number of detected counts. In reality, each event needs a finite time for processing, during which the system is not available to record other incoming events. This "dead time" depends largely on the decay time of the scintillator used in the detectors and characteristics of the electronics (e.g., shaping or integration). It is important that the dead time of the system be low for typical amounts of radioactivity in the field of view; otherwise system sensitivity is effectively decreased by the dead time losses.

9.3 HIGH RESOLUTION LABORATORY ANIMAL PET SCANNERS

Since the early 1990s, interest in the use of PET imaging in laboratory animal models has been growing. PET imaging already has an established role in studies of non-human primates. Ethical and economic considerations make imaging an attractive tool in such animals, and their brains are large enough that the resolution of existing PET systems designed for human imaging is often adequate. Some of the primary uses of PET in nonhuman primates include evaluation of new drugs and imaging tracers for the central nervous system,[9,10] in particular establishing drug concentrations at the target of interest, pharmacokinetics, determining appropriate dosing intervals for initial studies in man and, in the case of imaging tracers, dosimetry. Other important applications are studies of drugs of abuse and monitoring of novel restorative or protective therapies for neurogenerative disorders, particularly Parkinson's disease. While many of these types of studies are carried out with conventional clinical PET scanners, several dedicated scanners have been developed to achieve higher spatial resolution and/or sensitivity for imaging of nonhuman primates.[11,12]

Many more researchers have access to small laboratory animal models. Rats and mice are widely used and the combination of the ease of genetic manipulation (primarily in mice) and well characterized surgical and interventional models (primarily in rats) suggest a continued and probably expanded role for these laboratory animals in neuroscience. Although invasive procedures in these animals are more widely accepted, imaging studies still offer significant advantages, as described in the introduction.

PET imaging in smaller laboratory animals poses significant challenges, the most obvious of which relates to spatial resolution. Figure 9.3 shows images of a rat brain and a human brain generated on a PET scanner with a spatial resolution of ~4 mm, the best possible resolution in today's clinical systems. The loss of information due to the reduction in volume from ~1800 cc for the human down to ~5 cc for the rat brain is immediately apparent. Nonetheless, the first small animal PET scanner developed at the Hammersmith Hospital (London) in the early 1990s was based on the same detector technology found in clinical PET systems.[13] Despite the limited spatial resolution, this system, when used in conjunction with highly specific radiolabeled ligands for dopaminergic systems, was capable of resolving the striata in the rat brain and was used for a number of groundbreaking studies.[14]

Building on this early work, several groups across the world embarked on developing much higher spatial resolution PET systems, specifically for imaging small laboratory animals. Several academic groups developed their own systems based on a range of different detector technologies.[15–19] The majority of these systems produced an image resolution in the 1.5 to 3 mm range, and several groups are now pursuing prototype small animal PET systems with a spatial resolution approaching 1 mm.[20–22] A very different approach uses multiwire proportional chamber technology containing stacks of lead laminated boards that convert the incident gamma-rays into electrons that are then multiplied into a detectable signal within the gas. Multiwire chambers can achieve very high spatial resolution and a working system with ~ 1 mm resolution has been constructed.[23]

In 2000, the first commercial small animal PET scanners became available and now several companies are offering such systems[11,23] (Figure 9.4). The most widely distributed system is currently the microPET system manufactured by Concorde Microsystems (Knoxville, TN) based on a prototype originally developed at UCLA.[24] A description of this system will serve as a representative example of the features of dedicated small animal PET systems. The detector modules in the microPET scanners are multielement scintillation detectors, using a finely cut array of LSO scintillator material, coupled via a 5 cm long coherent bundle of optical fibers, to a position-sensitive photomultiplier tube (PMT). Each LSO block is cut into an 8×8 array of elements, with each element measuring $2 \times 2 \times 10$ mm on a 2.2 mm center to center spacing. The 200 µm cuts between the elements are filled with a reflective material to help prevent optical crosstalk between elements. The microPET R4 system consists of 168 of these detector modules arranged in four axially contiguous rings of 42 detectors each. The ring diameter is 24 cm and the axial field of view is 8 cm. A computer controlled bed and laser alignment system complete the basic hardware. The system is controlled by a dual processor Pentium PC with a large disk to accommodate the data.

The 511-keV annihilation photons interact in the dense scintillator material, producing a brief (~40 ns) and faint (~15,000 photons) flash of visible light. Roughly 5 to 10% of this light passes down the optical fiber bundle and into the PMT where it is converted with ~15% efficiency into electrons at the photocathode. These electrons are accelerated by a high potential through the ten electronic stages of the PMT, each electron generating three to four new electrons at each stage. A signal of $>10^6$ electrons is produced over a period of <100 ns at the PMT output for each interacting annihilation photon. This constitutes a substantial and easily detectable current that is passed on to amplifying electronics and to fast timing circuitry where

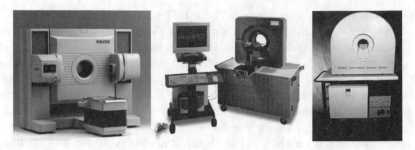

FIGURE 9.4 PET scanners designed for imaging laboratory animals: Left: Hamamatsu SHR 7700 primarily designed for studies in nonhuman primates. (Courtesy of Dr. Takaji Yamashita. With permission.) Center: Concorde microPET scanner designed for studies in small nonhuman primates and rodents. (Courtesy of Robert Nutt. With permission.). Right: Oxford Positron Systems Quad HIDAC. (Courtesy of Dr. Alan Jeavons. With permission.)

the arrival times of photons from all detectors are compared to determine annihilation photon pairs.

Valid event pairs (two photons detected within a few nanoseconds of each other) are written to disk and binned into a matrix known as a sinogram. The sinogram constitutes the raw PET data and each element in the sinogram represents the total number of events detected by a specific detector pair during the scanning time. This value is also directly proportional to the amount of radioactivity along the line between that detector pair. To obtain the image, these so-called line integrals (collected for all possible detector pairs) must be reconstructed using analytic (filtered backprojection) or iterative reconstruction algorithms. Iterative algorithms can include sophisticated models of the physics of the PET scanner and the statistical nature of the data[25] that often lead to significant improvements in image quality over analytic reconstruction techniques. After reconstruction, the final result, assuming that appropriate corrections have been applied for photon attenuation and scatter in the body, individual detector efficiency variations, detector dead time, and chance or random coincidence events, is a volumetric image dataset in which the intensity at each voxel is proportional to the radioactivity in the voxel.

The microPET R4 system produces images with a spatial resolution of ~2 mm in each direction. The peak sensitivity of the system is ~900 counts per second per μCi of activity at the center of the scanner, with an average sensitivity of ~500 cps/μCi in the rat brain and 685 cps/μCi in the mouse brain, assuming the brain is placed at the center of the field of view. The system is capable of reaching count rates >100,000 cps without significant dead time in brain imaging studies. The temporal resolution of the data is selectable by the user and is a trade-off with signal-to-noise (increases with longer acquisition times). Frame times as short as 0.5 seconds have been used to track the initial bolus of radioactivity after injection, with high quality images of the brain distribution of a radiotracer typically requiring 5 minutes for injected doses of ~150 μCi in the mouse and ~500 μCi in the rat. Figure 9.5 shows images of the rat brain obtained with the original microPET prototype scanner.

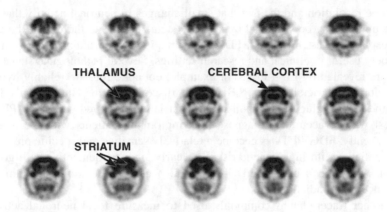

FIGURE 9.5 [^{18}F]-FDG images obtained in normal rat brain with a microPET scanner (resolution is approximately 1.5 mm). Coronal sections are shown running caudal (top left) to rostral (bottom right).

9.4 PET IN CLINICAL NEUROSCIENCE STUDIES

Clinical PET scanners have been used for a number of years to conduct studies in brain development, brain pathology, and neuroplasticity in humans and, to an extent, in nonhuman primates. The most common PET tracer for these purposes is [^{18}F]-fluorodeoxyglucose (FDG). This molecule is an analogue of 2-deoxyglucose (2-DG), a common substrate used to measure metabolic activity.[26] FDG and 2-DG are taken up by cells and phosphorylated by hexokinase, a step that traps the tracer inside the cell. Unlike glucose, however, FDG is not metabolized to pyruvate and does not contribute to the formation of ATP.

The amount of FDG taken up by a cell is proportional to the amount of glucose it utilizes. In the nervous system, while the precise cellular substrates for FDG uptake are not clear, the amount of FDG taken up within a particular brain region is proportional to the amount of synaptic activity.[27–29] This glucose utilization can be quantified in a relative way based on normalization to the amount of tracer injected or the signal in another brain region, or in an absolute way as the local cerebral metabolic rate for glucose.[26] This absolute measurement requires calculation of an input function based on measurements of blood FDG during the course of tracer uptake in arterial or "arterialized" capillary blood.

FDG has kinetic properties that are important to consider. After an intravenous bolus injection, approximately 30 to 45 minutes elapse before the tracer reaches a steady state in the brain. Usually after this time the subject is placed in the PET scanner. Additional time ranging from 5 to 60 minutes is required to obtain sufficient counts to generate optimal images. The image obtained, however, is a result of the summed neural activity that occurs during the uptake period, with the largest component represented by the interval between 5 and 15 minutes (depending on species). An advantage to this peculiarity of FDG is that neuronal activity can be measured during the awake state or during performance of a task. The difficulty lies in the poor time resolution and the fact that small changes in neuronal activity that occur during uptake may be swamped by activity occurring during the rest of the time.

Despite this last misgiving, FDG-PET imaging of the brain has proven to be extremely useful in clinical and research settings. Several pathological states of the brain are revealed by FDG-PET. For example, epileptic foci are reliably hypometabolic during interictal periods.[30] Before the discovery of the Huntington's disease gene, the lack of glucose metabolism in the striatum observed with FDG-PET was the best way to accurately diagnose presymptomatic patients with the disease.[31] More recently, FDG-PET has become a relatively sensitive and specific predictor of which patients with high genetic risks[32] or early signs of dementia[33] will go on to develop Alzheimer's disease. FDG-PET is also useful to distinguish brain tumor recurrence from radiation damage.[34]

Another tracer that is commonly used to measure focal neuronal activity is [^{15}O]-labeled water. Unlike ^{18}F, ^{15}O has a very short half-life, and must be used almost immediately after creation in the cyclotron. Labeled water is rapidly distributed throughout the bloodstream and can be used to measure local cerebral blood flow. Changes of neuronal activity within a certain brain area are reflected in changes in cerebral blood flow. Studies using this tracer have been used to map normal brain function[35] and the rearrangement of connections following brain insults such as a ruptured arteriovenous malformation.[36]

Although numerous brain studies are still being performed on a clinical and research basis using FDG and [^{15}O]-water, functional MRI is largely replacing PET for brain mapping studies. These are studies in which the observer wishes to detect patterns of neuronal activation during a certain task or following surgical or other intervention. The true power of PET in clinical research and medicine is its ability to assay biochemical function noninvasively. For example, [^{18}F]-DOPA, a compound specifically taken up and metabolized by dopamine nerve terminals, can be reliably used to detect early loss of the terminals in the putamens of patients with idiopathic Parkinsonism.[37] The same compound is also used to assess the efficacy of implants of embryonic dopamine neurons into the brains of patients.[38] Other neurochemical functions can also be measured with PET, for example, assays of dopamine, opiate, and other neurotransmitter receptor densities, measurement of serotonin uptake capacity, measurement of benzodiazepine binding sites, etc. While most probes used to measure these functional properties are experimental, several are likely to be used on a routine clinical basis.

9.5 USE OF PET IN RAT MODELS OF INJURY AND NEUROPLASTICITY

The 2-deoxyglucose autoradiographic method has long been used as a measure of rearrangement of neuronal connectivity following injury in the brain. One example is the expansion of surrounding barrel receptive fields following whisker ablation.[39] Another example is in the case of large cortical lesions. Suction ablation of the neocortex results in a remarkable rearrangement of connections between the remaining (contralateral) cortex and subcortical structures in young animals but not in adults. This phenomenon has been studied in rats, cats, and nonhuman primates. The rearranged connections correlate with changes observed in glucose metabolism in cats.[40]

To assess whether age-dependent changes in glucose metabolism occurred in rats following cortical ablations, we used the microPET scanner to perform FDG-PET in animals lesioned on the sixth day of life (P6) or in adulthood.[41] We were able to scan adult animals 3, 10, and 30 days after injury. However, due to limitations of resolution, animals lesioned on P6 were only scanned 1 month following lesion. We assessed the relative uptake of FDG in the neostriatum and thalamus on the side ipsilateral to the lesion and compared it to uptake on the contralateral side. By using this relative quantification method, we were able to avoid the placement of the chronic in-dwelling arterial catheters that would have been necessary to establish fully quantitative measures. Of course, the use of relative measures obscured potential global effects of the lesion.

As reported[41] and demonstrated for the thalamus in Figure 9.6, both thalamic and striatal metabolism diminished following cortical lesions in adults and then recovered, with less recovery occurring in the thalamus. Animals lesioned on P6 appeared to have improved recovery of metabolism in the neostriatum, as compared to adults, but worse thalamic recovery (Figure 9.6C).

These studies demonstrated several principles. First, we were able to reliably and reproducibly assess changes in glucose metabolism following lesions in groups of animals. Second, the microPET system was able to assess time-dependent changes in glucose metabolism in serial studies of individual adult animals following lesion. Additionally, we observed age-dependent differences in response to lesion, consistent with prior studies using conventional histological methods. Using the results of these studies as a foundation, current studies are now directed toward microPET as a platform to test potential therapies such as neurotrophic factor or neural stem cell implantation. It is our hypothesis that effective therapies will result in improved glucose metabolism following injury. If that turns out to be the case, future clinical studies will be able to utilize FDG-PET as an outcome measure.

The microPET system was used also to study responses to blunt trauma. Clinical studies revealed that PET performed within hours of severe trauma revealed significant hypermetabolism around the area of injury, while subsequent scans showed hypometabolism.[42] Autoradiographic studies of animals demonstrated initial hypermetabolism followed by hypometabolism after blunt head trauma. Moore et al.,[43] examined glucose metabolism *in vivo* using the microPET following blunt head trauma at a time expected to reveal ipsilateral hypometabolism and indeed found that result. These studies, in which small animal PET results could be compared directly to autoradiography following a lesion, demonstrate the reliability of PET in small animal models of brain injury.

The examples cited above demonstrate two uses of PET in clinically relevant rat models of brain injury and, to an extent, repair. These studies will serve as foundations for future studies of injury and potential therapy. Certainly, other models of injury such as stroke or chemical neurotoxicity (see below) can be and are being evaluated with small animal PET. Along with FDG, other tracers that allow measurement of different functional aspects should be put into use.

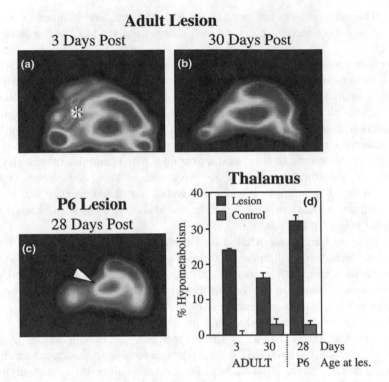

FIGURE 9.6 Effects of hemidecortication on thalamic metabolism studied by microPET. A and B are microPET images from an adult animal that underwent aspiration lesion of the left neocortex imaged 3 days (a) and 30 days (b) later. Note improvement in ipsilateral hypometabolism after 30 days. In an animal lesioned at 6 days of age and imaged 1 month later, imaging revealed severe hypometabolism in the ipsilateral thalamus (c). (d) Shows quantitative data demonstrating the degree of thalamic hypometabolism in adults 3 and 30 days postlesion and P6 animals scanned 28 days postlesion. See Color Figure 9.6 following page 210.

9.6 PET IN ANIMAL MODELS OF NEURODEGENERATIVE DISORDERS

One of the greatest areas of interest in neuroscience is the pathology and potential treatment of neurodegenerative disorders such as Alzheimer's, Parkinson's, and Huntington's diseases. Rodent models for these disorders exist and PET scanning has been used to evaluate pathology and treatment in at least two models.

9.6.1 PARKINSON'S DISEASE

Parkinson's disease results in a loss of dopamine neurons in the ventral midbrain and consequent elimination of dopaminergic input to the striatum. The loss of dopamine terminals in Parkinson's disease can be detected using [18F]-labeled DOPA (FDOPA), which is taken up and trapped by dopaminergic nerve terminals or by the use of [11C]-labeled ligands that label dopamine transporter sites (CFT). One of the

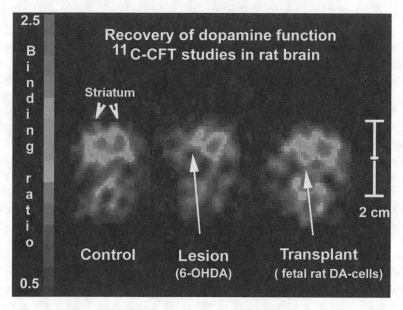

FIGURE 9.7 Imaging of dopamine terminals following 6-hydroxydopamine lesion and subsequent transplant using [^{11}C]-CFT. The left image shows uptake in the striatum of a control rat. The middle image shows loss of terminals following 6-hydroxy lesion. The right image demonstrates a return of function after transplantation of fetal dopaminergic neurons. Images were obtained on a PCR-1 tomograph. (Courtesy of Dr. A.L. Brownell, Harvard Medical School. With permission.) See Color Figure 9.7 following page 210.

most commonly used animal models of Parkinsons disease is the induction of unilateral loss of dopamine neurons by focal administration of 6-hydroxydopamine. Because of the very high specificity of these ligands and the anatomical limitation of dopamine terminals, one can visualize these terminals (and their absence) using even relatively low resolution animal scanners.

Cell transplantation strategies have been in therapeutic trials for Parkinson's disease. Following successful transplantation, the dopamine nerve terminals derived from transplanted cells can be visualized in patients using PET as described above. In an analogous manner, successful cell transplantation using either fetal midbrain (Figure 9.7)[44] or embryonic stem cells[45] can be detected with animal scanners, again using those scanners that do not have extremely high resolution or sensitivity.

9.6.2 HUNTINGTON'S DISEASE

FDG-PET has also been used to clinically evaluate Huntington's disease. Before genetic testing was available, loss of striatal glucose metabolism determined by FDG-PET was the most effective way to establish the diagnosis in early symptomatic patients and accurately predicted the onset of symptoms in presymptomatic individuals.[31] A number of animal models of Huntington's disease have been developed. In a model that reflects the pathological changes observed in the striatum, excitotoxins such as quinolinic acid are directly injected into the structure, with a subsequent loss of GABAergic projection neurons. Transgenic mouse models also exist[46] in which mice expressing varying portions of the abnormal human gene are generated. These mice have not yet been demonstrated to reproduce the striatal pathology of Huntington's disease.

PET has been used to study the effects of excitatory amino acid lesion in rats. Using a scanner with relatively low sensitivity and resolution, Hume et al. demonstrated a loss of dopamine D1 receptors in the striatum.[14] Subsequently, with a more modern scanner, Araujo et al.[47] found that FDG-PET readily demonstrates the loss of metabolically active neurons in the neostriatum following lesion. In addition, the loss of dopamine D2 receptors can also be detected with PET.[47] As with PET studies of brain injury described above, these studies will serve as the bases for study of interventions such as neural stem cell transplantation.

The study of glucose metabolism in transgenic mouse models of Huntington's disease has proven more difficult. Current rodent-dedicated scanners cannot easily resolve cortical and subcortical structures. Additionally, because transgenes are symmetrically expressed within the brain, fully quantitative studies need to be performed to evaluate functional deficits using PET. We anticipate that future high resolution scanners will be up to the task of performing such exacting imaging.

9.7 USING PET TO STUDY PATTERNS OF NEURAL ACTIVATION

As stated above, PET has been used in clinical studies to assess neuronal activation in clinical settings using either glucose metabolism or blood flow as a surrogate measure of neuronal activity. These clinical PET studies of neuronal activation patterns were largely supplanted by functional magnetic resonance imaging (fMRI), which has the advantage of allowing many repetitions of different conditions in a single experimental paradigm. In animal models, fMRI studies are likely to prove exceedingly difficult due to the need to maintain head immobility within a scanner during the performance of a task. FDG-PET has the theoretical advantage of allowing for uptake of tracer during an activation paradigm in an unrestrained animal prior to sedation for the scanning period.

We[41] used this fact to allow for the imaging of neuronal activation under two different paradigms (see Figures 9.8a and b). First, metabolic activation of limbic cortical structures was observed during seizures. Rats were injected with kainic acid and then FDG. After 45 minutes, seizures were terminated by sedation and the animals were placed in the microPET for imaging. Using such a paradigm, one might envision studies of the anatomical extent and intensity of hypermetabolism induced by seizures following several manipulations, such as during kindling or following lesions or pharmacological intervention.

In a demonstration of more subtle levels of neuronal activation, we performed unilateral whisker stimulation during the uptake period and found significant activation within the contralateral neocortex when visualized with microPET (Figures 9.8c and d). Future studies will address recovery of activation patterns following lesioning and therapeutic intervention.

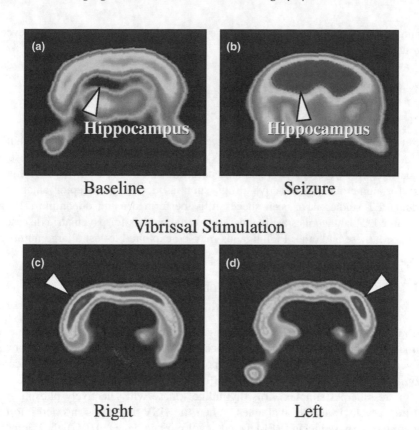

FIGURE 9.8 Detection of neuronal activation with FDG-microPET. (a) and (b) are images of an animal scanned prior to (a) and immediately following (b) kainic acid-induced seizure (uptake occurred during the seizure). Note the dramatic enhancement of signal in the hippo-campus (arrow). (c) and (d) are images of animals scanned following an uptake period during which the right (c) or left (d) moustachial vibrissae were stimulated. Note slightly enhanced uptake of tracer in the vicinity of the barrel field cortex contralateral to the stimulation (arrows). See Color Figure 9.8 following page 210.

Although the above examples demonstrate the utility of PET in studying patterns of neuronal activation in rats, some cautionary points must be stressed to those interested in such studies. The kinetics of FDG utilization creates a relatively extended uptake period and any neuronal activation paradigm would have to produce relatively prolonged epochs of activation, such as during a seizure or repetitive sensory stimulation. An activation paradigm that produces a brief burst of neuronal activity is unlikely to be visualizable using this technology, as the enhanced uptake during the activation will be averaged out by epochs during the uptake period in which no such activation takes place. Although [^{15}O]-water has been used to visualize neuronal activation successfully in human subjects, such studies may be too cum-bersome to practically perform in rodents, except under very special circumstances, given the need for the animals to remain still during uptake, the need to rapidly obtain isotope from the cyclotron, and the low resolution that would be achieved in any single scan.

9.8 EMERGING DIRECTIONS

9.8.1 PET IN MODELS OF PSYCHIATRIC DISEASE

The use of PET in rodent models of psychiatric disease has been limited, but the potential for rodent PET studies to assess animal models of psychiatric disease and evaluate psychiatric drugs is great. This potential can be seen now as PET ligands exist for numerous psychoactive drugs such as dopamine receptor antagonists. Rodent PET studies have been successfully performed using dopamine D1[14] and dopamine D2[47] antagonists as ligands. As animal models for psychiatric disease are developed, these and other PET ligands may be exploited to test a large number of appropriate neurotransmitter parameters within individual animals *in vivo*.

9.8.2 USING NOVEL TRACERS TO IMAGE GENE EXPRESSION AND BIOLOGICALLY RELEVANT MOLECULES

The major potential for PET in advancing scientific knowledge lies in its potential to image biochemical and molecular processes. One possible clinical use will be in the verification of gene therapy. PET reporter genes are DNA constructs encoding enzymes or other biomolecules that can be imaged with PET. For example, cells that express herpes simplex virus thymidine kinase will selectively phosphorylate and trap acyclovir and its analogues. When the HSV-tk gene is inserted into cells that are then exposed to an [18F]-labeled acyclovir analogue (FHBG), the compound is trapped and the cells become a source of signal in a PET scan. This has been performed *in vivo* using an adenoviral vector to deliver the HSV-tk gene.[48,49]

Dopamine D2 receptors have also been used as PET reporter probes.[50] In gene therapy trials, the effectiveness of delivery of a therapeutic gene can be monitored by the codelivery of a PET reporter gene. Such principles are potentially useful for imaging gene delivery in the CNS. The current constructs developed for PET gene imaging have not proven useful in the CNS. In the case of tk substrates, little or no blood–brain-barrier penetration occurs. In the case of dopamine D2 receptors, endogenous dopamine receptors would interfere with the signal. The development of other reporter constructs must occur before the successful use of these new methods in the CNS.

In addition to imaging exogenous genes, new generations of PET probes will be developed to image gene products of important biological pathways. The revolution in molecular biology and proteomics has tremendously expanded the number of potential targets for PET imaging, including receptors, signal transduction molecules, and transcription factors. The advent of combinatorial chemistry and rapid screening methods has allowed for the creation of huge libraries of potential reagents to selectively bind these macromolecules. With appropriate radiochemistry, these compounds will be turned into highly interesting PET tracers with the potential to dissect signalling pathways under a variety of conditions *in vivo*.

9.8.3 PET IN PRECLINICAL PHARMACOLOGICAL TESTING

The use of rodent PET has enormous potential for the preclinical pharmacological testing of new neuroactive agents.[9] PET will be utilized to test a variety of properties of pharmacological agents. It could be used to determine the biodistribution of a compound following injection. The pharmacologic and anatomical sites of binding within the brain can be discerned as well. The effects of a compound on glucose metabolism and other receptor and signaling systems could also be determined. PET could be used to test the effects of compounds in animal models of human disease. This has a particular appeal, because of the ability to use the same PET measures in animal and human subjects. If a compound has a positive effect on FDOPA uptake in the striata of lesioned rat models of Parkinson's disease, the hypothesis that it serves the same function in human patients can be directly tested with PET.

9.8.4 ADVANCES IN PET TECHNOLOGY

It appears likely that small animal PET systems routinely capable of submillimeter resolution imaging using low energy positron emitters such as carbon-11 and fluorine-18 will be available in 3 to 5 years. This will require innovations in detector design and image reconstruction techniques. Many of the essential elements are already in place or under development. The development of new solid-state detector technology may cause equipment costs to drop, putting small animal PET scanners in a cost category similar to confocal microscopes and digital autoradiographic systems. We also see a need to simplify dramatically all the data correction procedures so that the new PET systems can produce calibrated quantitative images in a transparent and robust fashion.

Finally, widespread use of PET imaging in the preclinical environment is limited primarily by the availability of positron-emitting radiotracers. Currently only centers with existing clinical or clinical research PET programs generally have access to sophisticated cyclotron and radiochemistry facilities, although several stand-alone small animal imaging facilities are beginning to appear. The key to improving accessibility to PET tracers will be a network of radioisotope distributors for medium and longer lived isotopes, particularly fluorine-18, and automated tracer synthesis modules that can be programmed to produce a wide range of tracers. These developments will depend on the continued clinical growth of PET and the development of tracers other than FDG for clinical use. Despite the inherent limitations for gaining access to positron-emitting tracers, most major neuroscience research centers in Northern America, Europe, and Japan already have access to positron-emitting radionuclides.

9.9 CONCLUSIONS

It is also important to acknowledge that the use of PET for neuroscience research will always have significant limitations despite the exciting technology. The limits of resolution of even the best scanners proposed will not allow for highly detailed functional analyses of small subregions of the rodent brain, such as differentiating between nuclei in the amygdala or dentate gyrus from CA1, unless these subregions are known to have completely differential uptakes of a particular tracer. Due to limits of both sensitivity and spatial resolution, it is also unlikely that the technology will reach the point where single cells or small groups (such as a few transplanted neural stem cells) will be visualizable *in vivo*. Other factors, such as relatively high cost, the need to use and shield radioisotopes, and the extensive training of qualified personnel will also place some limitations on the use of rodent PET scanners.

Successful use of PET will require that the technology be used wisely, addressing those questions for which it is well suited, and recognizing when other approaches are better employed. PET can provide unique information in the basic and translational neurosciences in many areas and we expect its use to grow. Although previous work in rodents focused on a few tracers under a limited range of conditions, future work will greatly broaden the number of biological molecules and disease conditions that will be visualizable in the brain *in vivo*.

REFERENCES

1. Cherry, S.R. and Phelps, M.E., Imaging brain function with positron emission tomography, in *Brain Mapping: The Methods*, 1st ed., Toga, A.W. and Mazziotta, J. C., Eds., Academic Press, San Diego, 1996, p. 191.
2. McCarthy, T.J. and Welch, M.J., The state of positron emitting radionuclide production in 1997, *Sem. Nucl. Med.*, 28, 235, 1998.
3. Fowler, J. S. and Wolf, A.P., Positron emitter-labeled compounds: priorities and problems, in *Positron Emission Tomography and Autoradiography*, Phelps, M., Mazziotta, J., and Schelbert, H., Eds., Raven Press, New York, 1986, p. 391.
4. Gambhir, S.S. et al., Imaging transgene expression with radionuclide imaging technologies, *Neoplasia* 2, 118, 2000.
5. Hume, S.P., Gunn, R.N., and Jones, T., Pharmacological constraints associated with positron emission tomographic scanning of small laboratory animals, *Eur. J. Nucl. Med.*, 25, 173, 1998.
6. Huang, S.-C. and Phelps, M.E., Principles of tracer kinetic modeling in positron emission tomography and autoradiography, in *Positron Emission Tomography and Autoradiography*, Phelps, M., Mazziotta, J., and Schelbert, H., Eds., Raven Press, New York, 1986, p. 287.
7. Cherry, S.R. and Phelps, M.E., Positron emission tomography: methods and instrumentation, in *Diagnostic Nuclear Medicine*, 3rd ed., Sandler, M.P. et al., Eds., Williams & Wilkins, Baltimore, 1996, p. 139.
8. Hoffman, E.J. et al., Quantitation in positron emission computed tomography 4. Effect of accidental coincidences, *J. Comput. Assisted Tomogr.*, 5, 391, 1981.
9. Burns, H.D. et al., Positron emission tomography neuroreceptor imaging as a tool in drug discovery, research and development, *Curr. Opin. Chem. Biol.*, 3, 388, 1999.
10. Fowler, J.S. et al., PET and drug research and development, *J. Nucl. Med.*, 40, 1154, 1999.
11. Tai, Y.-C. et al., Performance evaluation of the microPET P4: a PET system dedicated to animal imaging, *Phys. Med. Biol.*, 46, 1845, 2001.
12. Watanabe, M. et al., A high resolution animal PET scanner using compact PS-PMT detectors, *IEEE Trans. Nucl. Sci.*, 47, 1277, 1997.

13. Bloomfield, P.M. et al., Design and physical characteristics of a small animal positron emission tomograph, *Phys. Med. Biol.,* 40, 1105, 1995.
14. Hume, S.P. et al., The potential of high-resolution positron emission tomography to monitor striatal dopaminergic function in rat models of disease, *J. Neurosci. Methods,* 67, 103, 1996.
15. Cherry, S.R. et al., MicroPET: a high resolution PET scanner for imaging small animals, *IEEE Trans. Nucl. Sci.* 44, 1161, 1997.
16. Del Guerra, A. et al., High spatial resolution small animal YAP-PET, *Nucl. Instruments Methods,* 409, 508, 1998.
17. Lecomte, R. et al., Initial results from the Sherbrooke avalanche photodiode positron tomograph, *IEEE Trans. Nucl. Sci.,* 43, 1952, 1996.
18. Weber, S. et al., The design of an animal PET: flexible geometry for achieving optimal spatial resolution or high sensitivity, *IEEE Trans. Med.* Imaging, 16, 684, 1997.
19. Ziegler, S.I. et al., A prototype high-resolution animal positron tomograph with avalanche photodiode arrays and LSO crystals, *Eur. J. Nucl.* Med., 28, 136, 2001.
20. Chatziioannou, A. et al., Detector development for microPET II: a 1 μl resolution PET scanner for small animal imaging, *Phys. Med. Biol.,* 46, 2899, 2001.
21. Correia, J.A. et al., Development of a small animal PET imaging device with resolution approaching 1 mm, *IEEE Trans. Nucl. Imaging,* 46, 631, 1999.
22. Miyaoka, R.S., Kohlmyer, S.G., and Lewellen, T.K., Performance characteristics of micro crystal element (MiCE) detectors, *IEEE Trans. Nucl.* Sci., 48, 1403, 2001.
23. Jeavons, A.P., Chandler, R.A., and Dettmar, C.A.R., A three-dimensional HIDAC-PET camera with sub-millimetre resolution for imaging small animals, *IEEE Trans. Nucl. Sci.,* 46, 468, 1999.
24. Chatziioannou, A.F. et al., Performance evaluation of microPET: a high-resolution lutetium oxyorthosilicate PET scanner for animal imaging, *J. Nucl. Med.,* 40, 1164, 1999.
25. Qi, J. et al., High-resolution three-dimensional Bayesian image reconstruction using the microPET small-animal scanner, *Phys. Med. Biol.,* 43, 1001, 1998.
26. Kennedy, C. et al., Mapping of functional neural pathways by autoradiographic survey of local metabolic rate with (^{14}C)deoxyglucose, *Science,* 187, 850, 1975.
27. Schwartz, W.J. et al., Metabolic mapping of functional activity in the hypothalamo-neurohypophysial system of the rat, *Science,* 205, 723, 1979.
28. Greer, C.A. et al., Topographical and laminar localization of two-dimensionaleoxy-glucose uptake in rat olfactory bulb induced by electrical stimulation of olfactory nerves, *Brain Res.,* 217, 279, 1981.
29. Bruehl, C. and Witte, O.W., Cellular activity underlying altered brain metabolism during focal epileptic activity, *Ann. Neurol.,* 38, 414, 1995.
30. Engel, J., Jr. et al., Interictal cerebral glucose metabolism in partial epilepsy and its relation to EEG changes, *Ann. Neurol.,* 12, 510, 1982.
31. Mazziotta, J.C. et al., Reduced cerebral glucose metabolism in asymptomatic subjects at risk for Huntington's disease, *New Engl. J. Med.,* 316, 357, 1987.
32. Small, G.W. et al., Apolipoprotein E type 4 allele and cerebral glucose metabolism in relatives at risk for familial Alzheimer's disease, *JAMA,* 273, 942, 1995.
33. Silverman, D.H. and Small, G.W., Usefulness of positron emission tomography in evaluating dementia, JAMA, 287, 985, 2002.
34. Doyle, W.K. et al., Differentiation of cerebral radiation necrosis from tumor recurrence by [^{18}F]FDG and ^{82}Rb positron emission tomography, *J. Comput. Assisted Tomogr.,* 11, 563, 1987.

35. Fox, P.T., Burton, H., and Raichle, M.E., Mapping human somatosensory cortex with positron emission tomography, *J. Neurosurg.*, 67, 34, 1987.
36. Grafton, S.T. et al., Localization of motor areas adjacent to arteriovenous malformations: a positron emission tomographic study, *J. Neuroimaging*, 4, 97, 1994.
37. Barrio, J. R., Huang, S.C., and Phelps, M.E., Biological imaging and the molecular basis of dopaminergic diseases, *Biochem. Pharmacol.*, 54, 341, 1997.
38. Spencer, D.D. et al., Unilateral transplantation of human fetal mesencephalic tissue into the caudate nucleus of patients with Parkinson's disease, *New Engl. J. Med.*, 327, 1541, 1992.
39. Dietrich, W.D. et al., Metabolic alterations in rat somatosensory cortex following unilateral vibrissal removal, *J. Neurosci.*, 5, 874, 1985.
40. Hovda, D.A. et al., Cerebral metabolism following neonatal or adult hemineodecortication in cats: I. Effects on glucose metabolism using [^{14}C]2-deoxy-D-glucose autoradiography, *J. Cereb. Blood Flow Metabol.*, 16, 134, 1996.
41. Kornblum, H.I. et al., *In vivo* imaging of neuronal activation and plasticity in the rat brain by high resolution positron emission tomography (microPET), *Nature Biotechnol.*, 18, 655, 2000.
42. Bergsneider, M. et al., Cerebral hyperglycolysis following severe traumatic brain injury in humans: a positron emission tomography study, *J. Neurosurg.*, 86, 241, 1997.
43. Moore, T.H. et al., Quantitative assessment of longitudinal metabolic changes *in vivo* after traumatic brain injury in the adult rat using FDG-microPET, *J. Cereb. Blood Flow Metabol.*, 20, 1492, 2000.
44. Brownell, A.L. et al., *In vivo* PET imaging in rat of dopamine terminals reveals functional neural transplants, *Ann. Neurol.*, 43, 387, 1998.
45. Bjorklund, L.M. et al., Embryonic stem cells develop into functional dopaminergic neurons after transplantation in a Parkinson rat model, *Proc. Natl. Acad. Sci. U.S.A.*, 99, 2344, 2002.
46. Bates, G.P., Mangiarini, L., and Davies, S.W., Transgenic mice in the study of polyglutamine repeat expansion diseases, *Brain Pathol.*, 8, 699, 1998.
47. Araujo, D.M. et al., Deficits in striatal dopamine D(2) receptors and energy metabolism detected by *in vivo* microPET imaging in a rat model of Huntington's disease, *Exp. Neurol.*, 166, 287, 2000.
48. Tjuvajev, J.G. et al., Imaging herpes virus thymidine kinase gene transfer and expression by positron emission tomography, *Cancer Res.*, 58, 4333, 1998.
49. Gambhir, S.S. et al., Imaging adenoviral-directed reporter gene expression in living animals with positron emission tomography, *Proc. Natl. Acad. Sci. U.S.A.*, 96, 2333, 1999.
50. MacLaren, D.C. et al., Repetitive, non-invasive imaging of the dopamine D2 receptor as a reporter gene in living animals, *Gene Ther.*, 6, 785, 1999.

10 MRI and Novel Contrast Agents for Molecular Imaging

Michel M. Modo and Steven C.R. Williams

CONTENTS

10.1 INTRODUCTION

Mapping biological processes involved in development and pathology was largely confined to postmortem histological examinations or *in vitro* experimentation of cellular events. The ability to probe biological processes and anatomies of living systems was, to say the least, limited. The recent development of imaging technologies such as magnetic resonance imaging (MRI) that can scrutinize soft living tissue (such as brain and muscle) has allowed the investigation of anatomical structures and biological processes *in vivo*. Examination of the temporal progression of development and pathology will undoubtedly enhance our understanding of how structural changes relate to functional development and/or impairment. For example, in humans, the use of MRI and related imaging techniques has greatly enhanced our ability to diagnose a variety of pathologies.

The search for surrogate markers of disease requires investigation of the basic biological processes that lead to pathology. This search will involve molecular imaging technology — a technique that can monitor time-dependent molecular and cellular events in intact living organisms (Weissleder, 1999, Weissleder and Mahmood, 2001, Phelps, 2000). The techniques described in this chapter have the potential to probe these biological processes in human subjects and animal models of pathology.

Due to the recent proliferation of MRI procedures as clinical tools in diagnostic radiology, MRI has been applied primarily to human subjects. Humans do not require the same degree of spatial resolution necessary to image smaller animals, but ongoing hardware improvements have increased spatial resolution to a point where most imaging techniques are now well suited for the experimental investigation of animals (Chatham and Blackband, 2001, Krishna et al., 2001, Cherry and Gambhir, 2001, Green et al., 2001, Johnson et al., 1993). One advantage of preclinical studies is that controlled experimentation yields imaged tissue for subsequent, corroborative histological examination.

A wide variety of imaging techniques such as positron emission tomography (PET), computer tomography (CT), and single photon emission computed tomography (SPECT) are now used in addition to MRI to probe biological processes in laboratory animals (Green et al., 2001, Jacobs and Cherry, 2001, Balaban and Hampshire, 2001) These methods provide new information about intact organisms in three dimensions and unique data on the temporal evolution of this information (the fourth dimension). However, the important differences among the imaging techniques outlined herein make them apposite for different applications (Table 10.1).

10.2 MAGNETIC RESONANCE IMAGING OF MOLECULAR AND CELLULAR EVENTS

Recent work suggests that some of the most versatile molecular imaging methods may be developed from nuclear magnetic resonance (NMR) imaging. Increases in magnetic field strength and continued hardware improvements increased the spatial resolution obtainable by MRI. A recent article reported in-plane spatial resolution of approximately 1 μm (Lee et al., 2001). Such high spatial resolution MR imaging led to the development of an MR microscope to perform *in vivo* histology (Johnson et al., 1993). Such technology also offers dynamic information that provides a great advantage over *ex vivo* histology in the longitudinal study of biological events.

Two major challenges must be addressed as molecular imaging aims to investigate molecular or cellular events in intact tissues. First, the monitoring of molecular or cellular events requires *specificity* for the particular biological event (e.g., an antibody conjugated to a contrast agent allowing exclusive visualization of a particular receptor). Second, a hardware system that achieves enough *sensitivity* to detect a biological event is essential. MRI may afford satisfactory visualization (sensitivity)

TABLE 10.1
Molecular Imaging: Advantages and Disadvantages of Different Techniques

Technique	Advantages	Disadvantages
NMR-based		
MRI	High spatial resolution; noninvasive; high temporal resolution	No metabolic information; poor quantification; specificity
fMRI	Metabolic information; regional activity; noninvasive	Poor spatial resolution; poor quantification; specificity
MRS	Noninvasive; metabolic information; specificity	Poor spatial resolution; poor temporal resolution
EPR	Noninvasive; high spatial resolution; specificity	No metabolic information; poor temporal resolution
CT	Widely available; high spatial resolution	Radiation; poor temporal resolution
PET	Metabolic information; high specificity	Poor spatial resolution; invasive; on-site cyclotron
SPECT	High specificity	Poor spatial resolution; invasive; on-site cyclotron
Ultrasonography	Specificity; noninvasive; high temporal resolution	Limited depth penetration; limited specificity; poor spatial resolution
Two-photon microscopy	High resolution; high temporal resolution; freely moving animals	Craniectomy; limited depth; limited specificity
Confocal microscopy	High specificity; high spatial resolution	Mainly tissue sections; limited depth penetration; *in vitro* and *ex vivo* only

and discrimination (specificity) of such events via high resolution, contrast-enhanced imaging.

The hardware used for magnetic resonance imaging can be tailored to generate high spatial resolution images (magnetic resonance microscopy), provide information about the spatial distribution of particular metabolites (magnetic resonance spectroscopy), and localize functions (functional magnetic resonance imaging). Image acquisition protocols can be tailored to provide information about blood flow changes and differentiation between tissue types. No other current imaging technique can provide this diversity of information from the same hardware configuration.

The generation of contrast is essential in imaging and allows differentiation of the tissue, pathology, or function of interest. The discrimination of different types of tissue by MRI is dependent on the different physical characteristics of the imaged protons due to their local environment. Following radiofrequency excitation, the differential rate of return (relaxation) to equilibrium for white matter, gray matter, and cerebrospinal fluid (CSF) facilitates discrimination of tissue types (Figure 10.1) (Rattle, 1995, Tóth et al., 2001).

The discrimination of particular biological events can be enhanced by exogenously administered contrast agents. The most common type of contrast agent in neurological MRI is a lipophobic/hydrophilic compound that does not normally cross

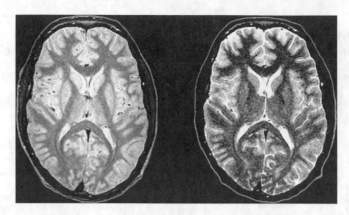

FIGURE 10.1 Natural contrast inherent within an axial MR image of the human head. Contrast can be obtained between the white and gray matter and cerebrospinal fluid by subtle manipulation of the timings of radiofrequency excitation and detection of the ensuing echo. The image on the left is regarded as a proton density (short echo time) image with good contrast between the darker (white matter) and the rest of the head, whereas the image on the right is deemed a T_2-weighted (long echo) scan with good contrast between the csf (bright) and the parenchyma. Both images were acquired simultaneously from the same subject and allow good delineation of brain anatomy without the need for contrast agents.

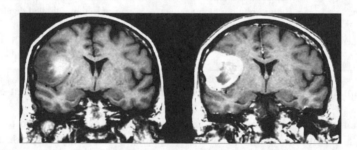

FIGURE 10.2 Contrast-enhanced MRI of a brain tumor before and after Gd-DTPA (Magnevist) administration. Although it is possible to differentiate certain tissue types and lesions by particular scanning sequences, further delineation can be gained by administration of MR contrast agents. Intravenous administration of an exogenous MR contrast agent makes it possible to alter the water relaxation characteristics in a region where the agent has leaked though a permeable brain barrier. In this case, the edges of a primary glioma are enhanced following the contrast injection (right), thus providing invaluable information to the oncologist and neurosurgeon.

the intact blood–brain barrier. In certain cases where the barrier is compromised, e.g., acute multiple sclerosis and brain tumors, the agent leaks into the brain and causes changes in the relaxation characteristics of the water protons as shown in Figure 10.2. Despite this rather crude specificity, such agents have been adopted widely in the clinic. We expect the combined specificity gained from increasingly sophisticated contrast agents and the improvements in spatial resolution (sensitivity) to render molecular MRI an increasingly attractive tool to neuroscientists.

10.3 DESIGNING NOVEL CONTRAST AGENTS

Several issues must be addressed in the design of novel contrast agents, notably safety, tolerance, and the specificity of image contrast.

10.3.1 SAFETY AND TOLERABILITY

Magnetic resonance imaging is a safe noninvasive technique, although the application of exogenous contrast agents to highlight specific biological processes or tissues requires an invasive procedure to administer the contrast agent. Furthermore, MR contrast agents generally involve the use of metal particles that are potentially toxic to cells. This toxicity must be minimized to prevent iatrogenic (treatment-induced) diseases such as renal nephropathies (Brücher and Sherry, 2001, Ray et al., 1996, Runge, 2000, 2001).

To determine the toxicity of a contrast agent, animal studies investigating possible side effects and toxicity are imperative preclinical determinants of how a compound will affect human beings. However, a direct extrapolation from animal to human data demands caution and should follow the parallel assessment procedure required in the development of novel pharmaceuticals (i.e., verification of results in at least two species by independent laboratories). For experimental studies with animals, the toxicity of contrast agents is perhaps less an immediate concern from the viewpoint of subject safety, but it is still important to minimize side effects that may confound experimental observations.

10.3.2 Ideal Contrast Agents

An ideal contrast agent is easy to synthesize, incurs low production costs, has low toxicity and low immunogenicity, is consistent in its mode of contrast, and is stable over time (see Table 10.2. for factors to be considered). The relaxation characteristics of a contrast agent should be strong enough to provide a high contrast-to-particle ratio to minimize the volume of the compound to be administered and reduce the amount of potentially toxic metal introduced to the organism (reduction of toxicity and increase in sensitivity). It is also important to consider whether the compound produces a negative charge (cleared through the kidneys), positive charge (accumulated in the heart), or neutral charge (necessary to cross the blood–brain barrier), to influence the *in vivo* behaviors of compounds (Anelli and Lattuada, 2001, Jacques and Desreux, 2001, Reichert et al., 1999, Reichert and Welch, 2001). Likewise, lipophilicity and hydrophilicity will also determine the types of tissues that will absorb the contrast agent. For instance, lipophobic contrast agents will not cross an intact blood–brain barrier.

Another desirable characteristic of metal particles used for contrast agents is the ability to bind with high affinity to other compounds such as dextran or albumin. Most ligands binding Gd^{3+} (gadolinium) form eight coordinate complexes, whereas

TABLE 10.2
Factors for Consideration in Designing Novel Contrast Agents

How easy is it to reliably synthesize the contrast agent?
What is the toxicity of the contrast agent?
How stable is the contrast agent over time?
What is the charge of the contrast agent?
What is the size/molecular weight of the contrast agent?
What system clears the contrast agent from the body?
What is the relaxivity of the contrast agent?
Is the contrast agent hydrophilic or lipophilic?
Does the contrast agent provoke an immune response?
How easily does the contrast agent cross the endothelial wall?
Does the contrast agent have any side effects?
Does the contrast agent cross the blood–brain barrier?
What is the range of applications of the contrast agent?
What is the most effective imaging protocol?
What is the best route of administration?
How much contrast agent is needed to produce a satisfactory signal change?

binding of Mn^{2+} (manganese) and Fe^{3+} (iron) forms six coordinate complexes. By forming robust, high stability complexes with a metal, it is possible to dramatically lower an agent's toxicity and increase circulation time in the blood stream. The metal particles function as contrast agents by increasing the relaxation rate of the imaged proton in the water molecules in the vicinity of the contrast agent. The observed contrast signal (R_{obs}) is the product of the outer sphere R_2 relaxivity (complex-based) and the inner sphere R_1 relaxivity (metal-based). The ligand used to bind the metal particles plays an important role indicating the main mechanism of relaxation, but major increases in the sensitivity of MR contrast agents are mainly influenced by inner sphere relaxivity conveyed by the magnetic properties of the metal particles (Reichert et al., 1999, Tóth et al., 2001).

A wide variety of contrast agents using metal particles mainly complexed with dextran are now available. The advantages of dextran-based over albumin-based contrast agents include good tolerance (i.e., lower toxicity), unlikely contamination by blood-borne infectious agents (a problem of albumin-based compounds), and better control over final molecular size (Wang et al., 1990). Controlling the size of the contrast agent is an important aspect of design. If a contrast agent is too large, it can cause ischemia by blocking the vasculature or reducing glomerular filtration through the kidneys leading to unacceptable renal side effects.

The tissue penetration of contrast agents is influenced by size. Larger compounds remain in the blood stream longer (Weissleder et al., 2001). A particle that is too small will perfuse into the parenchyma faster than a larger molecule, but larger molecules are more likely to be targets of the immune system or reticuloendothelial system (RES). Contrast agents in blood are removed by the RES which transports the contrast agent mainly through the liver or kidneys where it is cleared from the body (Tweedle et al., 1995).

Low immunogenicity is required to prevent phagocytosis of the contrast agent by immune effector cells such as macrophages. In some cases, phagocytic activity is a desirable property, as incorporation of the contrast agent into macrophages allows imaging of the infiltration of immune effector cells to central nervous system (CNS) lesions (Rausch et al., 2001, Zhang et al., 2000). Undesirable characteristics of a contrast agent for one application might be desirable for another.

Since the signal characteristics of a contrast agent are determined in part by the amount of bound water, the *in situ* relaxivity will change, depending on the water content of the surrounding tissue. The relaxivity of a contrast agent will be different in the blood and the parenchyma. To optimize the detection and hence the possibility of reducing the amount of contrast agent needed to produce a signal change, it is important to determine how the relaxivity characteristics will change depending on tissue localization of the agent. It is also appropriate to determine the temporal sequence of the relaxivity characteristics, since it may be possible to apply the same contrast agent to visualize different phenomena in longitudinal studies (e.g., soon after administration to increase the detection of the vasculature and at later time points as an enhancer of liver tissue).

10.3.3 RECENT DEVELOPMENTS

Materials that modulate signal contrast in MRI can be paramagnetic (weakly attracted to magnetic fields; unpaired electrons act as small magnets that align when a magnetic field is applied), ferromagnetic (individual magnetic moments align to produce larger overall local magnetic moment), or superparamagnetic (magnetic moments align within individual particles and produce very strong paramagnetic effects) (Rattle, 1995).

Contrast agents generally contain transition metals, such as Mn, Fe, Co, Ni, and Cu, or lanthanides, such as Eu, Gd, Tb, and Dy (Anelli and Lattuada, 2001, Jacques and Desreux, 2001, Muller et al., 2001, Reichert et al., 1999, Reichert and Welch, 2001). Due to its high relaxivity and relative safety, Gd is the most common contrast-generating particle (Roberts et al., 2000). A variety of Gd-based contrast agents are now used in experimental and clinical settings. Gd-DTPA (Magnevist) was the first widely available agent and played an important role in the contrast agent-mediated diagnosis of developing lesions and tumors of the CNS.

Several varieties of Gd-based contrast agents are under development. These complexes range in size from nanoparticles for rapid liver uptake (Reynolds et al., 2000) to large dextran-coated particles that promote longer blood circulation times or increase *in vivo* stability (Wang et al., 1990, Corot et al., 2000, Aime et al., 2000a), allowing potential enhancement of magnetic resonance angiograms (MRA). Also, sophisticated combinations of gadolinium particles with fluorescent moieties, such as rhodamine, linked to dextran chains that allow insertion into cell membranes have recently been developed (Hüber et al., 1998).

A variety of Fe-based contrast agents are gaining popularity (Muller et al., 2001). Ultrasmall superparamagnetic iron oxide particles (USPIOs) have recently been used in imaging studies in which Gd-based contrast agents might not be as suitable. The lower toxicity of unbound iron (an essential biological element of a normal organism)

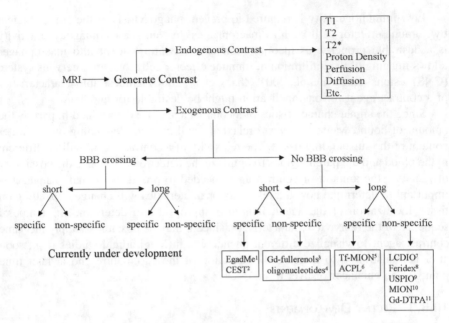

FIGURE 10.3 To detect different types of tissues or processes, MRI is dependent on the generation of a contrast that highlights a particular tissue type or process. Taking advantage of the different magnetic properties of certain biological processes or tissues, an endogenous contrast can be generated by MRI. The protocols used for the detection of different magnetic properties can also be generated by supplying exogenous contrast agents. Such agents typically shorten the T_1 (short relaxation time, short echo), T_2 (long excitation time, long echo), or more rarely the proton density (PD). To provide added contrast to brain tissue, these compounds must cross the blood–brain barrier. To date no contrast agent has been shown to cross the intact barrier, but current developments in contrast agent technology promise to provide novel compounds that might do so. [[1]Louie et al., 2000, [2]Ward et al., 2000, [3]Mikawa et al., 2001, [4]Hines et al., 1999, [5]Högemann et al., 2000, [6]Sipkins et al., 2000, [7]Moore et al., 2000, [8]Dubovitz, 2001, [9]Josephson et al., 1999, [10]Enochs et al., 1993, [11]Wang et al., 1990.]

compared to gadolinium is an attractive feature in studies where free metal could produce deleterious effects. Additionally, USPIOs have superparamagnetic effects and they can be used as T_2 contrast agents, whereas Gd is primarily used to modify T_1 signal contrast. Mikawa (2001) has indicated that paramagnetic water-soluble metallofullerenes provide greater changes in contrast than Gd-DTPA and might be attractive alternatives.

Novel contrast agents aim to provide better tissue differentiation, and at lower doses they may also provide greater specificity for a particular biological process. Apart from the chemical characteristics of the complex that affects the uptake and dispersion of the contrast agent, several targeting systems have been cited to achieve higher specificities. The conjugation of an antibody (geared toward a specific receptor or protein) with a contrast agent, such as monocrystalline iron oxide nanoparticles (MIONs), is believed to increase the specificity of the contrast agent (Högemann et al., 2000). The binding of antibodies to antigens is highly specific and therefore the generated contrast of a labeled antibody can provide a very efficient system to image a particular biological activity or distribution of proteins *in vivo*.

Furthermore, the widespread and well established immunohistochemical use of antibodies allows a direct and robust *ex vivo* cross-validation of *in vivo* imaging. A typical contrast agent requires a total of several thousand molecules of Gd-DTPA to provide a significant change in contrast. All amino acids of an antibody would be required to bind all of these molecules, rendering the antibody ineffective for binding to antigens (Unger et al., 1985). Perhaps, a more practical solution would be the use of polychelates of the contrast agent to bind to each labeling site (Sieving et al., 1999), thus maintaining the original binding properties of the antibody. These polychelates also show improved relaxivity compared to monomeric complexes (Reichert et al., 1999). The linking of polymeric compounds (Torchilin, 2000) with antibodies and different metal ions (Weissleder et al., 2001) shows great promise in experimental imaging. However, the large sizes of these constructs limit their effectiveness.

Targeting systems based on porphyrins (van Zijl et al., 1990), polysaccharides (Rongved and Laveness, 1991, Gibby et al., 1988), and oligonucleotides (Hines et al., 1999) might provide highly specific targeting systems while maintaining effective relaxivity despite their smaller size. A refinement of this targeting system uses antibody-conjugated paramagnetic liposomes (ACPL) to combine the properties of an MRI contrast agent, a specific antibody, and detection by fluorescence microscopy to visualize, for instance, the presence of adhesion molecules such as I-CAM on the surfaces of blood vessels (Sipkins et al., 2000). Further research endeavors that link different detection methods and increase the stability of such agents *in vivo* with different binding times may prove beneficial in our serial investigations of intact living systems. (Figure 10.3)

Another exciting development has been the use of antibody-conjugated MION contrast agent to image gene expression in transgenic animals (Högemann et al., 2000, Weissleder et al., 2000), thus demonstrating the potential of this system to screen transgenic animals for the particular localization of gene expression. To visualize gene expression without conjugation of an antibody to a metal ion, Louie et al. (2000) used a Gd-based contrast agent that produced a significant change in signal only if the compound binds to a particular gene product such as β-galactosidase. This "smart" contrast agent produces a more specific signal change compared to antibody-based contrast agents because the unbound smart contrast agent does not influence the MRI signal until it binds to the target protein. Although an antibody-based contrast agent can in principle provide high specificity, it may be compromised by concomitant signal contrast caused by unbound compounds in the blood circulation or freely moving in tissue without binding to a receptor. In comparison, the smart contrast agent will only produce a signal change if it binds to the target protein. A similar smart contrast agent that responds to intracellular Ca^{2+} has been described by Li et al. (1999).

The continued engineering of contrast agents for specific visualization of a biological process or environment will increase the ranges and applications of such imaging agents considerably. Recent developments in both MRI and contrast agent technology are on the brink of making huge impacts on our understanding of biological systems (Roberts et al., 2000).

10.4 APPLICATIONS OF MRI TO MOLECULAR IMAGING

Molecular imaging has provided information regarding cellular and molecular events in organisms during development, pathology, and treatment. Although the focus to date has been placed understandably on animal studies, the technology can be readily translated to humans, thus providing interspecies comparisons that can lead to substantive clinical benefits (Phelps, 2000).

10.4.1 NEURONAL DEVELOPMENT AND EMBRYOLOGY

Based on the different physical characteristics of different types of tissue, it is possible to develop an MR-based atlas of embryonic development (Figure 10.4). Dhenain et al. (2001) reported the creation of the first interactive MR-based atlas of mouse development differentiating bones, soft tissues, and arteries. Clearly, the use of such an atlas of development will be of paramount importance in characterizations of transgenic animals and allow us to understand the influences of certain genes in development (Smith et al., 1994, Beckmann, 2001, Budinger et al., 1999). No report to date has covered the application of repeated MRI to study the development of transgenic animals and a relationship to functional or physiological impairments. We believe that the ability of MRI to image a complete animal and hence probe all organs will provide biologists with important new tools in the comprehensive investigation of mammalian development.To understand how organisms develop, it is essential to perform repeated investigations of the same organism as it grows and magnetic resonance imaging is ideally suited to this task. To date, most imaging research of development has focused on chick growth by using optical techniques that penetrate eggshells. However, optical imaging does not effectively reveal the three-dimensional nature of development. The use of high field strength (17.5 T) magnets led to characterization of the development of the chick vasculature (Smith et al., 1992, Hogers et al., 2001). Recent successful efforts in imaging mouse development suggest that further research into mammalian development by MRI will ensue. For example, the noninvasive nature of MRI allowed the repeated imaging of mouse and rat development *in utero* (Hoydu et al., 2000, Smith et al., 1998a).

To probe the contributions of different neuronal populations to embryonic development, Jacobs and Fraser (1994) labeled a population of embryonic stem cells with a dextran-linked gadolinium contrast agent that was stably inserted into cell membranes before implanting the prelabeled cells into a developing frog embryo. The contrast agent allowed them to visualize how the labeled population contributed to the formation of different regions of the frog embryo. Investigating the influence of particular homeobox genes such as *Pax-6* in chimeric animals is well-suited for the *in vivo* investigation of how these genes and particular progenitor populations contribute to organogenesis (Hogan, 1999). Insertion of a reporter gene, such as lac Z, whose expression will be linked to the activation of a gene of interest, could be used

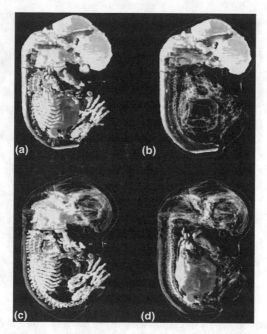

FIGURE 10.4 Three-dimensional "virtual mouse" embryo created from a volumetric *ex vivo* MR microscopic investigation. The computer model allows segmentation of all organs (a), the CNS (b), skeletal system (c), or a combination of systems (d). The ability to derive computer models of embryonic development and annotate these atlases will greatly benefit researchers investigating the influence of nature-versus-nurture developmental growth. (Adapted from Dhenain, M. et al., 2001. With permission.) See Color Figure 10.4 following page 210.

to image the spatial distribution and expression of a particular gene by using smart contrast agents, such as EgadMe (Louie et al., 2000, Figure 10.5). The conditionality of this contrast agent, based on the presence of the reporter gene lac Z, can be used as a surrogate marker for the expression of a particular gene linked to the expression of β-galactosidase. Since traditional histological methods exist to probe the expression of lac Z, corroborative evidence can be gained regarding the accuracy of the MRI detection of gene expression.

The combination of antibodies with contrast agents allows mapping of the temporal and spatial distribution of particular receptors or proteins in developing and adult organisms. Weissleder et al. (2000) described the visualization of the transgene expression of engineered transferrin receptors (ETRs) in transplanted tumors in mice by means of MION-conjugated antibodies against the ETRs. Optimization of targeted contrast agents geared toward a particular gene expression by bioengineering of novel chelating compounds and maximizing the relaxivities of these materials are important aspects in the development of novel *in vivo* molecular imaging strategies (Jacobs et al., 1999, Högemann et al., 2000, Bogdanov et al., 2001).

In utero imaging will also aid in the evaluation of a variety of pharmaceutical compounds and contrast agents for safe use during pregnancy. To determine the

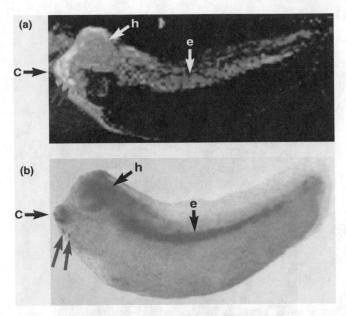

FIGURE 10.5 Detecting gene expression by MRI. The upper image (a) demonstrates a significant MR signal contrast change due to the presence of the smart contrast agent, EgadMe. This agent differentiates structures developed from cells modified to express the reporter gene lac Z from cells that did not carry the gene. The lower image (b) validates the presence of lac Z expression by traditional bright field histology. (Adapted from Louie, A.Y. et al., *Nature Biotechnol.*, 18, 321, 2000. With permission.) See Color Figure 10.5 following page 210.

effects of MR imaging and the use of contrast agents during embryonic and fetal development, a series of studies examined the exposure of laboratory animals to the stress of MR acoustic noise, exposure to high magnetic field strength, and potential toxicity of MR contrast agents (Magin et al., 2000). The development of *in vitro* MRI offers the possibility to directly investigate the more subtle effects of MRI on cells and its influence on the proliferation, altered gene expression, and maturation of different cell populations under various conditions involving exposure to magnetic fields (Magin et al., 2000, Rodegerdts et al., 2000).

With recent increases in spatial resolution due primarily to hardware improvements, studies using MRI can now be performed on *in vitro* samples. The development of a "hybrid" MRI microscope with an incubation chamber will provide the necessary hardware to probe three-dimensional cell aggregates such as neurospheres *in situ*. It will be possible also to investigate how both environmental and genetic manipulations can influence the formation and the structural integrity of such cells. A similar set-up can also be used to map developing embryos. We foresee that MR imaging can be performed continuously while embryos grow in incubation chambers.

A series of studies demonstrated the possibility of investigating single cells by MRI at a spatial resolution of approximately 10 μm (Aguayo et al., 1986, Schoeninger et al., 1994, Hsu et al., 1997), and by MRS (Posse and Aue., 1989, Grant et al., 2000). The possibility of obtaining spatial resolution required to image a single cell can provide important insights for tissue engineering. It will be possible to study how cells integrate into a matrix that forms biological tissue in a manner akin to current studies employing confocal microscopy (Thomas and White, 1998). Furthermore, the application of MRS simultaneously on the same sample can provide information about the metabolic status of the sample. As these studies can be performed *in vitro*, it will be possible to exert complete experimental control.

10.4.2 TRACT TRACING

In vivo assessment of axonal projections beyond the basic differentiation between gray and white matter has until recently proved to be elusive. One approach that involves adminstration of contrast agents transported in a anterograde (away from the cell body) or retrograde (in the direction of the cell body) manner along the axon allows the labeling of particular projection tracts connecting two distinct regions within the brain. An early study by Enochs et al. (1993) demonstrated that fluorescently tagged MION particles are transported bidirectionally (i.e., anterograde or retrograde transport depending on particle uptake at the cell body or synaptic cleft, respectively) with a 5 mm/day transport of particles along the axons. However, this study demonstrated tract tracing in the peripheral nervous system and is limited in its application to studying the brain because the contrast agent does not cross the blood–brain barrier. Nevertheless, it is possible to directly inject contrast agents into the brain parenchyma at sites of synaptic uptake to label projections.

Studies using manganese (Mn^{2+}) chloride indicate that tract tracing by contrast agent-enhanced MRI is also feasible. For instance, Pautler et al. (1998) traced the olfactory and visual pathways in rats by administering manganese that demonstrated selective change in T_1 relaxivity in neuronal tracts. Watanabe et al. (2001) mapped retinal projections from rat eyes using three-dimensional gradient-echo MRI. Manganese tract tracing has also been performed in nonhuman primates. Saleem et al. (2002) revealed sequential connections between the striatum and pallidum–substantia nigra leading to the thalamus. These data suggest that manganese is transported over at least one synapse *in vivo*. Therefore, important insights into lesion development in, for example, animal models of Parkinson's disease, in which the connections between substantia nigra and striatum are gradually lost, could ensue from manganese-enhanced imaging.

Manganese can trace axonal pathways and allows visualization of functional areas since it is taken up primarily by active cells which then transport it down the axonal projection to a connected area. Manganese-enhanced magnetic resonance imaging (MEMRI) permitted van der Linden (2002) to identify the vocal centers responsible for song in starlings. Pautler and Koretsky (2002) differentiated selective areas of the mouse olfactory bulb that respond to a variety of smells. Functional tract tracing via manganese administration will provide further insights into functional connections of different pathways involved in behavioral activities. Concerns remain regarding possible side effects of manganese (such as neurotoxicity) and investigations are limited to preclinical investigations (Ashner and Ashner, 1991). Possible new chelates of manganese that isolate exposure of the metal to organisms may make MEMRI-based methods interesting new vistas for human studies.

We must not forget parallel developments in diffusion tensor imaging (DTI) that also provide new opportunities to visualize pathways in the living brain noninvasively. Although this technique has been primarily used in human brain studies, it is used increasingly to answer basic biological questions. Combined with three-dimensional reconstructions, DTI provides a method to study different projection systems *in situ* without exogenously administered contrast agents. Xue et al. (1999) obtained three-dimensional representations of the eight major projection systems (genu and splenium of the corpus callosum, internal and external capsule, fimbria, anterior commissure, optic tract, and stria terminalis) in living rats within 2 hours of scanning, thus proving the applicability of DTI to tract tracing in animal studies.

We believe that these studies will provide invaluable information in the assessment of functional networks within the living brain. We can foresee that different behavioral tasks can be used to elicit activity of functional circuitry which could be complemented by tract tracing between functionally related areas. This would provide a better understanding of how the brain engages an integrative system aimed at solving particular tasks. Likewise, the effects of lesions could not only be assessed within the framework of a particular damaged area, but it would be possible to determine how damage to a particular area will impact functional networks.

10.4.3 IMAGING BRAIN DAMAGE

The most common application of MRI today is the noninvasive assessment of the CNS. Apart from the morphological changes associated with brain damage, changes in the signal characteristics of the lesion and surrounding tissue provide an opportunity to visualize an insult *in vivo*. A variety of MR imaging protocols have been developed to assess different aspects of brain damage.

Among the most commonly studied animal models of brain damage are rodent models of stroke. Rat models of stroke are believed to model accurately the proximal pathogenesis of a human focal ischemic lesion. Different MR imaging protocols take advantage of changes in the endogenous contrast produced by the ischemic tissue to visualize different aspects of the pathogenesis. Different protocols are useful at different stages of lesion evolution and can delineate certain aspects of an ischaemic insult. For instance, a T_2-weighted imaging protocol allows delineation of vasogenic edema about 4 hours after focal ischemia in rats (about 3 to 6 hours in humans), but will not be particularly helpful at earlier times (Hoehn et al., 2001). Also, perfusion imaging at an early stage can help delineate ischemic regions that will progress to infarctions in the absence of therapeutic intervention (van Doersten et al., 2002). A combination of *in vivo* MRI lesion assessment and *ex vivo* immunohistochemistry can help identify aspects of a pathogenic event revealed by a particular imaging protocol (Schroeter et al., 2001). Imaging may also yield surrogate markers for functional recovery (Rijnjtes and Weiller, 2002). Virley et al. (2000) demonstrated that impairments on the staircase test (which probes unilateral neglect) were primarily due to damage of the ipsilateral lower parietal cortex. This study also demonstrated the ability of serial MRI investigations to track changes in the ischemic brain from the progression of edema to necrosis and subsequent cavitation.

It is also possible to correlate behavioral deficits with changes in brain activity as assessed by a combination of functional MRI and histological analyses. A recent study by Tuor et al. (2001) demonstrated that activation of sensory motor areas by electrical forepaw stimulation was dramatically impaired at 4 months postischemia and that general behavioral performance also correlated negatively with the extent of ischemic brain damage. A recent report indicates that plasticity of adjacent ipsilateral regions and the contralateral homologue region of the infarct are fundamental to recovery of forelimb impairment (Dijkhuizen et al., 2001).

Sauter et al. (2002) indicated that treatment of ischemic animals with isradipine is cytoprotective and preserves proper activation of ipsilateral and contralateral activation of somatosensory areas by electrical forepaw stimulation. A consolidation approach by Harris et al. (2001) advocated the integration of several imaging modalities (including fMRI) to probe dysfunction after ischaemic damage in order to provide important insights into processes involved in lesion development including the potential prediction of functional outcome (Jacobs et al., 2001). In brief, the use of endogenous contrast methods, and especially the use of BOLD-based fMRI techniques under development for the objective assessment of functional impairment and recovery may be applied to patient management.

The use of exogeneous contrast agents can also provide an important avenue of information regarding ischemic brain damage, but care must be taken to limit possible side effects. In rare circumstances, Gd-based contrast agents can worsen neurological deficits and lesion volume due to the neurotoxicity of the unbound metal (Takahashi et al., 1996, Ray et al., 1996). Iron-based contrast agents such as USPIO may provide an attractive alternative without deleterious effects (Doerfler et al., 2000). The breakdown of the blood–brain barrier after some ischemic insults allows ingression of such contrast media into the locale of damaged tissue and can therefore provide enhanced detection of the infarct and surrounding area. de Crespigny et al. (2000) [based on pioneering work by Hopkins et al. (1991)] demonstrated that ^{17}O-enriched water acts as a T_2 shortening contrast agent that can be used to determine lesion location as reliably as diffusion and Gd-DTPA perfusion images. This approach highlights a potentially less toxic, freely diffusible contrast agent that might provide an attractive alternative to more conventional contrast media-enhanced imaging of ischemic lesions.

To determine the location of an embolus or thrombus causing an ischemic infarction, an MR angiogram may help detect changes in major vessel patency and therefore delineate the area of ischemia (Besselmann et al., 2001). The potential to detect such obstructions is further enhanced by contrast agents with long circulation times (blood pool agents). Although major blood vessels can be imaged without administration of exogenous agents, the use of contrast media to enhance the detection of blood vessels can substantially enhance the quality of the angiogram (Zheng et al., 2001). In a similar manner, specifically designed contrast agents with optimized characteristics for MRA, such as very small superparamagnetic iron oxide particles (VSPOs), are being developed to probe angiogenesis in laboratory animals and evaluate their potential clinical utility to investigate how blood supply to a lesion environment is restored (Taupitz et al., 2000). Flacke et al. (2001) demonstrated that a Gd-DTPA-BOA-based contrast agent that targets fibrin can increase the detection

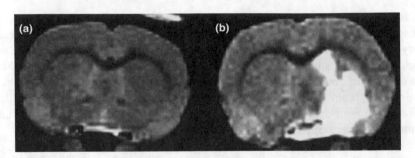

FIGURE 10.6 Focal ischemia in the rat. The possibility to repeatedly image the same subject by MRI allowed us to image a rat brain prelesion (a) and postlesion (b). A transient middle cerebral artery occlusion was imaged before and 4 months after occlusion. Hyperintensities in the right image reflect areas of ongoing damage in the CNS.

of blood clots *in vitro* and *in vivo*, helping to identify the presence and location of a thrombus (Yu et al., 2000).

Novel techniques in imaging science can, in general, also be applied to other disease areas. For example, novel MRA contrast media may also enhance the detection of brain tumors (see below) and can provide novel insights into other neurological disorders. The *in vivo* detection of immune effector cells from the blood to the site of a lesion can increase our understanding of the recruitment of macrophages or lymphocytes (Dodd et al., 1999, Dousset et al., 1999a, Rausch et al., 2001). Similar technology can also be applied to other diseases such as multiple sclerosis (Dousset et al., 1999b). Scanning sequences developed to detect different facets of an ischemic lesion can also be tailored to visualize different stages of excitotoxic brain damage during neurodegeneration (Ben-Horin et al., 1996). Studies using MRI and MRS have shown their effectiveness in animal models of disorders such as Parkinsonism (Chen et al., 1999), Huntington's disease (Chyi and Chang, 1999, Jenkins et al., 2000), multiple system atrophy (Schocke et al., 2000), Alzheimer's disease (Hauss-Wegrzyniak et al., 2000, Gilissen et al., 1999), multiple sclerosis (Ahrens et al., 1998), and spinal cord transections (Fraidakis et al., 1998). However, the lesions in these animal models can often only poorly mimic pathogenic events of neurological disorders observed in patients. Nevertheless, these models can provide useful insights into how a lesion affects behavior and responses to different treatment strategies. Jenkins et al. (1999) integrated various aspects of brain damage assessment into a neurofunctional examination that can be applied to a given neurodegenerative disease to determine etiology, natural history, and response to treatment.

Interest in animal models of psychiatric conditions has recently increased (Kahne et al., 2002), but a direct comparison of human and animal models is more difficult than comparing rat models of focal and global ischaemia or traumatic brain injury (Gregory et al., 2001, Hoehn et al., 2001, Smith et al., 1998b). The advent of tightly controlled, genetic modifications to laboratory animals, the potential to use MRI for phenotyping, and ongoing improvements in our ability to assess lesion progression and treatment will lead to a greater understanding of CNS disorders. (Figure 10.6)

10.4.4 DETECTION OF BRAIN TUMORS

The functional impairment of the brain is not always due to the loss of tissue; it can be the product of the neoplastic activity of CNS cells. The use of MRI to detect brain tumors has revolutionized the diagnosis and evaluation of treatments in human patients. Research in laboratory animals can provide important information regarding the progression and invasion of neoplastic cells. Typically, neoplastic cells are transplanted into the brains of animals and the formations of tumor masses can be followed by MRI. Due to the permeable blood–brain barrier in most tumors, contrast agents, such as Gd-DTPA, can be administered systemically to visualize tumor mass and aid differentiation from healthy tissue (Evelhoch et al., 2000). The difference in cell density and the infiltration of contrast media into tumor tissue (producing a different MR signal compared to signal from normal brain tissue) aid localization and resection of the neoplasm.

Animal studies are important in the evaluation of different treatment strategies and can be used in combination with MRI to evaluate changes in tumor size over time (Namba et al., 2000, Bogdanov et al., 1999, Chenevert et al., 2000) or success of surgical removal (Knauth et al., 2001). Although this approach helps to detect and treat primary tumors, extension to the amelioration of metastases and tumor invasion is, to the say the least, more challenging.

Novel contrast agents such as MIONs can be used to label neoplastic cells before transplantation and enhance detection of invading neoplastic cells at an early stage. Specific antibodies conjugated to particular contrast agents can directly target particular receptors (Tiefenauer et al., 1996) and differentiate between different types of neoplastic cells (see Figure 10.7). Fan et al. (2001) distinguished nonmetastatic and metastatic tumors based on the combination of contrast agent-enhanced image texture, tumor edge morphology, and changes in T_2*.

A further aspect of tumor ontogenesis and treatment is the increased angiogenesis and permeability of the endothelial wall that can be probed by contrast agents such as USPIO or Gd-DTPA (van der Sanden et al., 2001, Turetschek et al., 2001, Moore et al., 2000). As in a clinical setting, Gd-DTPA is routinely used to delineate brain tumors due to the enhanced uptake of the contrast agent into the tumor tissue. The imaging and visualization of the network of blood vessels within the tumor can be used as an outcome measure, especially in treatment strategies aimed at starving the tumor of nutrients (Kunkel et al., 2001). The spatial resolution and ability to visualize the microvasculature are important considerations when optimizing MRA (Jensen and Chandra, 2000).

Further sophistication of neuroimaging technology can also enhance the basic understanding of how tumors grow *in vivo*. Elongated T_1 and T_2 values are characteristics of highly proliferative tumor cell lines (Olsen et al., 1999). A significant correlation was found between the apparent diffusion coefficient (ADC) and the viability and density of some, but not all tumors (Lyng et al., 2000). To detect apoptosis in tumor cells, Zhao et al. (2001) applied a contrast agent conjugated to a protein recognizing synaptotagmin (binding to the membranes of apoptotic cells) and hence were able to distinguish apoptotic from viable cells *in vitro* and *in vivo*. Probing

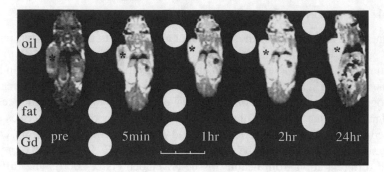

FIGURE 10.7 Tumor detection. Novel tumor-seeking contrast agents based on manganese metalloporphyrins with high specificity to the detection of a tumor implanted on the right flank of a mouse. Within 5 minutes of contrast agent administration, the tumor was easily distinguished from surrounding tissue. The enhanced contrast was maintained more than 24 hours after the administration. (Adapted from Takehara et al., *Mag. Res. Med.*, 47, 549, 2002. With permission.).

the development of a tumor and detection of early biochemical markers of tumor formation can also be followed over time (Foley et al., 2001), with the potential to investigate how treatment will affect tumor growth at different time points.

The abilities of MRI and its related technologies to investigate pathological states and response to treatment by noninvasive repeated measurements are ideally suited to investigate a number of pathological conditions. As with the study of oncology and carcinogenesis by grafting brain tumors to laboratory animals, the use of neural transplantation to remedy lesions of the CNS can be used to investigate clinical potential.

10.4.5 EVALUATION OF NEURAL TRANSPLANTS

Cell replacement therapy is a promising new treatment for a variety of neurological disorders (Björklund and Lindvall, 2000). Reports indicate that the transplantation of fetal tissue to ameliorate neurological symptoms in patients with Parkinson's or Huntington's disease has been functionally effective. Again, neuroimaging can provide important information about the survival, function, and integration of a transplant in a damaged brain (Schocke et al., 2000, Fricker et al., 1997, Piccini et al., 1999, Bachoud-Levi et al., 2000). Early rat studies by Norman and colleagues (1989a, 1989b, 1992) indicated that it was possible to define a fetal graft in a lesioned brain and distinguish it from a transplanted glioma. The blood–brain barrier in fetal transplants is permeable up to 35 days. Gadolinium will penetrate the transplant to differentiate it from host parenchyma (Isenmann et al., 1996)

Integration of complementary imaging modalities to study neural transplants *in vivo* provides a more holistic framework to determine transplant survival, integration, and function, leading to better preclinical development and understanding of brain repair. Chen et al. (1997, 1999) investigated *in vivo* effects of neural transplantation by determining graft survival by MRI, its functional significance by pharmacological MRI (phMRI), and its relationship and functional recovery with PET. Cichetti et al. (2001) further developed these complementary technologies to

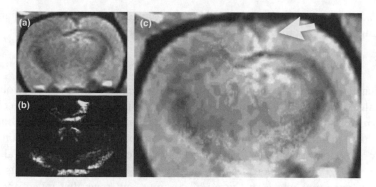

FIGURE 10.8 MRI visualization of a stem cell transplant in a rat with global ischaemic brain damage. The visualization of transplanted stem cells was feasible by prelabeling cells *in vitro* with a bifunctional contrast agent, GRID. This allowed us to detect the transplant on both MRI (a) and fluorescent microscopy (b). An overlay of both images (c) provides corroborative evidence that both imaging modalities visualized the stem cell transplant. (Modo, M. et al., *Neuroimage*, 17(2), 803, 2002. With permission.) See Color Figure 10.8 following page 210.

investigate the immunological responses (microglia/macrophages) to neural transplants. Clearly, the integration of different techniques to investigate particular aspects of transplants and cross-validate results is a powerful approach to improving our understanding of how neural transplants promote functional recovery.

Although fetal transplants have shown their effectiveness in experimental and clinical situations, the use of stem or progenitor cells has several advantages. Laboratory-grown cells pose fewer ethical concerns. Quality control procedures can be applied to provide consistent transplant material that poses little risk of contamination. Supplies are easily available. The cells do not aggregate and will seek out regions of damage (Gray et al., 2000). Due to the seamless integration and extensive migration, the challenge posed by such stem cells and progenitor cells transplanted into tissue such as the brain or liver will be the requirement for a different imaging strategy to discriminate between host and grafted cells.

To this end, grafted cells can be labeled with contrast agents before transplantation to produce a signal change of the transplanted cells compared to the host parenchyma. Several contrast agents, such as MIONs (Bulte et al., 1999), magnetodendrimers (Bulte et al., 2001), USPIO (Franklin et al., 1999), HIV/tat-derived superparamagentic nanoparticles (Lewin et al., 2000), and GRID (Modo et al., 2002, Figure 10.8) have been developed to allow the detection and migration of cell transplants. Prelabeling of stem cells with the bifunctional GRID agent permitted detection of transplanted cells by MRI and afforded direct corroboration of cell distribution via fluorescent, rhodamine subunit of the ligand (Modo et al., 2002). The advantage of using a bifunctional contrast agent detectable by MRI and fluorescence microscopy lies in the ability to identify the same cells by independent technologies without recourse to supplementary processing such as immunohistochemistry. It is, however, important to determine the stability, possible leakage, and reuptake of labels from transplanted into host cells (i.e., specificity of transplant detection). The ability to visualize grafted stem cells *in vivo* and determine the functional changes by functional and pharmacological MRI will greatly enhance our understanding of how these cells promote functional recovery.

10.4.6 PROBING BRAIN FUNCTION

Brain function can be assessed noninvasively by fMRI. This is typically observed as a localized increase in T_2*-weighted MR signal that reflects an increase in cerebral hemodynamics that goes in tandem with elevated neuronal activity. To date, rat fMRI studies have mainly probed the somatosensory response to the stimulation of the forepaw or hindpaw (Marota et al., 1999, Mandeville et al., 1998, Palmer et al., 1999, Spenger et al., 2000). Whisker stimulation may prove a better target due to its elegant cortical organization into a vast array of columns and rows that reflect the corresponding whisker barrel fields (Yang et al., 1997).

Since this field is still in its infancy, such fMRI studies have rarely been designed to investigate the plasticity or dynamics of the somatosensory system (Poldrack, 2000) (see Figure 10.9). They have been used to generally assess how different imaging protocols or experimental variables such as hyperventilation affect the detection of functional changes in the brain (Marota et al., 1999, Hsu et al., 1998, Nakao et al., 2001, Mandeville et al., 2001). Nevertheless, it has been possible to visualize the spatial pattern of odor discrimination (Xu et al., 2000) and the columnar organization following visual stimulation (Kim et al., 2000).

Although systems have been described for imaging conscious rats, (Lahti et al., 1998) movement artefacts and stress are major concerns; anesthesia therefore is commonly applied when performing animal fMRI. One potential confound in such fMRI studies is an anaesthetic that may modulate cerebral blood flow and metabolism and interact with any psychotropic agent (Wood et al., 2001). To date, only very basic sensory stimulation experiments have been reported in anesthetized rats. Nakao et al. (2001) compared the brain activation in conscious animals anesthetized with α–chloralose after vibrissal stimulation to demonstrate a down-regulation of the activation in anesthetized animals. Although anesthetics are generally assumed to affect the cardiovascular system and therefore influence parameters typically used to provide functional imaging data, it is unclear to what extent changes in functional activation are due to variations in neural activity or the cardiovascular system (Kalish et al., 2001, Hsu et al., 1998). The development of novel fMRI protocols can provide experimental manipulation of variables that could not easily be controlled in humans. By combining neurophysiological measures and fMRI (Brinker et al., 1999, Heeger et al., 2000), it is possible to determine how and to what degree functional activation measured by BOLD or cerebral blood volume relates to the firing of neurons within the region of interest.

A series of recent studies in monkeys by Logothetis et al. (1999, 2001) have indicated that the local field potential is the best predictor of the Blood Oxygenation Level Dependent (BOLD) contrast commonly used in human fMRI studies. It is currently a matter of debate as to what constitutes the neural correlates of the BOLD response and what may constitute the spatial and temporal characteristics of this response (Heeger et al., 2000, Logothetis, 2000, Menon, 2001).

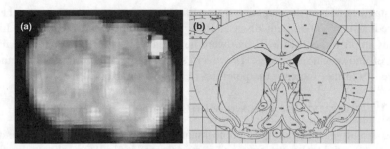

FIGURE 10.9 Detecting rodent brain function. Electrical stimulation of the rat forepaw was detected by BOLD-based fMRI in α-chloralose treated rats (a). The anatomical correlation of the functional activity corresponded to the area of the primary somatosensory cortex according to Paxinos' rat atlas (b). (Adapted from Lowe, A.S. et al., *Proc. 10th Annl. Mtg. Soc. Mag. Res. Med.*, 2002. With permission.) See Color Figure 10.9 following page 210.

Although a large proportion of fMRI studies focus on how a particular brain region or structure activates following stimulation, fMRI can also be adopted to provide information about activation of particular brain regions after pharmacological stimulation. This type of MRI (phMRI) holds promise in the investigation of pharmacodynamics, brain penetration, and dose-response in a manner that can be translated directly from experimental animal observations into man (Leslie and James, 1998). We believe that the development of a wide range of novel neuropharmaceuticals will be facilitated by phMRI. Such technology will allow us to determine which brain regions are affected by a particular drug and how this drug alters brain function (Houston et al., 2001, Marota et al., 2000). Pharmacological MRI may provide temporal and spatial indications as to the optimal target and dose of a particular drug that can then be refined for preclinical and clinical trials (Taylor and Reddick, 2000). In animal studies, cross-validation of different techniques providing corroborative evidence of a particular drug action can also be gained (Chen et al., 1997).

To enhance the signal contrast needed for fMRI and phMRI, it is possible to use blood pool contrast agents that will amplify signal change in a particular region in response to brain activation (Dubowitz et al., 2001, Chen et al., 1997, Vanduffel et al., 2001). MRA-based contrast agents can provide improved detection of brain activation which may require larger sample sizes or higher field strength systems when using BOLD based methods. With this in mind, it is highly likely that new contrast agents will be designed specifically for use in such fMRI studies. Contrast agents targeting particular processes in brain activity (such as glucose or oxygen consumption) may be engineered to provide alternative and possibly more refined methods of functional imaging (Aime et al., 2000b).

10.5 CONCLUSIONS AND FUTURE DIRECTIONS

Molecular imaging by MRI can be studied in organisms from neurodevelopment to neurodegeneration. The *in vivo* imaging of biological processes will allow a better understanding of how development over a lifetime occurs and what biological events are predictive of subsequent disease. Recent developments in contrast media and ongoing improvements in MRI hardware herald a new "golden age" for the *in vivo* study of biological processes. However, several important challenges must be resolved to further increase the potential of *in vivo* imaging.

10.5.1 INTEGRATION OF IMAGING MODALITIES

The possibility of integrating different imaging modalities can overcome the disadvantages of individual techniques and provide more information about a particular biological event. The combination of PET and MRI into one system will drastically increase the potential of molecular imaging by providing diverse information about particular biological events (Jacobs and Cherry, 2001). Integrating fMRI and PET will further elucidate the intricate relationship of brain and behavior. The corroboration of *in vivo* imaging by the integration of *ex vivo* confocal histology (Wind et al., 2000) with high spatial resolution and high specificity through immunohistochemistry will add an additional source of reliable information that can be used to link data to other scientific domains such as genetics or neuropathology. Apart from the development of multimodal imaging, increasing the selectivity and specificity of new contrast media are among the most important factors required to advance the contribution of molecular imaging by MRI to our understanding of the CNS.

10.5.2 RECENT ADVANCES IN CONTRAST AGENT DEVELOPMENT

The development of more sophisticated and specifically engineered contrast agents will increase the applicability of MRI to biological questions. Further development in three key areas of contrast agents will increase their research potential. First, optimization of metals producing the highest possible MR contrasts will reduce doses and therefore lower the toxicities. Second, increasing the specificities of contrast agents (by targeting receptors or proteins) to highlight particular biological processes will improve our understanding of how such processes modulate over time. Finally, the development of a broader range of contrast agents with different contrast mechanisms may allow better discrimination between the agent and any underlying contrast attributable to the biological state of the tissue.

In conclusion, molecular imaging provides the ability to monitor biological events *in vivo* and when used in combination with MRI, affords the possibility to perform repeated, three-dimensional measures over time. The recent development of novel contrast agents with improved specificities is an important contribution to the increasing use of MR as a tool for molecular imaging. Further diversity in the design and application of these new contrast agents offers huge potential for advances in both functional and structural neurobiology.

REFERENCES

Aguayo, J.B. et al. (1986). Nuclear magnetic resonance imaging of a single cell. *Nature*, 322, 190.

Ahrens, E.T. et al. (1998). A model for MRI contrast enhancement using T_1 agents. *Proc. Natl. Acad. Sci. U.S.A.*, 95, 8443.

Aime, S. et al. (2000a). [GdPCP2A(H$_2$O)$_2$]$^-$: a paramagnetic contrast agent designed for improved applications in magnetic resonance imaging. *J. Med. Chem.*, 43, 4017.

Aime, S. et al. (2000b). A p(O$_2$)-responsive MRI contrast agent based on the redox switch of manganese(II/III)-pophyrin complexes. *Angew. Chem. Int. Ed.*, 39, 747.

Anelli, P.L. and Lattuada, L. (2001). Synthesis of MRI contrast agents: acyclic ligands, in Merbach, A.E. and Tóth, E., Eds., *The Chemistry of Contrast Agents in Medical Magnetic Resonance Imaging*, John Wiley & Sons, Chichester.

Ashner, M. and Ashner, J. (1991). Manganese neurotoxicity: cellular effects and blood–brain barrier transport. *Neurosci. Biobehav. Rev.*, 15, 333.

Bachoud-Lévi, A.-C. et al. (2000). Safety and tolerability assessment of intrastriatal neural allografts in five patients with Huntington's disease. *Exp. Neurol.*, 161, 194.

Balaban, R.S. and Hampshire, V.A. (2001). Challenges in small animal noninvasive imaging. *ILAR J.* 42, 248.

Beckmann, N. et al. (2001). From anatomy to the target: contributions of magnetic resonance imaging to preclinical pharmaceutical research. *Anat. Record*, 265, 100.

Ben-Horin, N. et al. (1996). The ontogeny of a neurotoxic lesion in rat brain revealed by combined MRI and histology. *Brain Res.*, 718, 97.

Besselmann, M. et al. (2001). MR angiographic investigation of transient focal cerebral ischemia in rat. *NMR Biomed.*, 14, 289.

Björklund, A. and Lindvall, O. (2000). Cell replacement therapy for central nervous system disorders. *Nature Neurosci.*, 3, 537.

Bogdanov, A. et al. (1999). Treatment of experimental brain tumors with trombospondin-1 derived peptides: an *in vivo* imaging study. *Neoplasia*, 1, 438.

Bogdanov, A. and Weissleder, R. (2001). The development of *in vivo* imaging systems to study gene expression. *Trends Cell Biol.*, 16(1), 5–10.

Brinker, G. et al. (1999). Simultaneous recording of evoked potentials and T_2*-weighted MR images during somatosensory stimulation of rat. *Mag. Res. Med.*, 41, 469.

Brücher, E. and Sherry, A.D. (2001). Stability and toxicity of contrast agents, in Merbach, A.E. amd Tóth, E., Eds., *The Chemistry of Contrast Agents in Medical Magnetic Resonance Imaging*, John Wiley & Sons, Chichester.

Budinger, T.F., Benaron, D.A., and Koretsky, A.P. (1999). Imaging transgenic animals. *Ann. Rev. Biomed. Eng.*, 1, 611.

Bulte, J.W.M. et al. (1999). Neurotransplantation of magnetically labeled oligodendrocyte progenitors: magnetic resonance tracking of cell migration and myelination. *Proc. Natl. Acad. Sci. U.S.A.*, 96, 15256.

Bulte, J.W.M. et al. (2001). Magnetodendrimers allow endosomal magnetic labeling and *in vivo* tracking of stem cells. *Nature Biotechnol.*, 19, 1141.

Cicchetti, F. et al. (2001). Prevention of neuroinflammation of the nigrostriatal pathway during progressive dopamine degeneration. *Exp. Neurol.*, 170, 199. Abstr.

Chatham, J.C. and Blackband, S.J. (2001). Nuclear magnetic resonance spectroscopy and imaging in animal research. *ILAR J.*, 42, 189.

Chen, Y.C. et al. (1997). Detection of dopaminergic neurotransmitter activity using pharmacologic MRI: correlation with PET, microdialysis, and behavioral data. *Mag. Res. Med.*, 38, 389.

Chen, Y.I. et al. (1999). Detection of dopaminergic cell loss and neural transplantation using pharmacological MRI, PET, and behavioral assessment. *NeuroReport*, 10, 2881.

Chenevert, T.L. et al. (2000). Diffusion magnetic resonance imaging: an early surrogate marker for therapeutic efficacy in brain tumors. *J. Natl. Cancer Inst.*, 92, 2029.

Cherry, S.R. and Gambhir, S.S. (2001). Use of positron emmission tomography in animal research. *ILAR J.*, 42, 219.

Chyi, T. and Chang, C. (1999). Temporal evolution of 3-nitroproprionic acid-induced neurodegeneration in the rat brain by T_2-weighted, diffusion-weighted, and perfusion magnetic resonance imaging. *Neuroscience*, 92, 1035.

Corot, C. et al. (2000). Pharmacokinetics of three gadolinium chelates with different molecular sizes shortly after intravenous injection in rabbits: relevance to MR angiography. *Inv. Radiol.*, 35, 213.

de Crespigny, A.J. et al. (2000). MRI of focal cerebral ischemia using ^{17}O-labeled water. *Mag. Res. Med.*, 43, 876.

Dhenain, M., Ruffins, S.W., and Jacobs, R.E. (2001). Three-dimensional digital mouse atlas using high-resolution MRI. *Develop. Biol.*, 232, 458.

Dijkhuizen, R.M. et al. (2001). Functional magnetic resonance imaging of reorganization in rat brain after stroke. *Proc. Natl. Acad. Sci. U.S.A.*, 98, 12766.

Dodd, S.J. et al. (1999). Detection of single mammalian cells by high-resolution magnetic resonance imaging. *Biophys. J.*, 76, 103–109.

Doerfler, A. et al. (2000). MR contrast agents in acute experimental cerebral ischemia: potential adverse impacts on neurologic outcome and infarction size. *J. Mag. Res. Imaging*, 11, 418.

Dousset, V. et al. (1999a). *In vivo* macrophage activity imaging in the central nervous system detected by magnetic resonance. *Mag. Res. Med.*, 41, 329.

Dousset, V. et al. (1999b). Dose and scanning delay using USPIO for central nervous system macrophage imaging. *MAGMA*, 8, 185.

Dubowitz, D.J. et al. (2001). Enhancing fMRI contrast in awake-behaving primates using intravascular magnetite dextran nanoparticles. *NeuroReport*, 12, 2335.

Enochs, W.S. et al. (1993). MR imaging of slow axonal transport *in vivo*. *Exp. Neurol.*, 123, 235.

Evelhoch, J.L. et al. (2000). Applications of magnetic resonance in model systems: cancer therapeutics. *Neoplasia*, 2, 152.

Fan, X. et al. (2001). Differentiation of nonmetastatic and metastatic rodent prostate tumors with high spectral and spatial resolution MRI. *Mag. Res. Med.*, 45, 1046.

Flacke, S. et al. (2001). Novel MRI contrast agent for molecular imaging of fibrin: Implications for detecting vulnerable plaques. *Circulation*, 104, 1280.

Foley, L.M., Towner, R.A., and Painter, D.M. (2001). *In vivo* image guided $^{(1)}$H-magnetic spectroscopy of the serial development of hepatocarcinogenesis in an experimental animal model. *Biochim. Biophys. Acta*, 1526, 230.

Fraidakis, M. et al. (1998). High-resolution MRI of intact and transected rat spinal cord. *Exp. Neurol.*, 153, 299.

Franklin, R.J.M. et al. (1999). Magnetic resonance imaging of transplanted oligodendrocyte precursors in the rat brain. *NeuroReport*, 10, 3961.

Fricker, R.A. et al. (1997). The effect of donor stage on the survival and function of embryonic striatal grafts in the adult brain: correlation with positron emission tomography and reaching behaviour. *Neuroscience*, 79, 711.

Gibby, W.A., Bogdan, A., and Ovitt, T.W. (1988). Cross-linked DTPA polysaccharides for magnetic resonance imaging: synthesis and relaxation properties. *Inv. Radiol.*, 24, 302.

Gilissen, E.P., Jacobs, R.E., and Allman, J.M. (1999). Magnetic resonance microscopy of iron in the basal forebrain cholinergic structures of the aged mouse lemur. *J. Neurol. Sci.*, 168, 21.

Grant, S.C. et al. (2000). NMR spectroscopy of single neurons. *Mag. Res. Med.*, 44, 19.

Gray, J.A. et al. (2000). Conditionally immortalized, multipotential and multifunctional neural stem cell lines as an approach to clinical transplantation. *Cell Transplant.*, 9, 153.

Green, M.V. et al. (2001). High resolution PET, SPECT and projection imaging in small animals. *Comp. Med. Imaging Graphics*, 25, 79.

Gregory, L.J. et al. (2001). Diffusion-weighted magnetic resonance imaging detects early neuropathology following four-vessel occlusion ischemia in the rat. *J. Mag. Res. Imaging*, 14, 207.

Harris, N.G. et al. (2001). Cerebrovascular reactivity following focal ischemia in the rat: functional magnetic resonance imaging study. *Neuroimage*, 13, 339.

Hauss-Wegrzyniak, B., Galons, J.P., and Wenk, G.L. (2000). Quantitative volumetric analyses of brain magnetic resonance imaging from rat with chronic neuroinflammation. *Exp. Neurol.*, 165, 347.

Heeger, D.J. et al. (2000). Spikes versus BOLD: what does neuroimaging tell us about neuronal activity? *Nature Neurosci.*, 3, 631.

Hines, J.V. et al. (1999). Paramagnetic oligonucleotides: contrast agents for magnetic resonance imaging with proton relaxation enhancement effects. *Bioconjugate Chem.*, 10, 155.

Hogan, B.L.M. (1999). Morphogenesis. *Cell*, 96, 225.

Hoehn, M. et al. (2001). Application of magnetic resonance to animal models of cerebral ischemia. *J. Mag. Res. Imaging*, 14, 491.

Hogers, B. et al. (2001). Magnetic resonance microscopy at 17.6 Tesla on chicken embryos *in vitro*. *J. Mag. Res. Imaging*, 14, 83.

Högemann, D. et al. (2000). Improvement of MRI probes to allow efficient detection of gene expression. *Bioconjugate Chem.*, 11, 941.

Hopkins, A.L. et al. (1991). The stability of proton T_2 effects of oxygen-17 water in experimental cerebral ischemia. *Mag. Res. Med.*, 22, 167.

Houston, G.C. et al. (2001). Mapping of brain activation in response to pharmacological agents using fMRI in the rat. *Mag. Res. Imaging*, 19, 905.

Hoydu, A.K. et al. (2000). *In vivo*, *in utero* microscopic magnetic resonance imaging: application in a rat model of diaphragmatic hernia. *Mag. Res. Med.*, 44, 331.

Hsu, E.W., Aiken, N.R., and Blackband, S.J. (1997). A study of isotropy in single neurons by using NMR microscopy. *Mag. Res. Med.*, 37, 624.

Hsu, E.W., Hedlund, L.W., and MacFall, J.R. (1998). Functional MRI of the rat somatosensory cortex: effects of hyperventilation. *Mag. Res. Med.*, 40, 426.

Hüber, M.M. et al. (1998). Fluorescently detectable magnetic resonance imaging agents. *Bioconjugate Chem.*, 9, 242.

Isenmann, S. et al. (1996). Comparative *in vivo* and pathological analysis of the blood–brain barrier in mouse telencephalic transplants. *Neuropathol. Appl. Neurobiol.*, 22, 118.

Jacobs, R.E. and Fraser, S.E. (1994). Magnetic resonance microscopy of embryonic cell lineages and movements. *Science*, 263, 681.

Jacobs, R.E. et al. (1999). Looking deeper into vertebrate development. *Trends Cell Biol.*, 9, 73.

Jacobs, R.E. and Cherry, S.R. (2001). Complementary emerging techniques: high-resolution PET and MRI. *Curr. Opin. Neurobiol.*, 11, 621.

Jacques, V. and Desreux, J.-F. (2001). Synthesis of MRI contrast agents II. Macrocyclic ligands, in Merbach, A.E. and Tóth, E., Eds., *The Chemistry of Contrast Agents in Medical Magnetic Resonance Imaging,* John Wiley & Sons, Chichester.

Jenkins, B.G. et al. (1999). Integrated strategy for evaluation of metabolic and oxidative defects in neurodegenerative illness using magnetic resonance techniques. *Ann. NY Acad. Sci.*, 893, 214.

Jenkins, B.G. et al. (2000). Nonlinear decrease over time in N-acetyl aspartate levels in the absence of neuronal loss and increases in glutamine and glucose in transgenic Huntington's disease mice. *J. Neurochem.*, 74, 2108–2119.

Jensen, J.H. and Chandra, R. (2000). MR imaging of microvasculature. *Mag. Res. Med.*, 44, 224.

Johnson, G.A. et al. (1993). Histology by magnetic resonance microscopy. *Mag. Res. Q.*, 9, 1.

Kahne, D. et al. (2002). Behavioral and magnetic resonance spectroscopic studies in the rat hyperserotonemic model of autism. *Physiol. Behavior,* 75, 403.

Kalish, R. et al. (2001). Blood pressure changes induced by arterial blood withdrawal influence BOLD signal in anaesthetized rats at 7 Tesla: implications for pharmacological MRI. *Neuroimage,* 14, 891.

Kim, D.S., Duong, T.Q., and Kim, S.G. (2000). High-resolution mapping of iso-orientation columns by fMRI. *Nature Neurosci.*, 3, 164.

Knauth, M. et al. (2001). Monocrystalline iron oxide nanoparticles: possible solution to the problem of surgically induced intracranial contrast enhancement in intraoperative MR imaging. *Am. J. Neuroradiol.*, 22, 99.

Krishna, M.C. et al. (2001). Electron paramagnetic resonance for small animal imaging applications. *ILAR J.*, 42, 209.

Kunkel, P. et al. (2001). Inhibition of glioma angiogenesis and growth *in vivo* by systemic treatment with a monocloncal antibody against vascular endothelial factor receptor-2. *Cancer* Res., 16, 6624.

Lahti, K.M. et al. (1998). Imaging brain activity in conscious animals using functional MRI. *J. Neurosci. Methods*, 82, 75.

Lee, S.-C. et al. (2001). One micrometer resolution NMR microscopy. *J. Mag. Res.*, 150, 207.

Leslie, R.A. and James, M.F. (1998). Pharmacological magnetic resonance imaging: a new application for functional MRI. *Trends Pharm. Sci.*, 21, 314.

Lewin, M. et al. (2000). Tat peptide-derivatized magnetic nanoparticles allow *in vivo* tracking and recovery of progenitor cells. *Nature Biotechnol.*, 18, 410.

Li, W., Fraser, S.E., and Meade, T.J. (1999). A calcium-sensitive magnetic resonance imaging contrast agent. *J. Am. Chem. Soc.*, 121, 1413.

Logothetis, N.K. et al. (1999). Functional imaging of the monkey brain. *Nature Neurosci.*, 2, 555.

Logothetis, N. (2000). Can current fMRI techniques reveal microarchitecture of cortex? *Nature Neurosci.*, 3, 413.

Logothetis, N.K. et al. (2001). Neurophysiological investigation of the basis of the fMRI signal. *Nature,* 412, 150–157.

Louie, A.Y. et al. (2000). *In vivo* visualization of gene expression using magnetic resonance imaging. *Nature Biotechnol.*, 18, 321.

Lowe, A.S. et al. (2002). Positive contralateral and negative ipsilateral BOLD contrast changes during electrical stimulation of rat forepaw. *Proc. 10th Annl. Mtg. Int. Soc. Mag. Res. Med.*

Lyng, H., Haraldseth, O., and Rofstadt, E.K. (2000). Measurement of cell density and necrotic fraction in human melanoma xenografts by diffusion-weighted magnetic resonance imaging. *Mag. Res. Med.*, 43, 828.

Magin, R.L. et al. (2000). Biological effects of long-duration, high-field (4 T) MRI on growth and development in the mouse. *J. Mag. Res. Imaging*, 12, 140.

Mandeville, J.B. et al. (1998). Dynamic functional imaging of relative cerebral blood volume during rat forepaw stimulation. *Mag. Res. Med.*, 39, 615.

Mandeville, J.B. et al. (2001). Regional sensitivity and coupling of BOLD and CBV changes during stimulation of rat brain. *Mag. Res. Med.*, 45, 443.

Marota, J.J.A. et al. (1999). Investigation of the early response to rat forepaw stimulation. *Mag. Res. Med.*, 41, 247–252.

Marota, J.J.A. et al. (2000). Cocaine activation discriminates dopaminergic projections by temporal response: an fMRI study in rat. *Neuroimage,* 11, 13.

Menon, R.S. (2001). Imaging function in the working brain with fMRI. *Curr. Opin. Neurobiol.*, 11, 630.

Mikawa, M. et al. (2001). Paramagnetic water-soluble metallofullerenes having the highest relaxivity for MRI contrast agents. *Bioconjugate Chem.*, 12, 510.

Modo, M. et al. (2002). Tracking transplanted stem cell migration by bifunctional, contrast agent-enhanced, magnetic resonance imaging. *Neuroimage*, 17(2), 803–811.

Moore, A. et al. (2000). Tumoral distribution of long circulating dextran-coated iron oxide nanoparticles in a rodent model. *Radiology*, 214, 568.

Muller, R.N. et al. (2001). Particulate magnetic contrast agents, in Merbach, A.E. and Tóth, E., Eds., *The Chemistry of Contrast Agents in Medical Magnetic Resonance Imaging*, John Wiley & Sons, Chichester.

Nakao, Y. et al. (2001). Effects of anaesthesia on functional activation of cerebral blood flow and metabolism. *Proc. Natl. Acad. Sci. U.S.A.*, 98, 7593.

Namba, H. et al. (2000). Treatment of rat experimental brain tumor by herpes simplex virus thymidine kinase gene-transduced allogeneic tumor cells and gancilcovir. *Cancer Gene Ther.*, 7, 947.

Norman, A.B. et al. (1989a). Magnetic resonance imaging of rat brain following kainic acid-induced lesions and fetal striatal tissue transplants. *Brain Res.*, 483, 188.

Norman, A.B. et al. (1989b). A magnetic resonance imaging contrast agent differentiates between the vascular properties of fetal striatal tissue transplants and gliomas in rat brain *in vivo*. *Brain Res.*, 503, 156.

Norman, A.B. et al. (1992). Magnetic resonance imaging of neural transplants in rat brain using a supraparamagnetic contrast agent. *Brain Res.*, 594, 279.

Olsen, G. et al. (1999). Measurement of proliferation activity in human melanoma xenografts by magnetic resonance imaging. *Mag. Res. Imaging,* 17, 393.

Palmer, J.T. et al. (1999). High-resolution mapping of discrete representational areas in rat somatosensory cortex using blood volume-dependent functional MRI. *Neuroimage,* 9, 383.

Pautler, R.G., Silvia, A.C., and Koretsky, A.P. (1998). *In vivo* neuronal tract tracing using manganese-enhanced magnetic resonance imaging. *Mag. Res. Med.*, 40, 740.

Pautler, R.G. and Koretsky, A.P. (2002). Tracing odor-induced activation in the olfactory bulbs of mice using manganese-enhanced magnetic resonance imaging. *Neuroimage*, 16, 441.

Phelps, M.E. (2000). PET: the merging of biology and imaging into molecular imaging. *J. Nucl. Med.*, 41, 661.

Piccini, P. et al. (1999). Dopamine release from nigral transplants visualized *in vivo* in a Parkinson's patient. *Nature Neurosci.*, 2, 1137.

Poldrack, R.A. (2000). Imaging brain plasticity: conceptual and methodological issues: a theoretical review. *Neuroimage*, 12, 1.

Posse, S. and Aue, W.P. (1989). ^{1}H spectroscopic imaging at high spatial resolution. *NMR Biomed.*, 2, 234.

Rattle, H. (1995). *NMR Primer for Life Scientists*. Partnership Press, Fareham, Hants., U.K.

Rausch, M. et al. (2001). Dynamic patterns of USPIO enhancement can be observed in macrophages after ischemic brain damage. *Mag. Res. Med.*, 46, 1018.

Ray, D.E. et al. (1996). Neurotoxic effects of gadopentetate dimeglumine behavioural disturbance and morphology after intracerebroventricular injection in rats. *Am. J. Neuroradiol.*, 18, 785.

Reichert, D.E., Lewis, J.S., and Anderson, C.J. (1999). Metal complexes as diagnostic tools. *Coordination Chem. Rev.*, 184, 3.

Reichert, D.E. and Welch, M.J. (2001). Applications of molecular mechanics to metal-based imaging agents. *Coordination Chem. Rev.*, 212, 111.

Reynolds, C.H. et al. (2000). Gadolinium-loaded nanoparticles: new contrast agents for magnetic resonance imaging. *J. Am. Chem. Soc.*, 122, 8940.

Rijnjtes, M. and Weiller, C. (2002). Recovery of motor and language abilities after stroke: the contribution of functional imaging. *Progr. Neurobiol.*, 66, 109.

Roberts, T.P.L., Chuang, N., and Roberts, H.C. (2000). Neuroimaging: do we really need new contrast agents for MRI? *Eur. J. Radiol.*, 34, 166.

Rodegerdts, E.A. et al. (2000). *In vitro* evaluation of teratogenic effects by time-varying MR gradient fields on fetal human fibroblasts. *J. Mag. Res. Imaging*, 12, 150–156.

Rongved, P. and Laveness, J. (1991). Water-soluble polysaccharides as carriers of paramagnetic contrast agents for magnetic resonance imaging: synthesis and relaxation properties. *Carbohydrate Res.*, 214, 315.

Runge, V.M. (2000). Safety of approved MR contrast media for intravenous injection. *J. Mag. Res. Imaging*, 12, 205.

Runge, V.M. (2001). A review of contrast media research in 1999–2000. *Inv. Radiol.*, 36, 123.

Saleem, K.S. et al. (2002). Magnetic resonance imaging of neuronal connections in the macaque monkey. *Neuron*, 34, 685.

Sauter, A. et al. (2002). Recovery of function in cytoprotected cerebral cortex in rat stroke model assessed by functional MRI. *Mag. Res. Med.*, 47, 759.

Schocke, M.F.H. et al. (2000). *In vivo* magnetic resonance imaging of embryonic neural grafts in a rat model of striatonigral degeneration (multiple system atrophy). *Neuroimage*, 12, 209.

Schoeninger, J.S. et al. (1994). Relaxation-time and diffusion NMR microscopy of single neurons. *J. Mag. Res. B*, 103, 261.

Schroeter, M. et al. (2001). Dynamic changes of magnetic resonance imaging abnormalities in relation to inflammation and glial responses after photothrombotic cerebral infarction in the rat brain. *Acta Neuropathol.*, 101, 114.

Sieving, P.F. et al. (1990). Preparation and characterization of paramagnetic polychelates and their protein conjugates. *Bioconjugate Chem.*, 1, 65.

Sipkins, D.A. et al. (2000). ICAM-1 expression in autoimmune encephalitis visualized using magnetic resonance imaging. *J. Neuroimmunol.*, 104, 1.

Smith, B.R., Effmann, E.L., and Johnson, G.A. (1992). MR microscopy of chick embryo vasculature. *J. Mag. Res. Imaging*, 2, 237.

Smith, B.R. et al. (1994). Magnetic resonance microscopy of mouse embryos. *Proc. Int. Acad. Sci. U.S.A.*, 91, 3530.

Smith, B.R. et al. (1998a). Time-course imaging of rat embryos *in utero* with magnetic resonance microscopy. *Mag. Res. Med.*, 39, 673.

Smith, D.H. et al. (1998b). Magnetic resonance spectroscopy of diffuse brain trauma in the pig. *J. Neurotrauma*, 15, 665.

Spenger, C. et al. (2000). Functional MRI at 4.7 Tesla of the rat brain during electric stimulation of forepaw, hindpaw, or tail in single- and multislice experiments. *Exp. Neurol.*, 166, 246.

Takahashi, M. et al. (1996). Neurotoxicity of gadolinium contrast agents for magnetic resonance imaging in rats with osmotically disrupted blood–brain barrier. *Mag. Res. Imaging*,14, 619.

Takehara, Y. et al. (2002). Assessment of a potential tumor-seeking manganese metalloporphyrin contrast agent in a mouse model. *Mag. Res. Med.*, 47, 549.

Taylor, J.S. and Reddick, W.E. (2000). Evolution from empirical dynamic contrast-enhanced magnetic resonance imaging to pharmacokinetic MRI. *Adv. Drug Delivery Rev.*, 41, 91.

Taupitz, M. et al. (2000). New generation of monomer-stabilized very small superparamagnetic iron oxide particles (VSOP) as contrast medium for MR angiography: preclinical results in rats and rabbits. *J. Mag. Res. Imaging*, 12, 905.

Thomas, C.F. and White, J.G. (1998). Four-dimensional imaging: the exploration of space and time. *Trends Biotechnol.*, 16, 175.

Tiefenauer, X.L. et al. (1996). *In vivo* evaluation of magnetite nanoparticles for use as tumor contrast agent in MRI. *Mag. Res. Imaging*, 14, 391.

Torchilin, V.P. (2000). Polymeric contrast agents for medical imaging. *Curr. Pharm. Biotechnol.*, 1, 183.

Tóth, É., Helm, L., and Merbach, A.E. (2001). Relaxivity of gadolinium(III) complexes: theory and mechanisms, in Merbach, A.E. and Tóth, E., Eds., *The Chemistry of Contrast Agents in Medical Magnetic Resonance Imaging*, John Wiley & Sons, Chichester.

Tuor, U.I. et al. (2001). Long-term deficits following hypoxia-ischemia in four-week old rat: correspondence between behavioural, histological and magnetic resonance imaging assessments. *Exp. Neurol.*, 167, 272.

Turetschek, K. et al. (2001). Tumor microvascular characterization using ultrasmall superparamagnetic iron oxide particles (USPIO) in an experimental breast cancer model. *J. Mag. Res. Imaging*, 13, 882.

Tweedle, M.F., Wedeking, P., and Kumar, K. (1995). Biodistribution of radiolabeled, formulated gadopentetate, gadoteridol, gadoterate, and gadodiamide in mice and rats. *Inv. Radiol.*, 30, 372.

Unger, E.C. et al. (1985) Magnetic resonance imaging using gadolinium labeled monoclonal antibody. *Inv. Radiol.*, 20, 693.

van Doersten, F.A. et al. (2002). Dynamic changes of ADC, perfusion, and NMR relaxation parameters in transient focal ischemia of rat brain. *Mag. Res. Med.*, 47, 97.

van der Linden, A. et al. (2002). *In vivo* manganese-enhanced magnetic resonance imaging reveals connections and functional properties of the songbird vocal control system. *Neuroscience,* 112, 467.

van der Sanden, B.P. et al. (2001). Noninvasive assessment of the functional neovasculature in 9L-glioma growing in rat brain by dynamic 1H magnetic resonance imaging of gadolinium uptake. *J. Cereb. Blood Flow Metabol.*, 20, 861.

Vanduffel, W. et al. (2001). Visual motion processing investigated using contrast agent-enhanced fMRI in awake behaving monkeys. *Neuron*, 32, 565.

van Zijl, P.C. et al. (1990) Metalloporphyrin magnetic resonance contrast agents: feasibility of tumor-specific magnetic resonance imaging. *Acta Radiol.*, 374, 75.

Virley, D. et al. (2000). Temporal MRI assessment of neuropathology after transient middle cerebral artery occlusion in the rat: correlations with behavior. *J. Cereb. Blood Flow Metabol.*, 20, 563.

Wang, S. et al. (1990). Evaluation of Gd-DTPA-labeled dextran as an intravascular MR contrast agent: imaging characteristics in normal rat tissues. *Radiology*, 175, 483.

Ward, K.M., Aletras, A.H., and Balaban, R.S. (2000). A new class of contrast agents for MRI based on proton chemical dependent saturation transfer. *J. Mag. Res.*, 143, 79.

Watanabe, T., Michaelis, T., and Frahm, J. (2001). Mapping of retinal projections in the living brain using high-resolution three-dimensional gradient-echo MRI with Mn^{2+} induced contrast. *Mag. Res. Med.*, 46, 424.

Weissleder, R. (1999). Molecular imaging: exploring the next frontier. *Radiology,* 212, 609.

Weissleder, R. et al. (2000). *In vivo* magnetic resonance imaging of transgene expression. *Nature Med.*, 6(3), 351–354.

Weissleder, R. and Mahmood, U. (2001). Molecular imaging. *Radiology,* 219, 316–333.

Weissleder, R. et al. (2001). Size optimization of synthetic graft copolymers for *in vivo* angiogenesis imaging. *Bioconjugate Chem.*, 12, 213–219.

Wind, R.A. et al. (2000). An integrated confocal and magnetic resonance microscope for cellular research. *J. Mag. Res.,* 147, 371.

Wood, A.K.W. et al. (2001). Prolonged anaesthesia in MR studies of rats. *Acad. Radiol.*, 8, 1136.

Xu, F. et al. (2000). Assessment and discrimination of odor stimuli in the rat olfactory bulb by dynamic functional MRI. *Proc. Natl. Acad. Sci. U.S.A.*, 97, 10601.

Xue, R. et al. (1999). *In vivo* three-dimensional reconstruction of rat brain axonal projections by diffusion tensor imaging. *Mag. Res. Med.*, 42, 1123–1127.

Yang, X., Hyder, F., and Schulman, R.G. (1997). Functional MRI BOLD signal coincides with electrical activity in the rat whisker barrels. *Mag. Res. Med.* 38, 874.

Yu, X. et al. (2000). High-resolution MRI characterization of human thrombus using a novel fibrin-targeted paramagnetic nanoparticle contrast agent. *Mag. Res. Med.*, 44, 867.

Zhang, Y. et al. (2000). Magnetic resonance imaging detection of rat renal transplant rejection by monitoring macrophage infiltration. *Kidney Intl.*, 58, 1300–1310.

Zheng, J. et al. (2001). Contrast-enhanced coronary MR angiography: relationship between coronary artery delineation and blood T_1. *J. Mag. Res. Imaging*, 14, 348.

Zhao, M. et al. (2001). Non-invasive detection of apoptosis using magnetic resonance imaging and a targeted contrast agent. *Nature Med.*, 7, 1241.

11 The Future for Biomedical Imaging: Emerging and Alternative Technologies

Nick van Bruggen and Timothy P.L. Roberts

CONTENTS

11.1 INTRODUCTION: THE IMPORTANCE OF NONINVASIVE IMAGING

Studies of natural development, disease progression, response to external stimuli, and influences of new therapies and interventions share a common demand — the ability to characterize or determine some aspect of brain physiology at successive time points. Such studies are facilitated by serial or longitudinal examinations. If the nature of an examination (e.g., brain sectioning or immunohistologic staining) precludes repeated performance, alternative strategies involving large cohorts of similar preparations are required. Samples are drawn at certain stages and assumed to represent the population. To the extent that noninvasive imaging can offer information with sufficient physiologic specificity to serve as a reasonable alternative to invasive methods, we can reduce the number of animals required in our neuroscientific investigations while harnessing the statistical power of internal control.

Longitudinal studies allow us to monitor the development, progression, and responses of individual samples over time. They also allow us to probe interindividual variations in sample populations that invasive methods must assume are homogeneous. This approach has great importance when animal availability is restricted — as is often the case with transgenic or knockout animals. (Gene manipulation provides unprecedented ability to generate animal models of disease that closely mimic clinical conditions, but the techniques remain resource-intensive and costly.) Disease onset is often difficult to predict and highly variable. For efficient drug efficacy studies, screening to establish the baseline condition before treatment is necessary to avoid unmanageably large cohorts of animals. Thus heterogeneity issues can, in principle, be circumvented by image-based inclusion criteria.

Further improvement in the sensitivity to detecting biological response can be obtained by using inclusion criteria specific to the pathology of interest. For example, imaging tumor size may not be as relevant as the degree of apoptosis or even cellular necrosis. The endpoint chosen could be a marker of biological activity that does not necessarily provide a direct measure of drug efficacy. Monitoring tumor vessel permeability, for example, provides a surrogate marker of the biological activity of vascular endothelial growth factor (VEGF) action.[1,2] Such putative surrogates, while direct measures of biological activity, are not necessarily surrogates for ultimate efficacy, and establishing causality remains a challenge. Nevertheless, valuable insight into understanding pathologic processes can be obtained and online measures of tissue characterization must have physiologic specificity and sensitivity to change (progression and response).

In an ideal world, we would have noninvasive imaging techniques with unique physiologic specificities (the radiologist's equivalent of a biochemist's oxygen electrode or pH sensor). In practice, even advanced physiological imaging techniques have sensitivity to more than one physico-chemical feature of tissue. Inevitably, therefore, more than one technique is used to reveal the underlying pathophysiology. During the progression of ischemic damage resulting from occlusion of a major vessel in the brain, diffusion-weighted MRI is sensitive to an acute phase (minutes after vessel ligation) and a chronic tissue response (reperfusion injury, secondary energy failure, vasogenic edema).[3] In the absence of knowledge about the temporal response and in isolation, diffusion-weighted MRI alone is unable to define the pathological state of the tissue, for example, after putative therapy or in clinical presentation. To distinguish these stages, T_2-weighted imaging is included because it is sensitive only to chronic pathology resulting from reperfusion or vasogenic edema. In the acute phase, diffusion resolves a normal T_2 appearance (normal diffusion indicates healthy tissue and restricted diffusion reflects acute pathology as discussed in Chapter 3). At later stages when diffusion appears normal and successful therapy cannot be distinguished from true ischemic progression (combination of multiple pathologies including cytotoxic and/or vasogenic edema or even cellular necrosis), T_2 hyperintensity reflects pathology and T_2 normal intensity indicates recovery.

The concept of using multiple imaging approaches in a single exam can be extended to include a number of imaging sequences. While no single imaging sequence is definitively specific for any specific pathology, combinations of sequences can provide unique tissue characterization. Such multispectral techniques are now widely used for drug discovery and clinical diagnosis (see Chapter 3).

MRI provides a powerful imaging tool (or rather a suite of tools) of increasing physicochemical (and ultimately, by inference, physiological) specificity. MRI offers unique flexibility for investigating the disease state. MR techniques can provide information about a wide range of pathologies and physiologies including analyses of metabolic, cellular, and vascular integrity. Despite its obvious versatility and physiological specificity, MRI lacks the sensitivity to reveal biological processes at the molecular level. While MRS can provide insight into cellular metabolism, and has been used to monitor biochemical events within tissue, its lack of sensitivity and spatial resolution limit its utility. Consequently a real need for alternative imaging modalities with the sensitivity and resolution to probe cellular molecular events in live animals still exists.

This requirement motivated developments in the field of molecular imaging and led to rapid advances in the area of targeted MRI-based contrast agents and optical imaging techniques. While many of these approaches are in their infancy and remain restricted to a few specialized research laboratories, they hold great promise for CNS research and their full potential will be realized in the years ahead. The excitement and scope of this emerging field are, we hope, captured below.

11.2 MOLECULAR IMAGING USING NOVEL MRI CONTRAST AGENTS

As discussed in Chapter 10, the development of novel MRI contrast agents targeted to specific cellular processes has been achieved. The concept of using contrast-enhanced MRI to track specific cells or receptors *in vivo* has intrigued NMR scientists for many years.[4] Monoclonal antibodies targeted to disease-specific cell surface antigens (e.g., on cancer cells) can be labeled with a magnetic material (such as a paramagnetic metal ion) for *in vivo* localization and detection.

While this approach is very elegant in theory, few examples have been reported. The inherent low sensitivity of the MRI technique and its other limitations including agent clearance, limited binding sites, and low affinity of the modified antibody, restricted the application of this approach to a few specialized examples. Although conjugating paramagnetic liposomes to endothelial cell-specific integrin (αVβ3) can image regions of active angiogenesis in a rabbit cancer model,[5] the practicality of using MRI, especially compared with other imaging modalities such as radionuclide or optical imaging, remains to be fully established. Nevertheless, one area in which cell-specific targeting using MRI-based contrast agents has already been used to good effect in experimental neuroscience is detection of macrophage accumulation in CNS pathology.

Cells of the mononuclear phagocytic system internalize ultrasmall particles of iron oxide by absorptive endocytosis.[6,7] After systemic administration of iron-based MRI contrast agents (e.g., USPIO particles), macrophages laden with iron can be detected in regions of cerebral damage, including the border zone of an ischemic infarction in a rat model of stroke[8] and areas of chronic inflammation and demyelination in a mouse model of relapsing remitting experimental allergic encephalomyelitis.[9] These examples and others demonstrate the exciting ability of contrast-enhanced MRI to detect cell-specific processes in damaged tissues. Magnetic nanoparticles, by virtue of their magnetic susceptibilities, can produce relatively large signal changes on an MRI image, especially at high magnetic fields, and are attractive cell targeting contrast agents.

Paramagnetic contrast agents have also been used to tag progenitor cells in order to monitor their trafficking in the CNS. For example, Bulte et al.[10] demonstrated that cell migration of magnetically labeled, transplanted oligodendrocyte progenitor cells into regions of myelination in the spinal cords of myelin-deficient rats could be monitored with MRI. The transferrin receptor was used for internalization of magnetic nanoparticles but alternative approaches with different contrast agents may be possible.[11-13] The ability to monitor progenitor and stem cell migration, disruption, and fate noninvasively in the brains of experimental animals will help elucidate their role in tissue repair following trauma.

One of the most exciting developments in the arena of targeted contrast agents is the development of so-called "smart" agents.[14] The term implies that the contrast agent only becomes active in response to physiological or biochemical change. Smart agents change their conformational structures, and in so doing induce MR-detectable changes (i.e., become "switched on") in certain tissues. The "switch" can be, for example, increased enzymatic activity induced by upregulation of a gene product.

The best example is an agent called EGad ([4,7,10-tri(acetic acid)-1-(2-β-galactopyranosylethoxy)-1,4,7,10-tetraazacyclododoecane] gadolinium). When exposed to the β-galactosidase marker gene, EGad removes the galactopyranose from the cage of chelators surrounding the Gd^{3+} ion, thereby allowing water molecules access to the now-exposed metal ion and enhancing its MRI-detectable relaxation properties. β-galactosidase is commonly used as a marker gene since catalytic reaction of a single substrate results in a precipitate that is easily visualized as a blue stain and is used in cell-based assays and in tissue sections to regionally monitor gene expression. As illustrated in Chapter 10, the contrast-enhanced, MRI-based approach was used to image gene expression in living *Xenopus laevis* embryos.[15]

11.3 OPTICAL IMAGING

While macroscopic approaches to molecular imaging with novel MRI contrast agents (Chapter 10) and nuclear medicine techniques (Chapter 9) provide invaluable insights, fundamentally different imaging acquisition strategies are in development. They take advantage of the high sensitivity and spatial resolution inherent to, for example, optical imaging. They exploit intrinsic changes in the optical properties of tissue directly (e.g., the reflectance of light is used to image brain activity; near-infrared light absorption reveals the oxidation states of hemoglobin and cytochromes) or use exogenous light-emitting probes (as in fluorescent optical imaging — chemiluminescence and bioluminescence).

The application of optical imaging to neuroscience research is covered in another book in this series (*In Vivo Optical Imaging of Brain Function*, edited by Ron Frostig of University of California at Irvine, CRC Press, 2002) so only a brief introduction is included here.

11.3.1 Brain Activity Monitoring with Intrinsic Optical Signals

Brain activity measurement often relies on monitoring changes in tissue perfusion or alterations in blood flow and metabolism that occur in response to neural activity. An alternative strategy uses changes in tissue reflectance of visible light that occurs with cortical activity, that is, optical imaging based on intrinsic signals (OIS). OIS offers high spatial (μm) and temporal resolution (ms) and is a less costly alternative to MRI and PET. Visible wavelength light emission is, however, significantly attenuated by biological tissue and OIS is restricted to superficial cortical structures in the exposed brain. Using endogenous signal changes to monitor metabolic and hemodynamic changes associated with cerebral activity is not a new idea.[15a]

One of the earliest reports on the use of intrinsic signal changes that occur upon cerebral activation was published in *Science* in 1962.[15b] The functional architecture associated with neuronal activation has fascinated neuroanatomists for many decades. The explosion of interest in human brain mapping with fMRI and PET — techniques that can provide a mechanistic understanding of brain activation — led to a resurgence of interest in the last few years.

The experimental set-up necessary to perform OIS experiments is fairly straight-forward, but the practical implementations are technically demanding and such experimentation is restricted to a few laboratories. Optical imaging is performed through a cranial window — a stainless steel chamber with a "viewing window" fixed to the skull with dental cement to ensure rigidity. The chamber is placed over the region of interest above the exposed brain surface with the dura open. The chamber is equipped with inlet and outlet flow systems for the introduction of test substances and maintenance of a normal physiological environment. Since the received optical signals are sensitive to changes in blood flow and the oxygenation state of hemoglobin, it is important to maintain and monitor the basal physiological state of the animal. Fluctuations in peripheral blood pressure, depth of anesthesia, core temperature, and oxygen content of the blood can all cause misleading changes in signal responses. Choice of proper anesthetic and careful maintenance of systemic physiology are imperative.

The precise physiological mechanism underlying the intrinsic signal changes seen under cortical activation remains unclear and a number of physiological responses may contribute to the observed signal. Neuronal activity is coupled to cerebral blood flow. This forms the basis for the functional mapping studies obtained from MRI and PET (as discussed earlier). One component of the intrinsic signal response arises from an increase in local blood volume (from local vasodilatation of arteries or increased capillary recruitment). These changes presumably reflect a change in local hematocrit since the optical properties of hemoglobin influence the intrinsic signal. Another source of signal response is altered light scattering that may result from changes in water and ion homeostasis and cell volume changes. The scattering is more pronounced at longer wavelengths. A third component of the intrinsic signal changes reflects the oxygenation state of hemoglobin. The absorption spectra from heme reflect its oxygenation state. In many ways, the signal responses are analogous to the signal changes seen in the BOLD fMRI experiment. The increases in metabolic demand of the tissue and in the level of deoxyhemoglobin are compensated for by the increase in cerebral blood flow known to occur upon cerebral activation.

11.3.2 BIOLUMINESCENCE

Bioluminescence is an alternative to *in vivo* monitoring of cellular processes that exploits endogenous signal responses. The measurement of luminescence, i.e., emission of absorbed energy as light that results from a chemical reaction (chemiluminescence) or a physiological process (bioluminescence), is used routinely in biomedical research in a wide range of assays. Many organisms ranging from bacteria to fish and fireflies have the ability to emit light. The chemical reaction resulting in bioluminescence is due to the presence of an oxygenase that catalyzes the oxygenation of the substrate (a luciferin) to produce a molecule in an electronically excited state. In fireflies, for example, luciferase uses molecular oxygen and ATP to produce light with spectral characteristics suitable for detection with conventional microscopes and has found extensive utility in molecular biological applications.

Recombination DNA techniques allow the incorporation of the *luc* gene into cells so that selective expression of luciferase as a reporter gene can be observed with the addition of luciferin as substrate. This technique is used extensively in cellular biology *in vitro* and has applications for smaller whole organisms like Drosophilae or zebra fish, in which light penetration is not an issue. The increased need for noninvasive investigations of mammalian systems, in particular, genetically manipulated mice, created a resurgence of interest in the potential utility of monitoring bioluminescence from an *in vivo* source. The major limitation to using light-emitting probes for *in vivo* studies is the signal attenuation resulting from tissue absorption and scatter of photons at interfaces due to changes in refractive index.[16,17]

The degrees of scatter and absorption are dependent on many factors and are influenced by light wavelength. At longer wavelengths (>600 nm), scatter dominates. While the detection of light originating in deep tissues is possible, its emission will be highly diffuse. Longer wavelength dyes allow for greater tissue penetration of the laser light excitation and emission signal. To observe signals from deep structures inside tissue, it is desirable to have high sensitivity in the red or near-infrared range. This led to the use of fluorescence-tagged proteins conjugated to chromophores that excite in the near-infrared. Despite the tissue penetration limitations associated with bioluminescence, the availability of highly sensitive, cooled, back-thinned, intensified cameras suitable for detection of bioluminescence created many possibilities for *in vivo* detection of luciferase expression.

Among the first applications of this approach was to follow the course of infectious disease. In pioneering studies, bacteria containing luciferase expression together with accessory genes for substrate biosynthesis were infected into susceptible strains of mice and the progression of the infection was followed *in vivo*.[18–20] The technique was used to assess neoplastic disease in mouse models. Human mammary cancer cells transfected to expression *luc* were inoculated subcutaneously as xenografts or directly into target organs of nude mice. The resulting bioluminescence was used to track the development of the primary tumor and its regression in response to therapy.[21,22] In addition, it is possible to assess tumor tissue burden and occurrence of metastasis *in vivo* noninvasively over time with bioluminescence imaging.[23]

The signal attenuation of light emission from luciferase-mediated bioluminescence is especially problematic in the CNS and may limit its utility for *in vivo* imaging unless the skull is thinned or the brain exposed through a cranial window. Despite this limitation, bioluminescence has been used for monitoring and screening cancer treatment responses in an orthotopic rat brain glioma model.[24] Spatial and temporal resolutions were not issues. Rather, the focus was to develop a luminescence-based screen to monitor drug therapy. 9L gliosarcoma cells genetically engineered to stably express luciferase were implanted into rat brains. The resulting bioluminescence was measured at several time points following inoculation with and without therapeutic intervention and quantified in terms of total photon counts. Tumor volume was assessed at the same time points using MRI. A good correlation was observed between the two parameters, suggesting that quantitative bioluminescence is feasible and can provide accurate and rapid measure of tumor burden. This study illustrates the potential application of bioluminescent detection of reporter gene expression for CNS studies.

11.3.3 FLUORESCENT PROBES

The use of green fluorescent protein (GFP) as an alternative reporter gene to luciferase has been explored for *in vivo* imaging. GFP, identified from the jelly fish (genus Aequora) emits green light ($\lambda = 508$ nm) when irradiated with blue light ($\lambda = 395$ nm). GFP is widely used as a partner in gene fusion experiments and, like luciferase, due to its strong fluorescence and no apparent toxicity, is an ideal marker for cell-based assays. Since no cofactor or substrate is required, GFP has many advantages over, for example, luciferase. With the advent of highly sensitive CCD cameras and the increasing need for noninvasive molecular imaging in mice, GFP-mediated fluorescence has been successfully used for *in vivo* imaging. Most experiments involved GFP-transfected cells inoculated subcutaneously in nude mice and produced only superficial tumors. This technique has also demonstrated and tracked the occurrence of metastasis and internal orthotopic tumors but lacks spatial and temporal resolution. At these wavelengths, tissue attenuation, scatter, and absorption of light limit detection and spatial resolution, especially for deep structures, and restrict the use of GFP to superficial structures.

Tumor metastases in mouse models can be detected to a depth of 0.5 mm if the metastasis size is greater than 60 μm in diameter; the size must be greater than 1800 μm at a depth of 2.2 mm.[25] This clearly illustrates the depth limitation of the technique. Reversible skin flaps or cranial windows have been used to improve tissue penetration of internal structures.[26] This "intravital" approach can include conventional microscopes fitted with CCD cameras for fluorescence detection and offers the possibility of near-field high resolution detection of GFP expression (albeit invasive) in whole animals.

Signal attenuation from skull and surrounding structures has limited the utility of GFP-mediated fluorescence imaging in the intact brain and the majority of studies performed in the CNS have the intravital imaging techniques. An elegant example of the application of GFP- fluorescence imaging was performed in a study aimed at evaluating whether bone-marrow derived stem cells could give rise to neuronal phenotype. In these experiments intravital microscopy was used to demonstrate the appearance and occurrence of engrafted GFP-expressing bone marrow in the brain.[27]

11.3.4 IMAGING IN NEAR-INFRARED RANGE

Signal attenuation due to limited photon transmission through tissue has limited the use of light-emitting probes for *in vivo* research. Tissue penetration is a function of the wavelength used and significant advantage is offered by light-emitting probes that excite and emit at longer wavelengths, especially into the near-infrared. This is the concept of clinical near-infrared spectroscopy (ivNIRS) outlined in the next section. The transmission and reflectance of light in biological tissue are influenced by many parameters, including tissue type, heterogeneity, absorption, attenuation, and scatter.[17,28] Light scatter is likely to be the resolution-limiting factor at longer wavelengths. Since it decreases as the fourth power of the wavelength, significant advantage is afforded by probes that excite and emit at wavelengths >650 to 700 nm.

Blood and tissue absorption due to heme groups at these longer wavelengths is relatively low. For this reason, much interest in the development and use of fluorophores with spectral properties in the near-infrared range emerged over the last few years and has already shown great promise for noninvasive investigations of pathophysiology in mice.

One of the first applications of *in vivo* imaging with far-red emitting fluorochromes was the assessment of uptake and biodistribution of tumor-specific fluorescent labeled antibodies. Since radionuclide labeled antibodies could be localized *in vivo* in nude mice[29] and in humans,[30] similar protocols were adopted by replacing the radionuclide with a fluorescent tag. In the early studies, monoclonal antibodies directed against squamous cell carcinomas were conjugated with a fluorescent dye (indocyanin) that emits at 667 nm after excitation with laser light at 640 nm. Twenty-four hours following injection, specific binding was seen in the xenograft tumors in nude mice. A number of studies have since been published using cyanine-conjugated monoclonal antibodies for tumor localization in nude mice.[31,32]

The targeting potential for antibody-based cancer therapies can be easily monitored in nude mice with the addition of a fluorochrome conjugate to the therapeutic antibody of interest. The ability to provide information about uptake and biodistribution as part of an efficacy evaluation is now possible. Early and specific tumor localization and detection are clearly important for clinical diagnosis and prognosis and thus imaging techniques based on nuclear medicine are developing tumor-specific radiopharmaceuticals.

Certain tumor types including, for example, pulmonary malignancies and pancreatic endocrine tumors, have high rates of expression of somatostatin receptors. A synthetic peptide analogue (octreotate) of somatostatin radio-labeled with technetium (Tc) is used for identification of pulmonary malignancies using SPECT imaging. SPECT systems suitable for small animal research are only now becoming available, so the small animal equivalent of this receptor targeted-imaging device is not widely available. A more accessible approach for small animal research is to use a near-infrared fluorescence probe in place of the radionuclide. A dye–peptide conjugate that uses a cyanine dye derivative conjugated to octreotate has been synthesized and successfully used as a contrast agent for optical imaging in mouse xenograft models.[33] Dye accumulated in tumor tissue with a long retention time and was significantly greater than fluorescence from normal tissue.

Another exciting variant on the theme of near-infrared imaging for the study of tumor biology has come from the pioneering work of a group at Massachusetts General Hospital, Harvard Medical School. They developed a number of enzyme-activated probes for *in vivo* targeting of tumors in small animals. These elegant experiments use protein substrates containing near-infrared fluorochromes quenched by the nature of their proximity when attached to polymer background used as a delivery vehicle. Proteinase expression is characteristically much higher in tumor tissue than normal tissue. It has been shown to play an important role in tumor pathophysiology including angiogenesis and metastasis and represents a potential therapeutic target. Enzyme cleavage results in loss of fluorochrome quenching and a 15-fold increase in the near-infrared signal when measured in a mouse xenograft model.[34,35]

Near-infrared *in vivo* imaging with exogenous fluorescent probes is still in its infancy. Most studies were planar. True tomography is only now being tested.[36] Nevertheless, noninvasive imaging using near-infrared fluorescence probes has already proven its utility in small animal research. This field is rapidly expanding and includes studies ranging from tumor localization by specific-targeting antibodies, molecular targeting with activated NIR agents, specific agents that mimic the radionuclide pharmaceutical SPECT imaging now established clinically (including the imaging of osteoblast activity[37]), and octreotate conjugates.[33]

Several challenges still face investigators, including improved resolution and quantitation offered by tomographic imaging systems and increased availability of specific probes with spectral characteristics in the near-infrared and beyond.[36] Since this technology is a relatively recent addition to *in vivo* imaging studies, its use has been restricted to imaging outside the brain. It is clear, however, that targeting and specific near-infrared fluorescent imaging will become a powerful tool for neuroscience research.

11.4 NEAR-INFRARED SPECTROSCOPY

No discussion of optical techniques for *in vivo* investigation in neuroscience research would be complete without an explanation of the theory and application of near-infrared spectroscopy. Near-infrared wavelengths (750 to 1000 nm) achieve greater tissue penetration than visible light and show specific absorption by compounds of biological interest such as oxy- and deoxyhemoglobin and intracellular respiratory cytochrome oxidase enzymes. A number of articles have been dedicated to biological applications of near-infrared spectroscopy. Only a brief description to illustrate its use in small animal neuroscience research is provided here. Readers are referred to comprehensive reviews for details of the technique and its applications.[28,38–40]

The theory of oximetry, i.e., use of light absorption to assess the oxygen state of tissue and blood, originated early in the 20th century. Jobsis et al. recognized in the 1970s that near-infrared light transmission through biological material could provide information about essential physiological parameters including cerebral circulation and oxygen sufficiency.[41] These early experiments established the feasibility of measuring various indices of oxygenation in blood and tissue across the heads of small animals without surgical intervention. In essence, the spectral analysis of near-infrared absorption contains information about the oxygenation state of hemoglobin and the redox state of the terminal respiratory chain enzyme, cytochrome oxidase. From knowledge of spectral responses at specific wavelengths in the near-infrared spectra, it is possible to obtain quantitative information about the oxygenation state of hemoglobin, changes in blood volume and flow, and intracellular oxidative processes.

A main focus for the development of *in vivo* near-infrared spectroscopy was to monitor brain oxygenation levels in newborn babies. In particular, the assessment of hypoxic–ischemic brain injury associated with preterm delivery or traumatic birth was required for prognostic and clinical evaluation. Near-infrared spectroscopy provides a robust and sensitive technique for the assessment of cerebral metabolism and blood flow; it is suitable for intensive care environments. In general three wavelengths, typically 778, 813, and 867 nm, are employed to measure relative changes in CNS hemodynamics. Quantification is possible using a conversion scheme, such that absolute concentrations of total oxyhemoglobin, deoxyhemoglobin, and oxidized cytochrome aa3 can be determined. The cerebral blood volume in ml/100g tissue can be measured if a value for mean cerebral hematocrit is known. Monitoring cerebral hemodynamics and oxygenation continuously is now possible in neonatal studies and for fetal monitoring during delivery.[42]

The applications of near-infrared spectroscopy in small animal research remains restricted to a few specialized centers. Often the motivation for experimental studies is to interpret clinical findings. fMRI has been used to good effect in small animals at a spatial resolution sufficient to generate functional maps of specific somatosensory activation (discussed in Chapter 4). While near-infrared spectroscopy can provide similar information about the oxygenation state of blood and tissue, it is largely a global measure and therefore lacks the spatial resolution for functional activation involving discrete regions. Studies using experimental animals focused largely on technique development and/or validation of clinical measurements. Studies of physiological investigation are mainly restricted to global alteration in cerebral perfusion or metabolism, for example, monitoring brain oxygenation during hypotension[43] or in association with cerebral pathology.[44,45] Many recent studies using near-infrared spectroscopy in laboratory animals have been performed in conjunction with MRI to aid interpretation of fMRI response.[46]

11.5 MAGNETOENCEPHALOGRAPHY

While advances in high resolution and physiologically specific techniques in MRI may permit consideration of *in vivo* histology, approaches to studying electrical activities (ion fluxes, etc.) in the brain using noninvasive far-field sensing techniques, namely electroencephalography (EEG) and magnetoencephalography (MEG), can be described as avenues toward *in vivo* electrophysiology. Interestingly, advances in experimental techniques arrive in parallel with, and perhaps motivated by, clinical implementation and subsequent observation. Especially in the field of MEG, the attractive possibility of noninvasively accessing neuronal activity led to commercialization and adoption of human-sized biomagnetometer sensor arrays that allow a number of fundamental neuroscience issues to be addressed noninvasively in volunteers and patients.

Less emphasis has centered on small animal MEG research. Okada et al. demonstrated successful acquisition and source modeling of fields and potentials evoked by somatosensory stimulation, allowing a comparative study of EEG and MEG characteristics and revealing the independence of MEG recordings on tissue conductivity differences and the confounding influence such differences have on EEG potential recordings.[47] Teale et al.[48] succeeded in recording auditorily evoked neuromagnetic fields in macaque monkeys, analogous to the M100 response observed from superior temporal gyri in humans. Other studies[49] draw comparisons of invasive electrophysiological recordings (in cat or monkey preparations) and human observations. This is of key importance when realizing the high temporal resolution afforded by these techniques (submillisecond) that allow elucidation of temporal signatures characteristic of stimulus feature recognition extraction and processing.

11.6 CONCLUSIONS

The opportunities afforded by evolving molecular and cellular imaging techniques offer tantalizing prospects for noninvasive and physiologically specific characterization of diseases and therapeutic interventions. While MRI, due to its versatility and flexibility will remain the mainstay for small animals, clinical investigations, and diagnosis, new targeted techniques that have the capability of investigating the biology at the molecular level offer a new horizon for biochemically specific probes that will benefit from the higher sensitivity of radionuclide imaging and optical based techniques.

The range of biomedical imaging techniques available to the neuroscientist researcher is extensive. The scope and application of these rapidly evolving techniques, together with their limitations, are summarized in Table 11.1.

TABLE 11.1
Techniques of Biomedical Imaging Available for Experimental Research. Applications and Limitations

Modality	Resolution		Application Example	Limitations/Caveats
	Spatial	Temporal		
MRI				
Perfusion	≤mm	secs-min	μvessel flow.	Dynamic range - sensitivity.
Diffusion	≤mm	min	Cell vol/homeostasis, fiber tracking, mylination, necrosis.	CSF pulsitile flow. Spatial resolution for fiber tracking.
fMRI/phMRI	≤mm	secs-min	Mapping sensory/higher order function. Hemodynamic drug action. Blood gas manipulation.	Indirect. Anesthesia.
MRA	≈100 μm	secs-min	Vascular deficits. Quantitative flow.	Quantitation of stenosis and slow flow. Turbulence, spatial resolution.
MRS	≤cm	secs-min	Metabolic studies (energy metabolism and other nuclei).	Spatial and temporal resolution. Metabolite specificity.
Molecular	≤cm	min-hours	Cell tracking, embryogenesis.	Sensitivity and availability of appropriate agents. Time. Motion.
μMRI	≤100 μm	hrs	Morphology. Histology. Development.	
PET				
FDG	≥mm	min	Receptor binding. Plasticity. Biodistribution. Kinetics.	Radioactive material. Availability of ligands. Need for (local) cyclotron. Half-life (determines type of expt).
Labeled Agents			Neurodegeneration. Gene expression.	
Optical				
Intrinsic signal	≤10 μm	≥ms	Higher Order Functional Mapping.	Tissue penetration. Quantitation difficult. Indirect.
Bio-luminescence			Neoplasia gene expression and detection.	
Fluorescence				
MEG/EEG	≤cm	≤ms	Electrophysiological activity.	Source estimate. Orientation sensitivity (MEG). Conductivity sensitivity (EEG). Ensemble averaging.

REFERENCES

1. Brasch, R. and K. Turetschek, MRI characterization of tumors and grading angiogenesis using macromolecular contrast media: status report. *Eur. J. Radiol.*, 34, 148, 2000.
2. Pham, C.D. et al., Magnetic resonance imaging detects suppression of tumor vascular permeability after administration of antibody to vascular endothelial growth factor. *Cancer Invest.*, 16, 225, 1998.
3. van Lookeren, C.M. et al., Secondary reduction in the apparent diffusion coefficient of water, increase in cerebral blood volume, and delayed neuronal death after middle cerebral artery occlusion and early reperfusion in the rat. *J. Cereb. Blood Flow Metabol.*, 19, 1354, 1999.
4. Weissleder, R., Target-specific superparamagnetic MR contrast agents. *Mag. Res. Med.*, 22, 298, 1991.
5. Sipkins, D.A. et al., Detection of tumor angiogenesis *in vivo* by $\alpha V \beta 3$-targeted magnetic resonance imaging. *Nature Med.*, 4, 623, 1998.
6. Moore, A., R. Weissleder, and A. Bogdanov, Jr., Uptake of dextran-coated monocrystalline iron oxides in tumor cells and macrophages. *J. Mag. Res. Imaging*, 7, 1140, 1997.
7. Weissleder, R. et al., Ultrasmall superparamagnetic iron oxide: characterization of a new class of contrast agents for MR imaging. *Radiology*, 175, 489, 1990.
8. Rausch, M. et al., Dynamic patterns of USPIO enhancement can be observed in macrophages after ischemic brain damage. *Mag. Res. Med.*, 46, 1018, 2001.
9. Xu, S. et al., Study of relapsing remitting experimental allergic encephalomyelitis SJL mouse model using MION-46L-enhanced *in vivo* MRI: early histopathological correlation. *J. Neurosci. Res.*, 52, 549, 1998.
10. Bulte, J.W. et al., Neurotransplantation of magnetically labeled oligodendrocyte progenitors: magnetic resonance tracking of cell migration and myelination. *Proc. Natl. Acad. Sci. U.S.A.*, 96, 15256, 1999.
11. Lewin, M. et al., Tat peptide-derivatized magnetic nanoparticles allow *in vivo* tracking and recovery of progenitor cells. *Nature Biotechnol.*, 18, 410, 2000.
12. Bulte, J.W. et al., Magnetodendrimers allow endosomal magnetic labeling and *in vivo* tracking of stem cells. *Nature Biotechnol.*, 19, 1141, 2001.
13. Franklin, R.J. et al., Magnetic resonance imaging of transplanted oligodendrocyte precursors in the rat brain. *Neuroreport*, 10, 3961, 1999.
14. Moats, R.A., S.E. Fraser, and T.J. Meade, A "smart" magnetic resonance imaging agent that reports on specific enzymatic activity. *Angew. Chem. Int. Ed. Engl.*, 36, 726, 1997.
15. Louie, A.Y. et al., *In vivo* visualization of gene expression using magnetic resonance imaging. *Nature Biotechnol.*, 18, 321, 2000.
15a. Hill, D.K. and Keynes, R.D., Opacity changes in stimulated nerve, *J. Physiol.*, 108, 278, 1949.
15b. Chance, B. et al., Intracellular oxidation-reduction states *in vivo*, *Science*, 137, 499, 1962.
16. Rice, B.W., M.D. Cable, and M.B. Nelson, *In vivo* imaging of light-emitting probes. *J. Biomed. Opt.*, 6, 432, 2001.
17. Cheong, W.F., S.A. Prahl, and A.J. Welch, A review of optical properties of biological tissues. *IEEE J. Quantum Electr.* 26, 2166, 1990.
18. Contag, C.H. et al., Photonic detection of bacterial pathogens in living hosts. *Mol. Microbiol.*, 18, 593, 1995.

19. Contag, P.R. et al., Bioluminescent indicators in living mammals. *Nature Med.*, 4, 245, 1998.

20. Burns, S.M. et al., Revealing the spatiotemporal patterns of bacterial infectious diseases using bioluminescent pathogens and whole body imaging. *Contrib. Microbiol.*, 9, 71, 2001.

21. Contag, C.H. et al., Use of reporter genes for optical measurements of neoplastic disease *in vivo*. *Neoplasia*, 2, 41, 2000.

22. Sweeney, T.J. et al., Visualizing the kinetics of tumor-cell clearance in living animals. *Proc. Natl. Acad. Sci. U.S.A.*, 96, 12044, 1999.

23. Wetterwald, A. et al., Optical imaging of cancer metastasis to bone marrow: a mouse model of minimal residual disease. *Am. J. Pathol.*, 160, 1143, 2002.

24. Rehemtulla, A. et al., Rapid and quantitative assessment of cancer treatment response using *in vivo* bioluminescence imaging. *Neoplasia*, 2, 491, 2000.

25. Yang, M. et al., Whole-body optical imaging of green fluorescent protein-expressing tumors and metastases. *Proc. Natl. Acad. Sci. U.S.A.*, 97, 1206, 2000.

26. Yang, M. et al., Direct external imaging of nascent cancer, tumor progression, angiogenesis, and metastasis on internal organs in the fluorescent orthotopic model. *Proc. Natl. Acad. Sci. U.S.A.*, 12, 12, 2002.

27. Priller, J. et al., Neogenesis of cerebellar Purkinje neurons from gene-marked bone marrow cells *in vivo*. *J. Cell Biol.*, 155, 733, 2001.

28. Rolfe, P., *In vivo* near-infrared spectroscopy. *Annu. Rev. Biomed. Eng.*, 2000. 2: p. 715–54.

29. Mach, J.P. et al., *In vivo* localisation of radiolabelled antibodies to carcinoembryonic antigen in human colon carcinoma grafted into nude mice. *Nature*, 248, 704, 1974.

30. Buchegger, F. et al., Radiolabeled fragments of monoclonal antibodies against carcinoembryonic antigen for localization of human colon carcinoma grafted into nude mice. *J. Exp. Med.*, 158, 413, 1983.

31. Ballou, B. et al., Tumor labeling *in vivo* using cyanine-conjugated monoclonal antibodies. *Cancer Immunol. Immunother.*, 41, 257, 1995.

32. Ballou, B. et al., Cyanine fluorochrome-labeled antibodies *in vivo*: assessment of tumor imaging using Cy3, Cy5, Cy5.5, and Cy7. *Cancer Detect. Prev.*, 22, 251, 1998.

33. Becker, A. et al., Receptor-targeted optical imaging of tumors with near-infrared fluorescent ligands. *Nature Biotechnol.*, 19, 327, 2001.

34. Weissleder, R. et al., *In vivo* imaging of tumors with protease-activated near-infrared fluorescent probes. *Nature Biotechnol.*, 17, 375, 1999.

35. Tung, C.H. et al., Preparation of a cathepsin D sensitive near-infrared fluorescence probe for imaging. *Bioconjugate Chem.*, 10, 892, 1999.

36. Weissleder, R., Scaling down imaging: molecular mapping of cancer in mice. *Nature Rev. Cancer,* 2, 11, 2002.

37. Zaheer, A. et al., *In vivo* near-infrared fluorescence imaging of osteoblastic activity. *Nature Biotechnol.*, 19, 1148, 2001.

38. Wahr, J.A. et al., Near-infrared spectroscopy: theory and applications. *J. Cardiothorac Vasc. Anesth.*, 10, 406, 1996.

39. Cooper, C.E. et al., Measurement of cytochrome oxidase redox state by near infrared spectroscopy. *Adv. Exp. Med. Biol.*, 413, 63, 1997.

40. Cooper, C.E. et al., Near-infrared spectroscopy of the brain: relevance to cytochrome oxidase bioenergetics. *Biochem. Soc. Trans.*, 22, 974, 1994.

41. Jobsis, F.F., Noninvasive, infrared monitoring of cerebral and myocardial oxygen sufficiency and circulatory parameters. *Science*, 198, 1264, 1977.

42. Schmidt, S. et al., Animal experiments for the evaluation of laserspectroscopy in the fetus during labor. *J. Perinat. Med.*, 19, 107, 1991.

43. Tsuji, M. et al., Near-infrared spectroscopy detects cerebral ischemia during hypotension in piglets. *Pediatr. Res.*, 44, 591, 1998.

44. Park, W.S. and Y.S. Chang, Effects of decreased cerebral perfusion pressure on cerebral hemodynamics, brain cell membrane function and energy metabolism during the early phase of experimental *Escherichia coli* meningitis in the newborn piglet. *J. Korean Med. Sci.*, 15, 203, 2000.

45. van Rossem, K. et al., Brain oxygenation after experimental closed head injury: NIRS study. *Adv. Exp. Med. Biol.*, 471, 209, 1999.

46. Jezzard, P. et al., Comparison of EPI gradient-echo contrast changes in cat brain caused by respiratory challenges with direct simultaneous evaluation of cerebral oxygenation via a cranial window. *NMR Biomed.*, 7, 35, 1994.

47. Okada, Y., A. Lahteenmaki, and C. Xu, Comparison of MEG and EEG on the basis of somatic evoked responses elicited by stimulation of the snout in the juvenile swine. *Clin. Neurophysiol.*, 110, 214, 1999.

48. Teale, P. et al., Magnetic auditory source imaging in macaque monkey. *Brain Res. Bull.*, 33, 615, 1994.

49. Biermann, S. and P. Heil, Parallels between timing of onset responses of single neurons in cat and of evoked magnetic fields in human auditory cortex. *J. Neurophysiol.*, 84, 2426, 2000.

Index

O

P